Physiotherapy in Orthopaedics

For Elsevier

Senior Commissioning Editor: Heidi Harrison
Project Development Manager: Siobhan Campbell
Project Manager: Andrew Palfreyman
Illustration Manager: Bruce Hogarth
Design Direction: George Ajayi

Physiotherapy in Orthopaedics

A problem–solving approach

Karen Atkinson   MSc MCSP CertEd DipTP

Senior Lecturer, Department of Health Sciences, University of East London, London

Fiona Coutts   MSc MCSP SRP

Lecturer, Queen Margaret University College, Edinburgh

Anne-Marie Hassenkamp   MMACP MSc

Superintendent Physiotherapist, Royal National Orthopaedic Hospital, Stanmore

SECOND EDITION

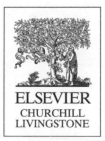

ELSEVIER
CHURCHILL
LIVINGSTONE

EDINBURGH LONDON NEW YORK OXFORD PHILADELPHIA ST LOUIS SYDNEY TORONTO 2005

First edition 1999
Second edition 2005
   Reprint 2006

ISBN 0 443 07406 2

British Library Cataloguing in Publication Data
A catalogue record for this book is available from the British Library

Library of Congress Cataloguing in Publication Data
A catalogue record for this book is available from the Library of Congress

Note
Knowledge and best practice in this field are constantly changing. As new research and experience broaden our knowledge, changes in practice, treatment and drug therapy may become necessary or appropriate. Readers are advised to check the most current information provided (i) on procedures featured or (ii) by the manufacturer of each product to be administered, to verify the recommended dose or formula, the method and duration of administration, and contraindications. It is the responsibility of the practitioner, relying on experience and knowledge of the patient, to make diagnoses, to determine dosages and the best treatment for each individual patient, and to take all appropriate safety precautions. To the fullest extent of the law, neither the publisher nor the authors assumes any liability for any injury and/or damage.

The Publisher

 ELSEVIER | your source for books, journals and multimedia in the health sciences
www.elsevierhealth.com

Working together to grow
libraries in developing countries
www.elsevier.com | www.bookaid.org | www.sabre.org
ELSEVIER   BOOK AID International   Sabre Foundation

The Publisher's policy is to use paper manufactured from sustainable forests

Printed in China

Contents

Preface

It was a great compliment to be asked by Elsevier to produce a second edition of *Physiotherapy in Orthopaedics*. Our reasons for producing this text, as outlined in the preface to the first edition, remain unchanged. It has, however, been a challenging exercise for us to review our previous work in the light of the developments within physiotherapy practice and more widely in the field of orthopaedics during the last few years. We believed that it was important to retain the core elements of the text. We have listened carefully to feedback from students, educators and clinical physiotherapists when producing this new edition. We have been pleased to note that the overall message is that our approach to this area of practice has met many of the needs of our main target group: undergraduate physiotherapists.

Physiotherapists are working within an increasingly complex environment. This relates in part to the evolving scope of practice of the physiotherapy profession as well as to nationally developed standards required as part of clinical governance to provide evidence-based interventions. We believe that an important foundation for enabling physiotherapists to provide high levels of clinical care is the ability to use problem-solving and clinical-reasoning skills in order to focus on patients as individuals. Background knowledge, an awareness of current research, the ability to apply, appropriately, the principles of assessment and treatment together with the self awareness to reflect upon and modify practice based upon experience are all key factors in successful problem solving. Working in co-operation with the patient, carers and other

members of the healthcare team in the light of the available evidence are addressed within the text, aiming to ensure that the outcomes of physiotherapy intervention are functional and meaningful to the client group. We hope this book will provide one medium through which undergraduate physiotherapy students will begin to develop these abilities, rather than unquestioningly accepting 'recipes' or 'formulae' for patient management.

There are some changes to the new edition. All except one of the existing chapters have been updated. The specific information that comprised the chapter on the paediatric client group has been subsumed within the remaining sections. We have added two new chapters. First, as a result of feedback from the user group, we have written a chapter on gait. Many people with orthopaedic problems present gait abnormalities as a consequence of disease processes, or resulting from trauma or surgery. These patients often require some physiotherapy to facilitate the improvement of their gait patterns. Assessment and rehabilitation of gait are difficult concepts to grasp and the new chapter attempts to address these issues and to provide the novice practitioner with an overview pertinent to this area of practice. The chapter also suggests links to resources which the reader can access to obtain more specific information where required. The second additional chapter focuses on hydrotherapy. Currently, few undergraduate courses deal with the subject of hydrotherapy in what we consider to be adequate detail to enable a novice practitioner to work safely in this different clinical environment. The chapter deals with the basic principles of hydrotherapy and applies them within the discipline of orthopaedics. Although there is no substitute for practice, we hope that the chapter will provide an adequate theoretical and practical background in hydrotherapy to enable the novice physiotherapist to feel more confident when treating orthopaedic patients in the pool for the first time.

Physiotherapy courses require students to undertake intense amounts of study and work-based learning in a complex and diverse range of specialities. We hope this book will help these students to focus on the patient and to realize that they have many and varied transferable skills upon which they can draw in any situation.

Karen Atkinson
Fiona Coutts
Anne-Marie Hassenkamp

Preface to first edition

Orthopaedics is a very wide-ranging and complex area of patient management. It encompasses conditions due to both trauma and disease which present within different client groups. Patients with orthopaedic problems are encountered throughout the physiotherapist's working life. They may present with a primary condition for the physiotherapist to treat specifically, or with problems requiring physiotherapy which have developed as a result of other pathologies. However, despite the importance of orthopaedic conditions to physiotherapy practice, it seems that orthopaedics is often perceived as a 'basic' subject which physiotherapy students should get to grips with early on in their programmes of study. Not surprisingly, given the wide variety of orthopaedic disorders which a physiotherapist may encounter, many students are daunted by the prospect of absorbing the knowledge and learning the skills necessary to work in this area.

As the authors of *Physiotherapy in Orthopaedics* we firmly believe that a good knowledge of orthopaedics is fundamental to sound physiotherapy practice. In preparing this text we have drawn on our many years of experience of clinical work in various orthopaedic settings and of teaching at both undergraduate and postgraduate levels. Its development was prompted after observing the difficulties that students (and some junior physiotherapists) have with their clinical reasoning when faced with apparently diverse patient problems. There is a tendency to rely on treatment 'recipes' so that when encountering patients with a particular injury or condition the student falls back on rote learning. We believe it is important that the therapist should learn to examine the person in front of them and then make decisions based on the information gathered. Although injuries and conditions vary, within the range of orthopaedics many of the signs and symptoms will be the same. Similarly, the physiotherapeutic interventions used in these situations are the same. The difficult part is being able to decompartmentalise them and this is where clinical reasoning and decision making are so important. It is for this reason that we have taken a problem-solving approach to the subject throughout the book.

The content of the book moves from normal to abnormal and from simple to complex. We have used case studies and self-assessment sections to encourage participation by the reader. The authors hope that this text will go some way towards helping undergraduate physiotherapy students to develop a reasoned and logical approach towards the management of their orthopaedic patients.

Introduction

How to use this book

Karen Atkinson

OBJECTIVES

By the end of this section you should:

- Understand the approach that we use in this book and be aware of the format. This will make the book easier for you to use
- Understand the aims and objectives of the book
- Be aware of the general framework that we use within the text (moving from normal to abnormal, simple to complex and so on) and understand why we use this method.

THE NATURE OF PHYSIOTHERAPY

Physiotherapy is a science-based healthcare profession in which principles from biological, physical and behavioural sciences are integrated and applied. It involves the identification and maximization of the individual patient's functional ability and potential and is concerned with health promotion, prevention of disease or injury, treatment and rehabilitation. With this focus on the individual, it is essential that physiotherapists are effective communicators able to understand and take account of situations from the perspective of the patients and the people in their support networks such as family members, friends and carers.

Physiotherapy is also concerned with enabling patients to maintain and restore maximum movement and functional ability throughout the lifespan. This is particularly important in circumstances where the process of ageing or that of injury or disease threatens movement and function.

Although sharing techniques and knowledge with other professionals and practitioners, the sum total of the physiotherapist's approach to movement is unique. Using this approach, physiotherapists are able to assess movement potential and capability through interaction with the patient and carers, so working towards agreed goals (World Confederation for Physical Therapy 1998).

Given these issues, and the fact that the great majority of patients with orthopaedic problems will be experiencing difficulties with movement, we believe that the movement continuum theory of physical therapy (Cott et al 1995) is a particularly appropriate model on which to base our approach in this textbook. A key concept in this theory is movement occurring at different levels on a continuum. This ranges from the microscopic level – transport of molecules around the body, activation of muscle contraction and so on – to the other end of the continuum, which relates to the macroscopic level of movement of the individual in society.

The main principles of the theory can be seen in Box I.1.

The overall approach that we use to look at orthopaedics in this textbook is one of problem solving. We believe that this method of presenting orthopaedics is quite different from most of the books about this area of practice that you may have come across so far. This approach could also be somewhat different from the usual way in which you deal with particular areas of knowledge or clinical practice.

In many, more traditional, orthopaedic textbooks, each condition is dealt with in turn and the specific management is described. The information you find in these books is extremely relevant but it can be quite repetitive, providing little stimulation or encouragement for you to think or to actively apply the things that you learn during your reading. They often still have their basis in the medical model, whereby the focus is very much on the pathology with any impairment being considered as a deficit that needs to be cured. The patient plays very little part in this process and the therapist can be seen as the powerful diagnostician and healer (Hassenkamp 1998). For the novice practitioner, the medical model tends to be very attractive as it puts the therapist into a powerful position in relation to the patient.

Box I.1   Principles of the movement continuum theory of physical therapy (Cott et al 1995)

General principles

I   Movement is essential to human life

II   Movement occurs on a continuum from the microscopic level to the level of the individual in society

III Movement levels on the continuum are influenced by physical, psychological, social and environmental factors

Physical therapy principles

IV   Movement levels on the continuum are interdependent

V   At each level on the continuum there is a maximum achievable movement potential (MAMP) which is influenced by the MAMP at other levels on the continuum and physical, social, psychological and environmental factors

VI   Within the limits set by the MAMP, each human being has a preferred movement capability (PMC) and a current movement capability (CMC) which in usual circumstances are the same

VII Pathological and developmental factors have the potential to change the MAMP and/or to create a differential between the PMC and CMC

VIII The focus of physical therapy is to minimize the potential and/or existing PMC/CMC differential

IX   The practice of physical therapy involves therapeutic movement, modalities, therapeutic use of self, education and technology and environmental modifications

---

Practice is very predictive and the effects of intervention can often be anticipated and controlled. It allows you to use technical terms and to think very diagnostically.

While this is not 'wrong,' it means that the whole interaction is very therapist-led and 'the patient's voice is not heard' (Thomson 1998). We try to encourage you to look at the patients and their orthopaedic problems in a more global way. The approach to patients in rehabilitation settings has moved on from being predominantly medical to one in which psychological and socio-cultural aspects are equally important (Wade & deJong 2000). Our main focus is on problem solving in physiotherapy and as part of this process you will be encouraged to consider the roles of the patients in their own rehabilitation as well as those of the people in their support networks. In line with the International Classification of Functioning, Disability and Health we view function as 'a complex interaction between the health condition of the individual and the contextual factors of the environment as well as personal factors' (ICF 2001). This also sits well with the movement continuum model of physical therapy mentioned earlier.

In order for rehabilitation in the orthopaedic setting to be effective, it is essential that all relevant services and agencies work together (Wade and deJong 2000). As a physiotherapist, generally you will not work with your patients in isolation. We do therefore, include the roles that other health-care professionals play in the overall approach to patients with orthopaedic problems. Prevention and education are also key elements of physiotherapy patient management and these are considered at appropriate points in various chapters.

Having made the point that we are not working from a medical model, we will still be presenting some information about the pathological changes that occur in the body as a result of ageing, injury and disease. It is important for you to feel secure in your knowledge base before you can go on to view your patients in a more holistic manner. As you build up your clinical experience you will find that the management of different 'conditions' is often similar or may at least overlap in many areas, and this means that each one does not necessarily need to be considered as a totally separate unit. It would seem reasonable, therefore, to suggest that the knowledge you gain from dealing with one type of problem could, where appropriate, be transferred to the management of others.

In the light of these points, the aim of this book is to tackle the subject of orthopaedics from a

different angle: you will consider groups of conditions in which patients present with similar problems. For each group, particular problems that may be experienced by patients with that type of condition are highlighted. A range of possible interventions that physiotherapists often use in their overall management of these issues and problems is then presented and discussed. The key point here, however, is that you will be encouraged to take part in the problem-solving process. A number of methods are used throughout the book to help you to think about the different scenarios and to come up with ideas and strategies that you might use when dealing with patients in these sorts of situation. For ease of reference, the groups of conditions are considered in separate sections and we try to avoid unnecessary repetition. It is important to remember, however, that the knowledge base you gain from working through the different chapters is often transferable to other areas of practice covered in the book.

We intend that by the time you have finished reading this book you will have a good idea of how you might approach the management of a large range of patients who have problems due to orthopaedic conditions. You will also be in a position to consider the role of the physiotherapist within the healthcare team and how each member of the team can contribute to patient management.

STRUCTURE OF THIS BOOK

General

Before you start to look at orthopaedics, it is a good idea for you to:

- think about what 'problem solving' actually means
- think about what the process of problem solving involves
- consider your individual style of problem solving.

Chapter 1 introduces you to these concepts in a general sense and includes some examples from clinical practice. It encourages you to consider flexible and creative methods of problem solving. Further thoughts about the way that problem solving feeds into decision making and clinical reasoning are presented in Chapter 4.

The first four chapters are introductory in nature, laying the foundations and providing the background necessary for you to be able to use the rest of the book successfully. They are also designed to encourage you to think about a range of issues concerned with problem solving, the normal and abnormal changes occurring in the body throughout the lifespan, assessment and clinical practice.

Key words

Under each chapter heading you will find a list of key words. These highlight the major points that are covered in that section.

Objectives and prerequisites

At the beginning of each chapter there is also a list of objectives that provide an indication of what you can learn from reading and working through that section. Where appropriate, we note some prerequisites that indicate what you 'should know' before beginning that chapter. If you make use of these prerequisites, the background knowledge will enable you to get the most out of each section.

Review points

At intervals within chapters you will find Review points. Some of these indicate stages where you should review what has been covered before moving on to the next section. This will help you to keep a check on your progress. Other Review points ask you to explore your own approach to a situation or problem, so stimulating your own thought processes about each subject.

Problem-solving exercises

As you work through the chapters of the book you are presented with a number of problem-solving exercises. In the first chapter they deal with general issues to do with problem solving and creative thinking. Later on they are related to clinical scenarios and specific patient case studies.

The exercises will be indicated as follows: Problem solving exercise 1.1 – the first number signifies the chapter you are in and the second number gives the sequence of the exercises (in this case 1.1 denotes Chapter 1 and the first exercise within that chapter). Some of the problem-solving exercises have questions associated with them. These are designed to direct you towards the areas you ought to be considering. Where the problem-solving exercises concern case studies, you are asked to consider each case in the light of the knowledge you have gained from earlier sections and to decide how you might manage them. It is envisaged that you will gradually develop some idea of clinical decision-making skills from this process. An example of this is prioritization, which may involve the following types of question: 'Which of the patient's problems are the most important and need to be dealt with first?', 'Which problem does the patient consider to be the most pressing?', 'Will other members of the healthcare team be involved, and if so, which ones and when?' and so on.

The Case studies are used to illustrate important points about the problem-solving approach and the management of particular client groups. Suggested solutions to the problem-solving exercises are either presented in the following text or given at the end of the appropriate chapter.

Self-assessment questions

A number of self-assessment questions (SAQs) are included in each chapter. They are numbered as follows: in Chapter 1 – SAQ 1.1, SAQ 1.2., in Chapter 2 – SAQ 2.1, SAQ 2.2 and so on. These questions will help you to monitor your understanding of the preceding sections. Solutions to the self-assessment questions are also given either in the text or at the end of the chapter.

The summary

Just before you reach the solutions for the exercises and questions in each chapter you will find a summary. This provides you with an overview of the areas you have covered and, when used in conjunction with the list of objectives at the beginning of the chapter, can indicate how much information you have absorbed.

AIMS AND RATIONALE OF THE BOOK

It is intended that, as you read, you will become an active participant in the process of problem solving with a special emphasis on orthopaedics. You will gradually begin to understand, and feel ready to apply, the concepts presented in the text. We have designed the book with a pyramidal framework in mind (Fig. I.1). It tackles issues by addressing simple concepts and conditions and gradually expands to encompass those that are more complex. Initially, this takes the form of transition from the normal condition of the body through to abnormal, i.e. when do normal changes in the tissues start to cause problems for the individual? An example of this is the natural ageing process – most older people will complain of some aches and pains but at what point do these become severe enough to warrant them approaching health professionals for advice or treatment? Following on from this, you are introduced to straightforward case studies, which gradually progress by the addition of extra facets for you to consider, e.g. different age groups or possible complications. Later on, the case studies deal with more complex conditions, and the extra aspects and differences involved in short- and long-term management are brought in. So you start at the point of the pyramid and work your way down, gradually broadening your approach and considering more and more aspects in relation to the cases presented. This process will involve the transference of knowledge and problem-solving skills that you have obtained in the earlier sections.

Research has shown that people rely heavily on 'worked out' examples in solving exercise problems (Kahney 1993), especially in new areas. In accordance with this, you are initially provided with lots of information, help and guidance. As you work through the book, you will gradually be given less help and so have the opportunity to carry out more independent problem solving. If you do run into difficulties, however, remember you can find the solutions either at the end of the chapters or within the text.

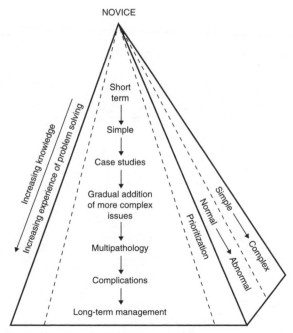

Figure I.1   The pyramidal framework.

SUMMARY

This section has introduced you to the general framework of the book, and the format of the chapters has been briefly explained. This includes Key words, Objectives, Prerequisites, Review points, Problem-solving exercises and Self-assessment questions. The background to our approach to orthopaedics has been explained and the aims and rationale of the book have also been briefly presented.

By working through the chapters and using the various methods described above to monitor and analyse your progress, you will become familiar with the problem-solving process and how this can be applied in the clinical orthopaedic setting.

References

Cott CA, Finch E, Gasner D et al (1995) The movement continuum theory of physical therapy. Physiotherapy Canada 47: 87–95

Hassenkamp AM 1998 Clinical reasoning: a student's nightmare. British Journal of Therapy and Rehabilitation 5: 75–77

ICF 2001 International Classification of Functioning, Disability and Health. World Health Organization, Geneva. Available on line at: www.who.int/icf/ (accessed 8 May 2003)

Kahney H 1993 Problem solving: current issues, 2nd edn. Open University Press, Buckingham

Thomson D 1998 Counselling and clinical reasoning: the meaning of practice. British Journal of Therapy and Rehabilitation 5: 88–94

Wade DT, deJong BA 2000 Clinical review: recent advances in rehabilitation. British Medical Journal 320: 1385–1388

World Confederation for Physical Therapy 1998 Description of physical therapy (draft). WCPT, London

Chapter 1

Introduction to problem solving

Karen Atkinson

OBJECTIVES

By the end of this chapter you should:

- Grasp the basic concepts of problem solving
- Be aware of the ways that you approach problem-solving activities
- Begin to appreciate how the problem-solving approach relates to clinical orthopaedic practice
- Have some ideas about how you can use creative thinking to enable more effective problem solving.

KEY WORDS

Problem solving, blocks, decision making, clinical reasoning, creative thinking.

Prerequisites

You should have read the Introduction, 'How to use this book', before starting this chapter.

PROBLEM SOLVING

Psychologists have been studying problem solving for over 100 years. As you may imagine, this work has produced extensive literature and our intention, therefore, is not to cover all angles of the subject in this book but to address some of the key issues. You need to be aware of the importance of problem solving in physiotherapy clinical practice. Problem-solving approaches are presented in many physiotherapy texts as innovative ways to deal with patient management in the clinical setting. This book also presents you with a problem-solving approach. In order to put this into perspective, however, we want to introduce you to it by linking it to your own everyday experiences. As you are aware, many of our daily routines involve problem-solving activities – for example, when we decide what to wear in the morning, how we will get to work or college, which job- or study-related activities we will carry out and in which order, and so on. We are, therefore, already extremely familiar with problem solving but generally the underlying processes that we use when dealing with different situations occur on a subconscious level; that is, we rarely think about 'how' we solve problems.

Not all problem solving is alike. According to Frensch & Funke (1995) some problems can be solved with a few mental steps and others require extensive thinking; there are some problems that we have never encountered before and there are others with which we are familiar; some problems have very clear goals and some have goals that are far from clear. Problems can, therefore, be distinguished in a range of meaningful dimensions and the solution processes may differ widely for different types of problem.

Our experience of solving problems begins very early in life. For a small child an initial problem such as 'How can I reach that colourful toy?' must seem very complex and difficult to solve, particularly if that child is not physically developed enough to move around independently. This problem becomes much simpler to deal with later on in life; that is, what may be problematic for a young child may not be so for an older child or an adult. Reaching the toy will be a dilemma the first few times it is encountered but it ceases to be a difficulty once the child learns how to do it.

For a physiotherapy student, discovering how to use an ultrasound machine could be a problem the first time. It may appear complex and not easy to understand. It does not remain so for long, however, because there is one fairly straightforward solution. This differs from the situation where a student has to decide on the appropriate physiotherapy

intervention for a patient with rheumatoid arthritis. The problems encountered here are much more complex and multifactorial. To make things even more interesting, the factors that need to be considered will change with each patient as everyone is so different (May & Newman 1980). This type of problem is more difficult to manage and it is not possible to learn just one, straightforward solution.

Evidence from developmental studies demonstrates that a child's abilities to solve problems emerge spontaneously as he acquires more knowledge, and superficial concepts are replaced with deeper ones (Kahney 1993). These skills improve with maturity as they are learned through experience. It is unlikely that anyone can get through a day without having to go through the problem-solving mechanism at some point. Even though this process begins from birth and continues throughout life it is interesting to note how little thought we give to what is actually going on in our minds at the time.

People vary in their problem-solving styles, some being quite systematic, working through step by step, whereas others appear to find solutions by intuition. Alternatively, there can be different approaches for different types of problem (May & Newman 1980). By the time you reach the stage of reading this book, you will have already developed your own approach to solving problems. If you are able to solve them with no difficulty, you probably never consider the process. Now you are starting to think about problems in the clinical setting, however, where you have less, if any, experience, you will need to develop different strategies to apply in your physiotherapy practice. Before we get into that, let's try to make the process a little simpler by considering the more general problems in the list below:

- How can I pass my anatomy exam?
- What is the best route to work tomorrow if there's a bus strike?
- If I have three different-sized rings on pole one, how can I move them to pole two and not break the rules?
- How do I go about performing a literature search for my project?
- How do I go about writing a classic novel?
- Where did I put my keys?

- How can I make something of my life?
- How will I manage to live for the rest of the term/month when my grant/salary runs out?

Some of these problems may be things that you have to deal with regularly, or perhaps have dealt with in the past. The rest, you may never have to tackle yourself, but hopefully you can see that they could be problems for other people. Using the terminology of cognitive research a problem exists when 'you want something and do not know immediately what series of mental operations you can use to get it' (Soden 1994). This description of 'a problem' allows a task to be a problem for one person but not for someone else who has encountered the situation previously.

Review point

In cognitive research terms your ability to problem solve has two key factors:

1. Your previous experience of the same or similar problems
2. Your knowledge base including what you learned and stored in memory about solving problems on previous occasions.

Think about a problem you have had to deal with lately – do these two factors seem appropriate to your way of problem solving?

It is widely recognized that there is a need for problem solving in physiotherapy as well as in medical and other allied health professions (Morris 1993). May & Newman (1980) state that 'problem solving is an integral part of effective physiotherapy practice'. If students or clinicians cannot recognize patients' problems then it will be difficult, if not impossible, to formulate the goals and appropriate treatment plans necessary for successful patient management. We will come back to this later.

Two other high-level cognitive skills, decision making and clinical reasoning, are intimately related to problem solving. These have been intensively investigated over the last 40 years by psychologists, philosophers and others.

Human beings have desires and needs, and they use their knowledge to decide what to do and to infer how best to achieve their goals. They reason in order to make decisions and to justify them both to themselves and others; they reason in order to determine the consequences of their beliefs and of their hypothetical actions; they reason to work out plans of action. They make decisions about what values to treat as paramount; they make decisions about what actions to take; and they make decisions about what information to base their reasoning on. Hence, there is an interdependence between reasoning and decision making.

Johnson-Laird & Shafir 1993

The 'reasoning' aspect is extremely important for us as it refers to the thinking processes associated with clinical practice. According to Higgs (1992) this includes the ability to utilize thinking skills, reflection, review and evaluation. It also entails metacognition which involves an awareness of the thinking processes, and the ability to access data already stored in long-term memory.

Decision making is something that everyone does on a regular basis, but the making of decisions, whether they are large or small, is often complicated and difficult because of uncertainty and conflict. We might be uncertain of the exact consequences of the actions we take as a result of our decisions. We may also experience conflict about how much of one attribute (e.g. time saving) to trade off against another (e.g. quality of the result) (Shafir et al 1993).

Lindsay & Norman (1977) state that decision making is 'choice among complex issues involving combining psychological impressions of the issues and comparing these'. So psychological impressions are formed, then compared, and the positive and negative factors are weighed to determine the final decisions made. It is important to realize, however, that the availability of data stored in memory will also play a large part in this process; that is, what is already known influences the decisions made. This relates directly to the problem solving and reasoning skills mentioned earlier. Considering the influence of the existing 'database' may give us some clue to the individual differences found between problem solvers when they are faced with exactly the same issues and information. Even more fascinating is that one person may arrive at different decisions if the same issues and information are considered, but in a different order (Lindsay & Norman 1977).

SO, WHAT IS PROBLEM SOLVING?

Look back briefly at the list of general problems given earlier. According to Kahney (1993) all problems have two things in common:

- a goal – for example, something a person wants or wants to do/achieve, such as finding the keys or performing a literature search
- something stopping them from immediately reaching that goal; that is, some kind of block, which could be due, for example, to lack of resources or lack of knowledge.

This then provides the basis for the concept of problem solving: whenever our desired goals are blocked, we are faced with problems; and whatever we do to achieve our goals is problem solving. The block keeping us from our goal has to be dealt with in some way, and this could involve mental or physical processes, or elements of both (Fig. 1.1).

Much of the work that has been carried out into problem solving has been in-depth study of what are known as transformational problems; that is, where an initial state is transformed into a target state by certain moves. A simple example of this would be changing yellow into green by adding blue. If the resulting shade of green were too dark then it could be lightened by adding more yellow and so on, until the desired shade was achieved.

So that you don't get too bored with reading for a long period, it's now time for you to have a go at problem solving. The intention of this is twofold:

- to show you a slightly more complex example of a transformational problem (the exercise below is one commonly used by psychologists)
- to let you 'have a go' at solving a problem, which should aid in your appreciation of some of the mental operations involved, which will be discussed later.

In order to get the most out of this exercise, it is important that you observe yourself as you go through the stages of reaching a solution. Note:

- what you do
- the difficulties you have
- the points of the problem that give you clues to move on.

Quite a useful way of doing this is to jot down what you do as you go along – or even better, tape it. Say everything you think out loud as you work on the problem, and why you decide on certain moves. You can then look back on the stages you went through. This type of verbal record is known as a protocol.

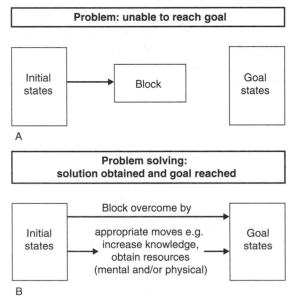

Figure 1.1 A: A problem: some block preventing solution. B: Problem solving: processes that allow goal achievement.

Problem-solving exercise 1.1

The Towers of Hanoi

There are three poles labelled 1, 2 and 3. On pole 1 there are three rings, a large, a medium and a small. You must transfer all the three rings from pole 1 to pole 2 (largest on the bottom, then the medium and then the smallest on top). Both these states – i.e. the initial state and the goal state – are shown in Figure 1.2. These are the rules:

- You can only move one ring at a time
- You must not place the rings anywhere except on one of the other poles (e.g. not on floor or table)

- You may not place a larger ring on top of a smaller one.

If you have access to poles and rings, you can use these to help you, if not, three different-sized coins can be used, or draw it out on a piece of paper.

1. How many moves did it take you to solve the problem? (It should take seven – see end of chapter.) Look back at your notes or listen to the tape you made while solving the Towers of Hanoi.
2. Do you think you recorded everything that you thought?
3. Do you think everything you did was accompanied by a specific thought?

You will probably find that there are some gaps; there could even be times when you did not know what you were thinking. If this is the case with such a well-defined problem then imagine the difficulties in describing the processes occurring

when we try to reason through a more complex problem. According to Johnson-Laird & Shafir (1993), we are often not aware of how we reason through a problem and in fact probably only glimpse some parts of the process. We are aware of the results but not the mechanism and often what we say about our reasoning does not compare closely with its real nature. In fact, we are often not aware of the real basis of our decisions. Because of these issues the 'protocol analysis' technique of looking at the process of problem solving can be rather controversial. It is fully effective only when two specific conditions are met:

- the person must describe what they are doing at that moment, not what they previously did
- what the person says they are doing must be reflected in their actual behaviour (Banyard & Hayes 1991).

As we said at the beginning of the chapter, our intention here is not to go into all aspects of problem solving, either positive or negative. What we want to encourage you to do is to start thinking about how you problem solve already and how you might develop these skills. The purpose of the exercise above is to begin this process.

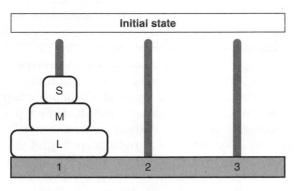

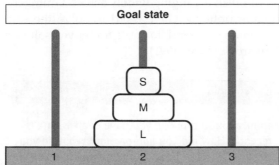

Figure 1.2   The Towers of Hanoi.

Review point

You have just had the experience of producing a protocol and trying to analyse it. How easy or difficult did you find it in relation to the two conditions above? Do you think you always described what you were doing at the time? Did your behaviour reflect what you said?

As mentioned earlier, it is important to remember that if you were presented with the same problem a second time you would almost certainly tackle it differently – this is because of your previous experience of it and the data that you effectively stored in your memory. Even if there was quite a protracted period of time between the first and second tries, you would probably remember the overall successful approach that you eventually came up with in the initial instance. Undoubtedly, experience changes the nature of the problem-solving task.

When studying the process you went through when solving the Towers of Hanoi, you probably found that you broke the overall goal down into a number of smaller steps.

This is quite a common technique. The difference between the beginning of the problem and the problem being solved is sometimes known as the 'problem space'. Even for fairly simple problems the problem space might be quite large and so exploring all possibilities is too cumbersome. A 'means–ends' analysis involves breaking the problem down into a number of smaller stages, which reduces the problem space. The problem can then be solved in a stepwise manner, working towards each sub-goal in turn (Banyard & Hayes 1991). People presented with a problem will try out a variety of simple strategies, hoping that each will yield relevant information. Some strategies work, which gives more data, some do not and so backing up occurs, followed by a different line of approach (Lindsay & Norman 1977).

The Towers of Hanoi is one type of problem that has been used by psychologists to study the processes involved in problem solving. There is, however, dissatisfaction with these sorts of task being used in such studies because they are seen as being too one-sided. This refers to them being too simple, fully transparent and static in contrast to real life situations, which tend to be complex, intransparent and dynamic (Buchner 1995). These tasks are said to lack 'ecological validity', i.e. they have little to do with problem-solving situations in everyday life (Kluwe 1995). That being said, however, for those people who are novices at problem-solving analysis, this type of task can be a useful starting point.

So why is there such a fascination with problem solving? Well, the ideal situation would be to put all problems into groups or categories, and then to work out and understand the mental operations used by successful problem solvers while reaching their solutions. If this were possible, the next step, within the context of this book at least, would be to teach you the successful strategies used by expert clinicians in dealing with the management of their patients. You would then be good at problem solving in that situation yourselves – well at least you might be better at it! Unfortunately, because of the extremely wide range of problems and differences in context, complexity and content, this is unlikely to happen. It is often difficult to see the common elements and similarities between two apparently simple problems. This suggests, therefore, that even the categorization itself would be impossible.

This does not mean however, that you cannot become a better problem solver. Education systems have a tendency to emphasize the use of our minds for storing information instead of developing their power to produce new ideas (Lumsdaine & Lumsdaine 1995). By participating in exercises and activities such as those presented in this book (and also those in many creative problem-solving texts) you can build your problem-solving skills. Working on problems in groups can also help in this process as you can explore, discuss and brainstorm the relevant issues. The ability to think in creative and flexible ways will enable you to become a more effective physiotherapist.

Convergent and divergent thinking

This is one way of trying to think about how you might address a problem – your 'cognitive style'. It might also explain to some degree why you find some types of problem easier to solve than others. Convergent thinkers tend to be very logical, adopting linear and focused styles of reasoning when asked to solve a particular problem. They work consistently towards a defined solution, generally assuming that there is a 'right answer' and that the best way to reach it is to work directly towards it. Divergent thinkers are often more intuitive and impulsive, ranging widely across a number of different options when asked to solve the same problem. They tend to look for novel solutions (Banyard & Hayes 1991).

Think about a problem you have dealt with recently. How did you approach it? What do you think your cognitive style might be? Are you a convergent or a divergent thinker?

Problem-solving exercise 1.2 Uses for a brick

On a piece of paper write down as many uses (both usual and unusual) that you can think of for a brick, and then do the same for a cup.

How many did you come up with? Was it hard or easy to do this? If you get a few friends to do this too (without any prompting), how do your lists compare?

Divergent thinkers may find this sort of exercise easier and come up with many more uses than convergent thinkers. In fact, they often suggest uses that their more convergent colleagues regard as quite bizarre (Banyard & Hayes 1991).

Convergent and divergent thinking as discussed above are at the opposite ends of a continuum and most of us sit somewhere in between. Also, just because we tend towards one end of the spectrum or the other does not mean that we are unable to develop our abilities in the other way of thinking. We believe that it is useful to have elements of each of the approaches when considering patient problems. This may be why healthcare teams can work so well if you have a mixture of convergent and divergent thinkers in the group who will look at the issues from different angles.

MENTAL SETS, FIXED THINKING AND MENTAL BLOCKS

Research has shown that we can develop mental sets in our approach to problem solving. If we have enough experience of solving one type of problem in a particular way, we will tend to choose that method even if there is an easier and quicker way of finding a solution. A mental set can be positive, as it may mean the way we have learned is the fastest and most efficient method of solving the problem. Alternatively, it can be negative because it can block us from seeing more effective possibilities (Banyard & Hayes 1991). Fixed thinking of this type can result in us mistakenly assuming that there are boundaries or limits to problems that do not actually exist, which can also be known as a conceptual block. This may happen

particularly when someone is presented with a new scenario (Banyard & Hayes 1991, Soden 1994, Fogler & LeBlanc 1995). The Nine Dot Problem is a simple example of this.

Problem-solving exercise 1.3

Join up all nine dots with four straight lines or fewer. You must not take the pencil off the paper or go over the same line twice.

Try this exercise on a separate piece of paper before looking at the solutions overleaf.

How did you do?

This puzzle is very difficult to solve if you do not cross the imaginary boundary created by the eight outer dots. There are a number of solutions, some more creative than others. The rules said nothing about the lines needing to stay within the square formed by the dots (see solution 1 – Fig. 1.4) or about the lines having to go through the centre of each dot (see solution 2 – Fig. 1.5) but many people constrain themselves by applying these non-existent rules when trying to solve this problem. The purpose of this type of exercise is to show that putting too many constraints (conscious or unconscious) on the problem statement narrows the range of possible solutions. This tendency is more common in novice problem solvers, who will not cross perceived imaginary limits (constraints formed unconsciously in the mind of the problem solver), even though these are not part of the original problem (Fogler & LeBlanc 1995). Next time you are faced with a difficult problem, think of the nine dots to remind yourself to challenge the boundaries.

In order to do something about mental blocks, you need to identify or recognize them in the first place and understand how they can interfere with the problem-solving process. A range of mental

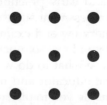

Figure 1.3   The Nine Dot Problem.

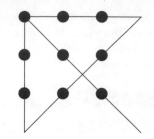

Figure 1.4   One solution to the Nine Dot Problem.

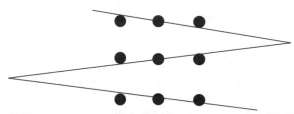

Figure 1.5   A second possible solution to the Nine Dot Problem.

blocks has been described (Fogler & LeBlanc 1995), many of which we can examine in relation to the clinical setting.

Perceptual blocks

These are obstacles that prevent us from perceiving either the problem itself or the information needed to solve it. Stereotyping, limiting the problem unnecessarily and/or information overload can cause this sort of block to problem solving. For example, if you learn 'recipes' of physiotherapy treatment interventions for patients with particular conditions (as is very tempting for a novice practitioner), this will cause you to have a stereotyped and limited approach to the problems with which they may present. This 'mental set' may work for some situations but will fall down eventually if you do not start to look beyond your subconscious boundaries.

For students and early practitioners, overload can occur at the assessment stage of patient management. You interview and examine the patient, only to find that you have so much information it is difficult to know what to do with it. Guidance from your clinical educator and more experience will gradually enable you to pick out the essential information and to challenge the boundaries. These

are necessary elements in the problem-solving process.

Emotional blocks

These can interfere with your abilities to solve problems in many ways. They can prevent you from exploring ideas, can reduce flexibility in your thinking and can prevent you from communicating clearly. This can be the case for students, especially at the beginning of clinical placements when confidence levels are often low. There are elements here that relate to risk taking and dealing with confusing and contradictory information. Sometimes it is tempting to latch on to the first apparently feasible solution to a problem. This is a negative approach, where the situation is judged too quickly and can create blocks to finding a workable solution.

'Believing that you can't do something is a self-fulfilling prophesy' (Fogler & LeBlanc 1995). Most people fear failure and often feel unable to take risks but we can learn from mistakes and so should not be afraid to make them (Lumsdaine & Lumsdaine 1995). Risk taking is a scary business, you have to use good judgement to decide when to take a risk and it needs practice. You can start with mental practice; that is, think about the risk you might be taking and about why it is important, then imagine the best and the worst possible outcomes. If the result of taking your risk was poor, imagine what your options would be and how you would deal with the failure. When you actually try out risk taking, start with something small and relatively safe, for example, speaking out in a group when you have an idea. If the result of doing this is positive you can store the information (what you did and how it felt) for future reference. If the result is negative, however, again you can reflect on what you did and how it felt and feed the experience into your next attempt so starting from a more informed position. It is a good learning experience and, because you only took a relatively small risk, your confidence will not be too dented. Use your peers and the role models around you to get feedback on your thinking and also ask others how they reason their way through to solutions. By being positive and reflecting on your problem-solving experiences you will build your confidence and reduce emotional blocks.

Cultural blocks

Cultural blocks to problem solving are acquired by exposure to specific cultural patterns. This is a particularly important issue for physiotherapists working with patients from a wide range of minority ethnic and cultural groups. It is extremely important to be aware of differences in beliefs about health and wellbeing and how these might affect a patient's approach to your intervention.

Environmental blocks

This type of block can be due to both physical and psychological factors. If you are trying to concentrate but keep getting distracted by the telephone or other people, or if the environment is overly hot or cold, these relatively simple environmental factors can have a negative effect on your problem-solving ability. Psychologically, if you feel supported by your peers and your clinical educator and the working atmosphere is pleasant, you will feel safer and will be more likely to think and problem solve effectively and creatively. Conversely if you are working in conditions where you feel you are unsupported emotionally, physically and/or organizationally you are less likely to be an effective problem solver. It is unlikely that new and creative ideas will be welcomed in this type of environment.

Intellectual blocks

These can occur in two ways – as a result of lack of background knowledge in the particular area or a lack of and/or inflexibility in the use of problem-solving abilities. This again can be an issue for novice practitioners such as students or newly qualified therapists. You may need to increase your background knowledge and over time improve your problem-solving approach in the specific clinical setting. Make sure you ask for help when you need it but remember that problem solving is a transferable skill and previous clinical and life experience will be of help to you. Don't undermine your own confidence by thinking that just because you are a student or a newly qualified therapist you have no useful knowledge and experience to bring to a new situation.

Expressive blocks

These blocks can be due to an inability to communicate your ideas in verbal or written form. Most physiotherapists are good communicators but if you are a novice practitioner it may initially be more difficult to express your ideas clearly.

We have talked about a number of blocks to the problem-solving process and included some ideas for addressing these. Most of the blocks appear to centre on boundaries and limitations to thinking. They can be either internal (whether conscious or subconscious) or external. More and more writers are looking at ways to break free from these limitations by using lateral and creative thinking techniques. 'Lateral thinking' was a term coined by Edward de Bono and involves the ability to step outside the boundaries of a problem and to develop innovative and novel solutions (Banyard & Hayes 1991).

Fogler & LeBlanc (1995) cite an example that clearly illustrates blocks to effective problem solving. The majority of solvers put limitations in place that were not included in the problem statement. At an American Medical Association convention an X-ray of the upper body was displayed at the registration desk. The doctors were asked to diagnose the problem and put their answers in a competition box. A winner would be drawn from those giving the correct diagnosis and a valuable prize awarded. Because the X-ray showed the upper torso, every kind of lung pathology was suggested. Eventually there was no need to have a draw as only one doctor gave the correct diagnosis: a fractured left arm.

There are a number of principles that you can refer to if you are interested in improving your creative thinking abilities in order to facilitate your problem-solving skills. These are set out in Box 1.1.

MENTAL OPERATIONS FOR EFFECTIVE PROBLEM SOLVING

Alongside improvements in your creative thinking, which can facilitate your problem-solving skills, it is useful to consider some of the processes that might be going on in your mind while you are working towards your solutions. If you look at these carefully you will see quite a lot of parallels between them and the creative-thinking strategies.

Box 1.1 Improving your creative abilities

- Keep a note of your ideas – you will probably forget them if you don't write them down
- Be curious, have an inquiring mind – pose new questions to yourself each day
- Work on developing a solid foundation of knowledge and skills in physiotherapy and keep up to date
- Look outside physiotherapy – concepts from other specialities can be very useful
- Question conventional wisdom and be wary of rigid, set ways of doing things
- Actively look for new ways of doing things and be open and receptive to ideas
- Actively observe situations and problems to identify relationships – similarities and differences
- Be a risk taker, be persistent and don't let temporary setbacks undermine your confidence
- Keep your sense of humour – this can reduce tension and makes you more relaxed. It can help to put your problems into perspective
- Engage in creative hobbies. These keep your mind active and more receptive to new ideas. They can also help you to relax
- Be self-confident and courageous – believe in yourself, you know you can perform well, you are well prepared, you've done it before so you can do it again even in a new situation
- Increase your self-knowledge and understanding – strengths, weaknesses, likes, dislikes, biases, expectations, fears and prejudices. This will help you to understand how and why you react in certain ways.

(Lumsdaine & Lumsdaine 1995, Fogler & LeBlanc 1995)

Many psychologists have identified the following points as some of the mental operations that contribute to efficient problem solving:

- Generation of alternative courses of action, not just sticking to one set way of looking at a problem
- Identification of the future consequences of the proposed course of action. If I do this, or choose this method/treatment, or say that – what might the effect or result be? You do, however, have to be careful with this one. It is possible to get so bogged down with thinking through the consequences that you never act
- Describing the advantages and disadvantages of courses of action. This is closely linked to the previous point but is also associated with risk assessment
- Recalling similar problems and actions taken and being able to generalize these to the current problem. This point comes up over and again in the problem-solving texts. Previous experience and the database you build up as a result of this are of great importance in improving your problem-solving skills
- Finding a starting point in a problem that allows you to move forward. This is why physiotherapists carry out assessments when they first see their patients in order to establish a baseline from which to proceed. There is a lot of skill involved here when dealing with a complex problem and you need to guard against coming up against perceptual blocks such as overload
- Checking solutions against facts. If you have built your solid foundation of physiotherapy knowledge and skills along with bringing in ideas from other areas, this will enable you to carry out this checking activity. Remember that you don't need to have all the information in your head, but need to know where you can obtain it in a timely manner
- Looking for features of a problem that remind you of a problem previously tackled successfully. Again we return to previous experience and the strategy of actively observing your problem-solving processes to identify relationships.

These mental operations often take the form of questions that you can ask yourself during a problem-solving procedure (Soden 1994).

Review point

Think of a problem you have had to deal with recently at college or at work. How many, if any, of the above mental operations did you use when tackling the problem?

Familiar examples of mental procedures that may take place when addressing a task are decision making, planning, prioritizing and organizing. Effective problem solvers learn a wide range of mental procedures that they can call upon and modify as necessary with little conscious effort. They can also build new procedures by amalgamating parts of existing ones. This may mean that the task is not perceived as 'a problem' because there are few, if any, blocks in the way of achieving the goal state. It may only be when the solver becomes aware of the need to search for a procedure to deal with a task that it is deemed to be a problem (Soden 1994).

WELL-DEFINED AND ILL-DEFINED PROBLEMS

Some researchers have divided problems into two broad categories or classes:

- well-defined problems
- ill-defined problems.

Well-defined problems

This category of problem is one where there is a clearly stated goal. It is well structured and all the information necessary to solve the problem is provided. As you probably realize, you have had experience of solving a well-defined problem in the Towers of Hanoi example. It is necessary to have a goal, and ways to tell whether the problem solving is proceeding as hoped. Kahney (1993) divides the information needed to solve a well-defined problem into four sections:

- initial state of the problem
- goal state
- legal operators – things you are allowed to do to solve it
- operator restrictions – factors governing or constraining the use of legal operators. These could be seen as the 'rules' in some instances.

Self-assessment questions

- **SAQ 1.1** Go back to the Towers of Hanoi problem and work out the four parts mentioned above, i.e. the initial state of the problem, goal state, legal operators and operator restrictions.

- **SAQ 1.2** Work out the initial states and goal states for the following problems:
  1. A game of scrabble
  2. Solving a crossword clue.

A more general example of a well-defined problem may be something like the earlier ones: 'What is the best route to work tomorrow if there is a bus strike?' or 'How do I go about performing a literature search for my project?' It is possible to work out the initial state, what the goal is and how you can achieve it. It might also be appropriate to think about what constraints or restrictions there might be.

Ill-defined problems

In comparison to the well-defined problem, ill-defined problems have poor structure with little or no information regarding initial and goal states, or operators. If you try to analyse these problems, everything is rather vaguely defined. There was an example of this earlier: 'How can I pass my anatomy exam?'

So how can this be analysed?

- *Initial state*: anatomy paper containing questions. You know how many to answer and how much time you've got

- *Goal state*: the grade you want. So, if you want a good pass, your answers will have to be better than if you only want to scrape a pass. But how do you know whether your answers are worth a good pass? How do you know if your goal has been achieved? Presumably the only way you will know for certain is when you receive your results, by which time it could be a little late

- *Operators*: well there is really no information given here. You are not told about retrieving information from memory, making notes, doing essay plans, not including irrelevant material, division of time between questions and so on. All the things you are expected to know already about sitting an exam – but do you? Has anyone gone through the process with you to at least provide you with the opportunity for mental rehearsal?

- *Operator restrictions*: because you are in an exam situation, many of the ways you might normally obtain information are not available to you, such as asking your peers, looking at your notes, reading books, consulting a lecturer and so on. Even your time is restricted.

In this example, you have to take part in defining the problem. As we have discussed before, the degree of the problem structure depends on your knowledge and experience. If you are an experienced student who has taken many exams before and who is very familiar with the subject matter, you will augment the information given to you at the beginning with knowledge from long-term memory. So the problem of 'How can I pass my anatomy exam?' might be relatively straightforward, even though it is categorized as 'ill defined'. If, however, you are a mature student entering physiotherapy education after a long break, never having taken an exam before, with many external factors affecting your capacity to study, this piece of assessment may be a much more complex problem for you to solve.

EXPERIENCE OF THE PROBLEM SOLVER

It becomes clear that the boundary between well- and ill-defined problems becomes blurred when the solver's knowledge is taken into account. This suggests that the amount of structure that a problem has initially can be used to decide how it will be treated by the solver, rather than trying to put it into a particular category.

For those people interested in analysing the 'solving process', however, it is the ill-defined, more complex category of problem that comes up more frequently. Even though scientists try to analyse the operations going on in the problem-solving process, they are unlikely to be fully successful because each person tackling the problem will have his or her own internal representation of it. Furthermore, as the problem is worked on, those internal representations will change and these changes will not be the same for each person. The problem state may be exactly the same for each person at the beginning but, after a few individual solution steps, different people will face different problem states (Kluwe 1995). So again we come back to an individual's performance in problem solving being an amalgam of existing knowledge base and any strategies in place as a result of previous experience of solving similar problems.

Our knowledge, attitudes and abilities are controlled by neural networks that have been determined by experience. The older we get and the more experiences we have, the more 'hard wired' these networks become and it takes time and effort to change. Learning new habits and problem-solving skills takes effort because we have to establish new connections in the neural networks to override the old habitual patterns (Lumsdaine & Lumsdaine 1995).

Most of the studies into problem solving concentrate on the well-defined problems. The goal is to understand the processes people use in working through to the solution of problems. This involves the construction of internal models of the problem, the strategies used, the rules followed and the assessment of progress. Kahney (1993) gives some reasons for the use of the simpler, well-defined problems in research work. 'Toy worlds' are set up and examined as models of reality to help in the understanding of how people behave in real world situations, because the real world is extremely complex and 'messy' and therefore difficult to study. These studies can be done in the laboratory setting, in easily observable stages with subjects needing no prior knowledge. Problems can be presented in different ways with different 'cover stories'. They can be scaled up, for example by repeating the Towers of Hanoi but increasing the number of rings to five. This may then show how the subjects use their previous experience with similar problems to help in solving the present one. These experiments take a relatively short time. This makes them manageable in comparison to the real world, where problems may take anywhere from a few minutes, to more than a lifetime to solve.

How realistic it is to generalize the results from the above types of problem solving to real-world everyday activities has been discussed earlier. We would however, like to reassure you that we are including these activities and descriptions of problems to act as triggers for you to begin thinking about your own mental operations when problem solving.

Problem-solving exercise 1.4 The Chinese Tea Ceremony (adapted from Kahney 1993)

In a number of Himalayan villages, the innkeepers perform a very refined and civilized tea ceremony. It involves the innkeeper himself, who is the host, and two guests, never more or less. One guest holds a more exalted position than the other. The guests arrive and are seated comfortably at the table. The host then performs three services for them.

- Stoking the fire, which is the least noble task
- Pouring the tea, which is of medium nobility
- Reciting poetry, which is the most noble of the three.

    The 'rules' are as follows:

    As the ceremony proceeds any person present may ask another 'Honoured Sir, may I perform this onerous task for you?'

    He may only ask to perform the least noble task that the other is performing. Then, if someone is already performing any tasks, he cannot ask to take on a task that is nobler than the least noble task he is already doing. According to custom, by the time the ceremony is completed, all tasks must be transferred from the host to the most senior guest.

1. How can this be done?
    All of the information that you need to solve this problem is given to you.

    Here's a clue: it is exactly the same in underlying structure as the Towers of Hanoi.

2. Did you have any idea of the similarity between the two problems before you were given the clue?

This is an example of two problems that are identical in structure, but they have very different cover stories. It is quite common for problems to appear different superficially but to have similar solutions. As you've probably found, this is not always easy to detect. It can be useful to find analogies between present problems and ones for which the solution is known, to recognize similarities and differences. It is important, however, not to waste time and effort looking for similarities when there may not be any and what is really needed is a fresh approach (Lindsay & Norman 1977). This relates back to the earlier point about using creative and flexible thinking when problem solving. Psychologists can draw up plans of the structure of problems called state space diagrams. Some are quite difficult to work out, as certain problems have the possibility of a lot of 'illegal moves'. But the path taken through a state space diagram can be used to analyse a person's problem-solving behaviour.

An example of a simple state space diagram can be seen in Figure 1.6, which shows the possible steps in making a cup of tea (after Kahney 1993).

Many well-defined problems, for example those in mathematics, have direct and efficient solutions, i.e. algorithms. Use the rules properly and you will always get the right answer. But when people are asked to solve these problems they often use rambling trial and error methods. Why is this? Well, first, there could be difficulties in the person's understanding of the problem: not everyone will have perfect understanding of each one encountered. Second, algorithms and state space diagrams are very helpful if you can remember them, but each person will have a unique representation of the problem in his/her mind and each will also have a different amount of data stored in memory that can be brought to bear on it. Some people will have more and some will have less.

A side issue, which nevertheless needs to be briefly addressed, is that of the quality of each step taken when solving a problem. If making a cup of tea is used as an example, it may not seem very complex to you but it can still be difficult for someone who has never done it before. Any route taken through the state space diagram will result in a cup of tea being made – but will it be a good cup of tea?

Some people insist that a certain routine needs to be followed otherwise the result is poor. In other words, the milk should never be put in before the tea – and then of course, how much milk should be added? This is a simple illustration. It is not just a matter of following a route through to a solution. In order to ensure a quality

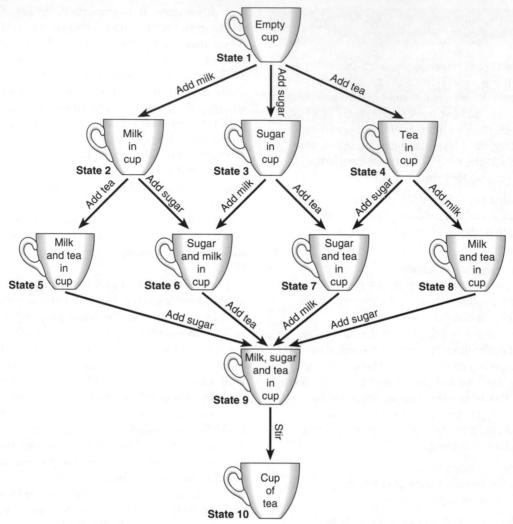

Figure 1.6 State space diagram for making a cup of tea. Any route through the plan will result in all the necessary constituents for a cup of tea being in the cup together.

result, it is also extremely important to consider the fine detail, i.e. the manner in which each step is performed.

THE ROLE OF MEMORY

Problem solving is limited by the constraints of short-term or working memory. It also depends on the information-processing system, the time involved in storage, and retrieval in long-term memory. It is only possible to think ahead effectively when there is already some experience with the topic. According to Lindsay & Norman (1977), the game of noughts and crosses is at the limit of human cognitive ability. For someone playing this game for the first time, there is no way that all the possibilities can be kept in mind, because of the limits of working memory. If it were played by sheer reasoning alone, it would not be possible to do it. But it is played, and in fact appears a very simple game, so why is this?

Well, again we return to people having previous experience. They have played the game and have learned certain structures that enable them to decide where to place the next symbol in the grid. If the first symbol is placed in the centre it will ensure a win, or at worst a draw. If the first player has already placed a symbol in the centre, then the second player must place his/hers in a corner, anything else guarantees a loss. Because it is possible to remember winning and losing configurations from previous games, it reduces the amount of forward planning necessary.

But is the human mind really as restricted as the noughts and crosses example suggests?

Yes and no.

Yes, because limitations of working memory do restrict performance – it is not possible to plan very far ahead when solving problems, especially those encountered in everyday life. But then, no, because it is possible to augment the limited amount of working memory with the following.

- *External aids to thought* such as writing, referral to notes, symbolic representation and so on.

- *Strategies to guide searches for solutions to problems.* Algorithms have already been considered, which, if followed, guarantee a solution. But they are not always helpful, particularly when dealing with complex problem-solving situations. Heuristics can be useful and are sometimes known as 'rule of thumb' problem-solving methods. A problem-solving heuristic is a systematic approach that helps to guide us through the process and to generate alternative solutions (Fogler & LeBlanc 1995). These methods often succeed by providing a uniform systematic approach for dealing with problems but they certainly do not guarantee success or prevent people from making mistakes. They involve taking the most probable options from a possible set rather than working through all the possible alternatives. They can be useful short cuts but they can go wrong too (Banyard & Hayes 1991). For example, if you are lost in a new city, your heuristic method of problem solving may be to ask someone the way. This usually works, but only if the person you ask knows the place you want to get to.

- *The capacity and flexibility of long-term memory.* This involves drawing on previous experience when confronted with a new problem. A person can become an 'expert' in a particular field

because of thousands of hours of practice, acquiring large amounts of structured knowledge that is stored in long-term memory. An example commonly used is that of expert chess players. They are often seen as having some sort of unique mental ability. This is, however, not so, because everyone has the same capabilities. The expert chess players have a large amount of knowledge of the game obtained through experience. They have organized this into clusters of meaningful, well-learned, structured information. These configurations can then be brought to bear on each new chess game. A novice, however, needs to use working memory just to remember the rules and moves. The experts have all this already stored in long-term memory and so they can use the working memory to concentrate on the problem in hand.

It is possible for anyone to use this strategy and in fact many people do so much of the time without being conscious of it. The key factor is that the configurations stored in long-term memory are meaningful, making them easier to retain and to work with than those that make no sense.

Problem–solving exercise 1.5

How well can you remember a sequence of letters? The limit for most people is about 10. Look at the following letters once and then try to repeat them without looking at the page:

F T P G I B J Z M U

1. Did you find them difficult to remember?
2. If so, why do you think this is?

Each letter is a separate unit and must therefore be stored separately in memory.

Now consider what happens if letters are organized into some meaningful configuration – repeat the exercise with the following sequence of letters:

P R O C E S S I N G

Not only is it easy, but in fact you probably do not even think of them as separate at all but as a contained unit, which is represented in memory as a single item. It is easy to remember even longer lists of letters in this way, try the one below:

The book *Physiotherapy in Orthopaedics – a problem-solving approach* introduces the reader to problem solving in the clinical setting.

Here, even though there are 112 letters, the exercise is relatively easy because the sequence of letters is meaningful to you.

The apparent skill of expert chess players deteriorates markedly when they are asked to remember meaningless configurations of pieces on a chess board, just as yours does when asked to remember meaningless sequences of letters. An efficient way of storing information or knowledge in memory is therefore based on meaning. Concepts that are meaningfully related to one another are stored together and this enables us to retrieve information that makes sense. Understanding develops as more meaningful information is collected or received and added to the existing concept structure. Depth of understanding can be thought of as the number of meaningful links made with other concepts. We all have huge numbers of these concept structures, enabling us to store a vast amount of knowledge in memory, and there are many links between these structures. As we gain more knowledge these links change. An important difference between novices and experts in a particular occupational area is that experts store their knowledge in larger concept structures with a greater network of links in place. This enables easier and more efficient retrieval of knowledge, as they don't have to spend time searching a great number of more haphazardly stored, unrelated concept structures. The larger structures used by experts tend to be built around core principles and concepts rather than specific facts (Soden 1994).

ANALOGICAL PROBLEM SOLVING

According to Kahney (1993), it has been shown that people actively use old knowledge in trying to understand new events or problems. This is known as analogical problem solving – analogies between old problems and new problems are identified. Most of the situations encountered in everyday life are fairly familiar and therefore analogous to previous experience. This means that each person already has a lot of the knowledge necessary to deal with each scenario. But it is not always easy to identify the analogy or to know how to apply the solution. Experiments have shown that subjects are good at using this method if they are given hints that this is what they should do; if the hints are not given, previous analogies are not so helpful.

This type of problem solving is useful in new situations, but again it does rely on retrieval of data from long-term memory. So if the original problem can be remembered, this will help in solving the present one. There are, however, some difficulties with this. If long-term memory fails and the old problem cannot be retrieved, then the new problem has to be solved from the beginning. It is also possible that false analogies may be used that will lead to the wrong solution. For example, meeting one person with rheumatoid arthritis (RA) who copes very well with the long-term symptoms may lead you to assume that 'all people with RA cope well with the condition'. This in turn may lead to an incorrect reaction in a new situation.

Even with the disadvantages discussed above, however, there is no doubt that past experience does help in present problem solving. Clear differences can be seen between novices, those with intermediate amounts of experience and experts. This is not to say that experts never have to problem solve or never come across unfamiliar situations. As discussed earlier, because of the highly structured amounts of information they have in long-term memory, they have a marked advantage over novices in many tasks. They probably have solutions memorized for many types of problem they come across, whereas the novice has a much smaller store of answers to fall back on. Even if there is not a direct answer available to the experts, they will have evolved general strategies for dealing with particular types of problem within their own field, which novices will not yet have developed. Novices tend to concentrate on the objects mentioned in the problem rather than relating back to underlying principles. If, however, experts are put into areas with which they are unfamiliar, their problem-solving skills revert back to those used by novices.

COMPLEX PROBLEM SOLVING

Most of the situations that you will come across in physiotherapy practice will involve what is known as complex problem solving (CPS). Frensch & Funke (1995) offer the following as a definition of CPS:

> CPS occurs to overcome barriers between a given state and a desired goal state by means of behavioural and/or cognitive, multistep activities. The given state, goal state and barriers between given state and goal state are complex, change dynamically during problem solving, and are intransparent (e.g. only knowledge about symptoms is available, from which one has to infer the underlying state (Funke 1991)). The exact properties of the given state, goal state and barriers are unknown to the solver at the outset. CPS implies the efficient interaction between a solver and the situational requirements of the task and involves a solver's cognitive, emotional, personal and social abilities and knowledge.

This definition is much wider and considers many more elements than those used in solving the previously discussed transformational problems. It is however, much more relevant to your situation when dealing with patients in the clinical setting. First it returns us to the mental operations that occur during problem solving that we considered earlier. Second, it adds in a behavioural element – thinking and doing; following a certain procedure to solve a problem in a real life context. Third, it brings in an affective dimension; emotional and personal elements that influence the abilities of the solver to address the problem. Fourth, this definition acknowledges the importance of the specific situation and how changes can occur during the problem-solving process. Lastly, it returns us again to knowledge, i.e. the database already in place, including background knowledge and previous experience of solving similar problems, which the solver can call upon in the current situation.

DECISION MAKING

Decision making is part of the problem-solving process. We have to tackle problems throughout life and so we regularly make choices between alternatives. These decision-making tasks involve choices between actions and normally involve commitment to particular acts at one time, the consequences of which only become clear later. An objectively good decision is one that would pay off best on average if the decision could be made under the same circumstances a large number of times (Evans et al 1993). The making of decisions, however, both big and small, is often difficult because of uncertainty and conflict. We are uncertain about the exact consequences of our actions, which could also depend on external factors (Shafir et al 1993). In the process of selecting our alternatives, we weigh and evaluate relative merits and consider the costs and benefits. As already discussed in relation to problem solving, however, the selection process is often done without any awareness of the steps we go through to come to the final decision.

The choices of a rational decision maker are determined by the expected values associated with possible decisions. The probabilities of events and the payoffs and penalties are related to various outcomes. There is a definite distinction, however, between the rules that ought to be followed and those that are. Studies highlight the differences between logical decision making and human decision making. It is clear that logic is not often a major factor in decision making (Banyard & Hayes 1991). People may make decisions that appear illogical to you but may be perfectly sensible from their position, in terms of the information they have available at the time and the situation in which they find themselves. We have to take into account past experience, social factors, emotions and personal choice. In general terms, the major principle of rational decision making is 'optimization' – everything else being equal, choose the alternative with the greatest value. This does not, however, work very well in human decision making as each person will view benefits and costs differently (Lindsay & Norman 1977). You may well have heard someone say: 'I know it's stupid and it probably won't work, but I'm going to do it anyway' or you might have had the experience of making this type of decision yourself. In fact our conspicuous failure to recognize or take any notice of the possible negative outcomes of certain decisions has led some researchers in the field to question human rationality (Legrenzi et al 1993).

Because of the limits of working memory, people are often forced into decisions that minimize 'cognitive strain'; that is, they are unable to consider all the important variables. They may use what appear to be logical strategies to come to their decisions but they will probably not be the optimal ones. Inevitably they are unable to take everything into account that may impinge upon the situation. Estimates of optimization can also change over time. A particular decision might be made at one time but then a very different one made when the same information is considered at a later date. It is also true that different people have different judgements of the value of the same events.

This makes it sound as though it should be impossible to make decisions at all. People are, however, constantly choosing between alternatives and are often successful and happy with their choice. Some choices that we make stem from affective judgements that stop us making a thorough evaluation of all the options. This type of decision is very difficult to analyse. Other choices that we make may follow standard 'operating procedures' and involve minimal reflective effort. There are decisions that we make however, that result from careful evaluation of options in which we attempt to arrive at what we believe is the best choice. We will often discard the least attractive options but may still be left with choices that are hard to resolve. In these cases we will look for a compelling reason for choosing one alternative over another. The reasons that enter into decision making are likely to be intricate and diverse (Shafir et al 1993).

Many of the so-called imperfections in human judgement and reasoning seem to come and go depending on a number of factors such as the wording of the problem, the goals of the individual, the person's level of expertise in the area, and so on. Sometimes people manage quite well by the standards that are important to them and sometimes they do not. On the whole we are all fairly well adapted to making decisions in the general environment but not as well adapted to each 'sub-environment' we encounter (Klayman & Brown 1993). This is particularly the case when we first enter a new area – for example, clinical practice.

In the clinical setting, therefore, your problem solving in relation to patients is inseparable from your reasoning and decision-making processes. The decisions you make and the reasoning you use to reach them will influence whether or not you reach a satisfactory solution. This will be explored further in Chapter 4, but for now a number of factors need to be kept in mind for successful problem solving and decision making:

- When you see patients with a large variety of orthopaedic conditions, you need to have an accessible, organized knowledge base from which to work, in order to reach effective solutions

- Work on improving your awareness of your own problem-solving processes, be flexible and creative and use previous experiences of problem solving to feed into current practice

- Take some risks and reflect on the results. Use role models to improve your problem solving and be proactive in asking for feedback

- Recognize that patients must be involved in decision making and that they should be encouraged to play a responsible role in their own healthcare (Higgs 1992).

SUMMARY

This chapter has introduced you to the general issues of problem solving and decision making. These are both processes that you use constantly on a day to day basis. You have been encouraged to start thinking about the mechanisms involved and your own thinking and problem-solving style.

Problem solving in clinical orthopaedic practice has been presented briefly and will be expanded upon later in the book.

On reading this summary, do you feel you have grasped the above points? If not, perhaps you should go back and re-read any appropriate parts of the chapter before moving on.

ANSWERS TO QUESTIONS AND EXERCISES

Problem-solving exercise 1.1 – The Towers of Hanoi (page 10)

Answer: It should take seven moves as follows;

1. Small ring to pole 2
2. Medium ring to pole 3
3. Small ring to pole 3
4. Large ring to pole 2
5. Small ring to pole 1
6. Medium ring to pole 2
7. Small ring to pole 2.

Problem-solving exercise 1.3 (page 13)

See Figures 1.4 and 1.5 in text.

Self-assessment question 1.1 (page 17)

● **SAQ 1.1** Go back to the Towers of Hanoi problem and work out the initial state of the problem, goal state, legal operators and operator restrictions.

Answer:

Initial state – three poles, number 1 on the left with three rings on it (small on top of medium on top of large), then two empty poles, number 2 in the middle and number 3 on the right.

Goal state – the three rings on pole 2 in the same order as above.

Legal operators – move rings from one pole to another.

Operator restrictions – (i) move one ring at a time, (ii) do not place rings anywhere except on another pole, (iii) do not place larger rings on top of smaller.

Self-assessment question 1.2 (page 17)

● **SAQ 1.2** Work out the initial states and goal states for the following problems:

a. A game of Scrabble

Answer:

Initial state – an empty Scrabble board, every player has several tiles each with a letter on, spare tiles in bag.

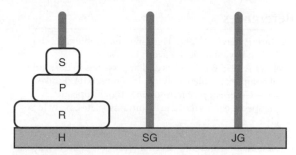

Figure 1.7 The underlying structure of the Chinese tea ceremony problem and its similarity to the Towers of Hanoi. Key: H = host; SG = senior guest; JG = junior guest; S = stoking fire; P = pouring tea; R = reciting poetry.

Goal state – the highest number of points (gained by placing letters down in a crossword pattern on the board in winning combinations).

b. Solving a crossword clue.

Answer:

Initial state – empty squares

Goal state – squares filled with letters making up the word(s) that correctly answer the given clue.

Problem-solving exercise 1.4 – The Chinese Tea Ceremony (page 19)

Answer: As stated in the text, this is identical to the Towers of Hanoi in underlying structure, which means that the solution is also the same.

If we arrange it in the same way, the solution becomes easier to work out: use host (H), senior guest (SG) and junior guest (JG) as the three poles (1, 2 and 3 respectively) and the three tasks – stoking, which is the least noble (S); pouring, of medium nobility (P) and reciting, most noble (R) as the three rings (small, medium and large respectively; see Fig 1.7).

It is now easy to work out the solution:

1. Stoking to senior guest
2. Pouring to junior guest
3. Stoking to junior guest
4. Reciting to senior guest
5. Stoking to host
6. Pouring to senior guest
7. Reciting to senior guest.

References

Banyard P, Hayes N 1991 Thinking and problem solving. British Psychological Society, Leicester

Buchner A 1995 Basic topics and approaches to the study of complex problem solving. In: Frensch PA, Funke J (eds) Complex problem solving: the European perspective. Lawrence Erlbaum Associates, New Jersey, ch 2, p28

Evans JStBT, Over DE, Manktelow KI 1993 Reasoning, decision making and rationality. In: Johnson-Laird PN, Shafir E (eds) Reasoning and decision making. Elsevier Science Publishers, Amsterdam, ch 7, p166–187

Fogler HS, LeBlanc SE 1995 Strategies for creative problem solving. Prentice-Hall PTR, Englewood Cliffs, NJ

Frensch PA, Funke J 1995 Definitions, traditions and a general framework for understanding complex problem solving. In: Frensch PA, Funke J (eds) Complex problem solving: the European perspective. Lawrence Erlbaum Associates, New Jersey, ch 1, p18

Funke J 1991 Solving complex problems: exploration and control of complex systems. In: Sternberg RJ, Frensch PA (eds) Complex problem solving: principles and mechanisms. Lawrence Erlbaum Associates, New Jersey, ch 6, p186

Higgs J 1992 Developing clinical reasoning competencies. Physiotherapy 78, 575–581

Johnson-Laird PN, Shafir E 1993 The interaction between reasoning and decision making: an introduction. In: Johnson-Laird PN, Shafir E (eds) Reasoning and decision making. Elsevier Science Publishers, Amsterdam

Kahney H 1993 Problem solving: current issues, 2nd edn. Open University Press, Buckingham

Klayman J, Brown K 1993 Debias the environment instead of the judge: an alternative approach to reducing error in diagnostic judgement. In: Johnson-Laird PN, Shafir E (eds) Reasoning and decision making. Elsevier Science Publishers, Amsterdam, ch 5, p97–122

Kluwe RH 1995 Single case studies and models of complex problems solving. In: Frensch PA, Funke J (eds) Complex problem solving: the European perspective. Lawrence Erlbaum Associates, New Jersey, ch 11, p270

Legrenzi P, Girotto V, Johnson-Laird PN 1993 Focussing in reasoning and decision making. In: Johnson-Laird PN, Shafir E (eds) Reasoning and decision making. Elsevier Science Publishers, Amsterdam, ch 3, p37–66

Lindsay PH, Norman DA 1977 Human information processing – an introduction to psychology, 2nd edn. Academic Press, London

Lumsdaine E, Lumsdaine M 1995 Creative problem solving: thinking skills for a changing world. McGraw-Hill, New York

May BJ, Newman J 1980 Developing competence in problem solving: a behavioural model. Physical Therapy 57, 807–813

Morris J 1993 An overview of and comparison among three current approaches to medical and physiotherapy undergraduate education. Physiotherapy 79, 91–94

Shafir E, Simonson I, Tversky A 1993 Reason-based choice. In: Johnson-Laird PN, Shafir E (eds) Reasoning and decision making. Elsevier Science Publishers, Amsterdam, ch 2, p11–36

Soden R 1994 Teaching problem solving in vocational education. Routledge, London

Chapter 2

Changes in the musculoskeletal system

Fiona Coutts

OBJECTIVES

By the end of this chapter you should:

- Have an awareness of the development of the musculoskeletal system and its relationship with the development of the cardiovascular and neural systems.
- Understand the changes that occur in the mature adult through the ageing process of the musculoskeletal system.
- Be able to differentiate between the changes due to ageing and those which occur in osteoarthrosis.

KEY WORDS

Development, ageing, physiological change, musculoskeletal system.

Prerequisites

Before reading this chapter you should revise the basic anatomy of muscle, bone, and synovial joints and the pathology of osteoarthrosis. The background knowledge you obtain from this reading will augment the information presented in this section and will help you to answer the questions posed.

INTRODUCTION

The musculoskeletal system provides the gross components of movement and function and is composed of two main sections: the skeletal structure, which provides a scaffolding for muscle attachment, protection for soft, sensitive organs and formation of moveable links (joints); and the muscular system, which gives a means of controlling the motion at the joints for function.

The musculoskeletal system cannot work in isolation and is totally dependent on the normal functioning of the other body systems, i.e. the central and peripheral nervous system and the cardiovascular system. These are also influenced by the psychological and emotional responses. The initiation and control of movement is governed by the central and peripheral nervous system and the cardiovascular system provides the nutrition and oxygenation to the bones, joints and muscles.

The main emphasis of this chapter will be on the development of the musculoskeletal system, particularly the changes associated with ageing. Where appropriate the related changes in the neural and cardiovascular systems will be considered, as this may clarify the overall picture.

As illustrated in Figure I.1 (p 5), a knowledge of the progression from the normal state, and its possible ranges, to the abnormal is essential to your understanding of problem solving in orthopaedics. This chapter identifies and defines 'normal' in relation to the changes that naturally occur in the body systems, thus providing you with a grounding from which to explore the 'abnormal'.

DEVELOPMENT

The body develops throughout childhood and adolescence, then reaching a point of maturity, after which it slowly declines towards death (Fig. 2.1).

Of course this is a very general overview and the timing of events will vary from person to person. However, there are definite stages in the developmental cycle during which the maturity of each of the body systems is altered (Bell et al 1980).

birth
puberty   (around 10–14 years)
adolescent growth spurt   (around 12–15 years)
menopause   (around 45–55 years)

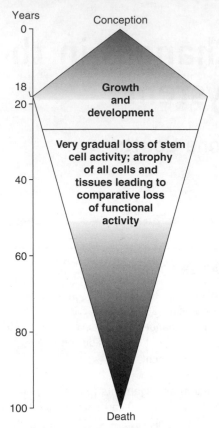

Figure 2.1   Growth, development and atrophy during the ageing process. (Adapted with permission from Govan et al 1991.)

For example, the adolescent growth spurt, which occurs at a slightly later age for boys (around 14–15 years) than girls (around 12–13 years), is responsible for many of the gross changes in body form and structure, which in turn are associated with changes to the cardiovascular system, so that the latter system does not reach maturity until after this time (Russo 1990). This may also be true for all the other systems.

You can see from Figure 2.1 that growth continues until around the age of 18 years and the maturation processes continue until the mid 20s.

This does not mean that a person cannot develop and refine skills after this time, but generally that the body systems have reached their point of maturation resulting in maximal control of motor performance. The level of this control is individual and the ability to perform maximally is also dependent on other factors such as; lifestyle, exercise and fitness (Govan et al 1991).

More specifically, there are recognizable patterns of change in muscle strength, which appear to be predetermined by hereditary factors, but the intervals at which they occur are variable (Hinderer & Hinderer 1993). It is also recognized that the ongoing control of motion is dependent on the parallel development of the musculoskeletal system and the neural systems, which should evolve in tandem, each acting as a precursor in the development of the other (Hinderer & Hinderer 1993).

In the infant, neuromuscular system development progresses in a predictable sequence, from the control of gross antigravity movements, enabling the growing child to gradually assume and maintain an erect posture, to the fine control of the extremities (Hinderer & Hinderer 1993).

Age, sex and body proportions have an effect on muscle strength throughout development but particularly after the onset of puberty (Methany 1941, Monotoye & Lamphiear 1977). There are other factors that influence strength, such as motor learning, and seasonal and diurnal variation, but these are as relevant to the mature adult as to the developing child.

It is important for therapists to know about the evolution of muscle strength in order to recognize these changes as normal, as opposed to those due to some pathology or abnormality.

Muscle changes during development

Skeletal muscle eventually constitutes 40–45% of total body weight, providing motion, strength and protection to the skeleton by absorbing forces and distributing loads (Nordin & Frankel 2001). Each muscle is composed of a large number of muscle fibres (each containing numerous myofibrils) that form bundles (fascicles), which are in turn surrounded by a sheath of connective tissue (perimysium). A fibrous connective tissue then overlies the whole muscle (epimysium) which, along with the perimysium, forms a continuation of the collagen tissue of tendons, the normal mechanism for attaching muscle to bone.

Each myofibril consists of fibrous filaments of actin and myosin in repeating bands called sarcomeres, throughout the length of the fibril, and it is the delicate strands that are the functional contractile units of the muscle.

Developmental muscle changes occur at a very early point, with the neuromuscular system developing from the fifth week after conception, when pre-muscle masses are formed. The muscles have well-established innervation by the eighth week and muscular movements can be detected in utero as early as the 16th week (Espenschade & Eckert 1980). Changes continue throughout the gestation period and so, at birth, the baby is able to perform reflex movements and some gross activity patterns but is unable to perform controlled voluntary movements. This is due to the immaturity of the nervous system; that is, the nerves and muscles are connected but much more refinement is needed before smooth controlled movement is possible (Thelen 1985).

After birth there is a large increase in muscle length and diameter, with the number of myofibrils rising markedly. This occurs because the existing myofibrils split longitudinally (Goldspink & Williams 1990). As muscle strength is known to be directly proportional to the cross sectional muscle area (Rutherford & Jones 1992, Young 1984, Young et al 1984, 1985) and the number of myofibril units (Goldspink & Williams 1990); this would explain the natural increase in strength during development.

The increase in length of the muscle is necessary to allow for the growth of long bones. This is accomplished by the addition of serial sarcomeres, enabling a continued overlap between the actin and myosin filaments (in myofibrils), thus retaining the ability to generate force (Goldspink & Williams 1990). These changes in the muscle must be accompanied by adaptations to the neural and vascular supply to permit normal function, i.e. control and initiation of muscle contraction and the removal of the resultant waste products.

The development of muscle in the growing child is dependent on the rate of development of the neurological system. During the first year of life, as myelination progresses, the child gains control of its body, first from the neck down and from proximal to distal areas. Thus gross control of the neck, scapula and shoulder movement occurs before control of the hands and all these are acquired before fine movement and precision is gained. Upper limb control is therefore gained before that of the lower limb, and gross antigravity control develops prior to accuracy (Hinderer & Hinderer 1993).

As the neural control increases, muscle strength is gained and refined but will only attain its full magnitude if this control is complemented by the addition of more myofibrils.

One other factor can influence muscle strength – the skill and coordination of a movement. In both developing and mature muscle the learning and repetition of a task can greatly influence the performance of it (Hinderer & Hinderer 1993). Thus muscle strength can be increased as a result of the learning of the task, with more complicated tasks, such as precision movements, walking, etc., demonstrating an even greater effect.

Self-assessment questions

- **SAQ 2.1** Which part(s) of a muscle constitute(s) the contractile unit?
- **SAQ 2.2** In general, which types of movements can be performed at birth?
- **SAQ 2.3** What does muscle strength directly depend upon?
- **SAQ 2.4** How does a muscle maintain the generation of force as it is lengthening, during the developmental sequence?

(Answers at end of chapter.)

Bone and joint changes during development

Bone is a specialized connective tissue that provides a solid but flexible structure for support and protection. It is high in inorganic material, i.e. mineral salts (such as calcium and phosphate), which provide the rigid structure, and of organic material (e.g. collagen fibres, glycosaminoglycans (GAGs) and water), which gives bone its flexibility (Nordin & Frankel 2001).

As bone stores a significant proportion of the body's mineral salt content, particularly calcium, it therefore plays a major role in the body's mineral homeostasis, but the true mechanism involved is not clear (Bland 1993). In general, the length and shape of bones are genetically determined but bone mass increases with activity and bone structure can alter to accommodate weight-bearing stresses (Nordin & Frankel 2001).

This constant response to the demands of weight-bearing by altering the infrastructure of bone and connective tissue to accommodate for the altered stress was first recognized by Wolff, who stated that 'bone will alter its size, shape and trabecular pattern in both the subchondral and cortical bone according to the lines of physical stress' (Wolff's law of bone remodelling; Bland 1993). Therefore, bone can constantly change shape to accommodate the structural demands made on it by weight bearing, muscle pull, stress, etc. during perpetual normal everyday activity.

Biomechanically, bone combines strength and stiffness, allowing a certain amount of load to be applied, within its elastic limit, with no permanent deformation taking place. During loading the bone stores the energy transferred and when the load is reduced the bone returns to its normal shape. If the load is taken past the elastic limit of the bone ('yield point'), then permanent deformation will take place. If the loading continues, then failure (fracture) occurs (Nordin & Frankel 2001).

Growth and development of bone occurs in two ways: the long bones (femur, humerus, tibia, etc.), vertebrae, sternum and ribs develop from rods of cartilage (endochondral ossification) and the shorter flatter bones such as the clavicle, skull (parietal, frontal bones), nasal bone, maxilla/mandible, etc. form from membranes (intramembranous ossification).

In the fertilized egg, two layers of tissue develop around the ninth day: ectoderm, which eventually becomes the superficial layers of skin, hair, nails, some glands and the central nervous system, and the endoderm, which develops into the lining of the pulmonary and digestive systems and so on. Cell proliferation from the ectoderm forms a loose connective tissue, which becomes the mesenchyme, a thin layer of tissue between the ectoderm and the endoderm (Shipman et al 1985).

From this mesenchyme, the mesoderm cell layer develops from the 16th day post-fertilization, and the gradual condensation or proliferation of these

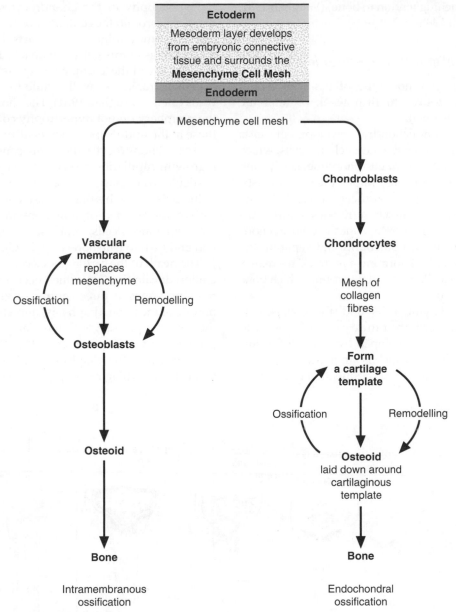

Figure 2.2   From mesenchyme to bone.

cells results in either endochondral or intramembranous ossification (Fig. 2.2).

Intramembranous growth and ossification

The proliferation of the mesenchyme eventually forms a highly vascular membrane. Three months after fertilization the mesenchyme cells progress to osteoblasts (major bone-forming cells responsible for producing large quantities of osteoid), which ossify and then remodel the already-formed membranous tissue. As the condensed mesenchyme is replaced by bone, the thick membrane is left surrounding the growing bone tissue, eventually becoming the periosteum (the outer fibrous cover of bone, which provides nutrition and the main means of attaching tendon to bone) (Vaughan 1981, Shipman et al 1985).

Endochondral growth and ossification

This is more common type of ossification and starts at the fourth to fifth week of fetal life (Shipman et al 1985).

Once again endochondral development starts from the formation of the mesenchyme cells, which proliferate and then turn into chondroblasts (young immature cartilage cells) rather than osteoblasts, as in intramembranous ossification (Fig. 2.2). The chondroblasts turn into chondrocytes (mature cartilage cells), which secrete a mesh of collagenous fibres, which in turn surround and separate the cells (Vaughan 1981), forming a matrix. This matrix is basically a cartilage template around which bone is generated.

The mesenchyme cells and the collagenous fibres together form the future centres for ossification and are again enveloped by a layer of tissue, the perichondrium, which is similar to the periosteum in intramembranous ossification (Fig. 2.3A).

Hypertrophy of the chondrocytes occurs and the matrix around the centrally positioned chondrocytes becomes thinner and starts to disappear, leaving large empty gaps ('lacunae'). Thus the cells in the centre of the 'cartilage template' enlarge and lose their transverse walls while the longitudinal walls calcify (Vaughan 1981). The chondrocytes on the periphery do not hypertrophy compared with those in the middle (Shipman et al 1985; Fig. 2.3B).

As the chondrocytes die in the constant cycle of regrowth, capillaries carrying osteogenic cells, in particular osteoblasts and osteoclasts, overrun the dying cells. From this time the osteoblasts lay down osteoid (uncalcified organic bone matrix) around the cartilaginous cells, which slowly become calcified and turn to true bone (Fig. 2.3C).

The death of the cartilaginous cells allows proliferation of calcification, which occurs especially in the long bones at three centres of growth: at the middle of the bone (diaphysis) and at either end of the bone (epiphysis), with the diaphysis being the primary centre (Shipman et al 1985; Fig. 2.4).

Even when the diaphysis and epiphyses are ossified, the cartilaginous epiphyseal plates are still

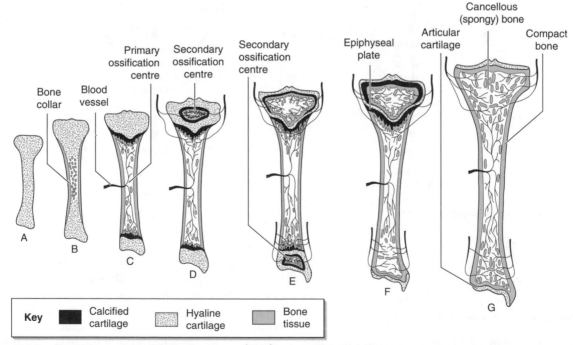

Figure 2.3   Formation and growth of a long bone (tibia) on a model of cartilage.

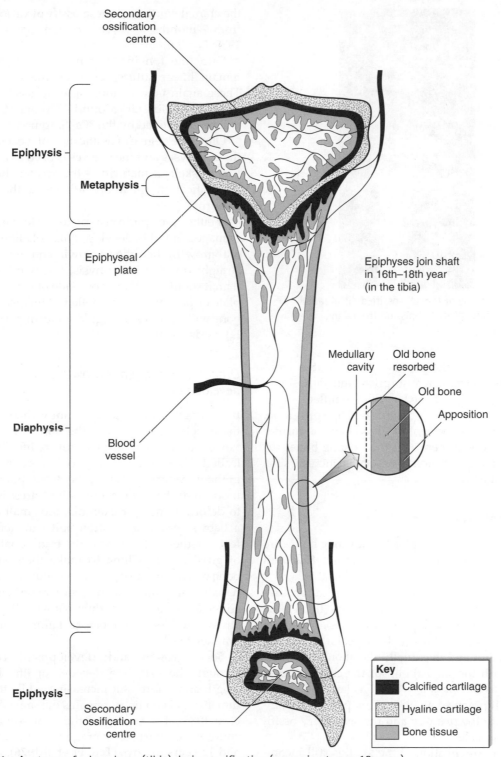

Figure 2.4   Anatomy of a long bone (tibia) during ossification (approximate age 12 years).

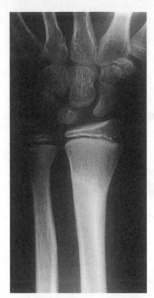

Figure 2.5 X-ray of the non-ossified distal radial epiphyseal plate. (With permission from Dandy & Edwards 2003.)

developing and the process of ossification continues, by constant reabsorption and deposition, until the growth in bone length is complete.

The width of bone is determined by apposition. In this process, osteoblasts lay down a further matrix of bone minerals on the existing bone surface, and the generation of new bone increases the width of the bone.

Patterns of ossification

At birth the epiphyseal plates of the long bones are still cartilaginous and some remain like this until bone maturity (Shipman et al 1985; Fig. 2.5).

The pattern of epiphyseal ossification has been identified as progressing from the elbow (13–15 years) to the hip (13–16 years), the ankle (13–18 years), the knee (14–18 years), the wrist (18–20 years) and eventually the shoulder (15–20 years), with the medial end of the clavicle being reported as incompletely fused as late as 30 years of age (Shipman et al 1985). This pattern encompasses both the primary and the secondary ossification timescales.

At birth, ossification of the skull is still incomplete, with much of the base remaining cartilaginous. Six large membranes – fontanelles – separate

the cranial vaults and these ossify at various times from 2 months to 2 years of age (Shipman et al 1985; Fig. 2.6).

Once the fontanelles have ossified there still remain linear sutures between the vault bones. These again take various times to ossify, but the process should start around 17 years of age and will be completed by the 30s (Shipman et al 1985).

Often, the degree of ossification of the fontanelles, the epiphyses and the sutures is used as an indication of skeletal maturity – the greater the degree of ossification the more advanced the skeletal maturity.

If either the epiphyseal plates or fontanelles are damaged or fail to develop, thus not allowing normal growth, then the bone will continue to grow straight (from the diaphysis) but will be shorter than it should be. If only one side of the epiphyseal plate or part of the fontanelle is damaged then the bone will develop an angular deformity (Dandy & Edwards 2003).

Other features of bone growth and development

Bone length and shape constantly change during the developing years but the bone remains both flexible and elastic throughout its life. This malleability does gradually reduce but is at its greatest in the very early years. In the developing skeletal tissue of the baby, then, only slight stress is needed to deform bone. For example, too small a size of a baby's elasticated cotton suit can deform the feet; another example was the traditional binding of girls' feet in China to make them small. As bone reaches maturity (25 years plus) its flexibility remains fairly high, 'with cortical bone being much stiffer than cancellous, thus withstanding greater stress but less strain before failure' (Nordin & Frankel 2001).

Bone growth and development continues through the first two decades of life, with the length and width still increasing while the three-dimensional geometry remains the same (Shipman et al 1985). The timing of the adolescent growth spurt, which starts on average at 10.3 years in girls and 12 years in boys (Tanner et al 1976), is crucial in determining skeletal height, and the delay of the growth spurt in males gives boys a full 2 years

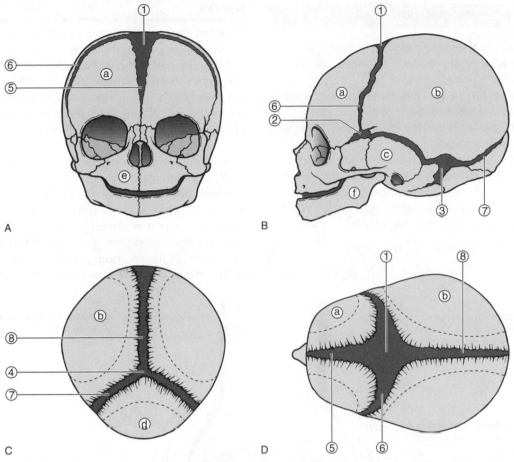

Figure 2.6 Skull of a full-term fetus. A: From the front. B: From the left. C: From behind. D: From above. a, frontal bone; b, parietal bone; c, temporal bone; d, occipital bone; e, maxilla; f, mandible; 1, anterior or bergamatic fontanelle; 2, spheroidal fontanelle; 3, mastoid fontanelle; 4, posterior or lambdoid fontanelle; 5, frontal suture; 6, coronal suture; 7, lambdoid suture; 8, sagittal suture.

to continue growing before the sudden growth spurt takes place. As a result the boys have a mean 28 cm further growth from the start to the end of the spurt, while girls only have a mean growth of 25 cm (Vaughan 1981). Bone growth stops some time after the peak velocity of growth: girls at around 12 years and boys at 14 years. However remodelling by reabsorption and deposition of bone still continues, ensuring the strength of the overall skeletal structure (Shipman et al 1985).

The main factors that will alter the normal skeletal balance, even after bone maturity, are:

- hormonal level changes of oestrogen, testosterone, parathormone, growth hormone and thyroxine

- mechanical changes from altered muscle pull or fracture: gradually, increased muscle pull will stimulate new bone growth and strengthen the bone; loss of muscle strength will reduce the pull on the bone and therefore diminish local bone strength
- stress and pressure changes: bone grows in areas of increased weight bearing and reduces in the areas where this is decreased.

As the child/adolescent develops, often the soft tissue and the bone growth do not advance at the same rate resulting in pain or aching, due to tissue being pulled at its extreme. Once all tissues catch up with each other the pain/ache will disappear.

Self–assessment questions

- **SAQ 2.5** Name the main functions of bone.
- **SAQ 2.6** What does Wolff's law state and what does this imply?
- **SAQ 2.7** Name the types of ossification of bone.
- **SAQ 2.8** Name the parts of a long bone.
- **SAQ 2.9** Describe the pattern of timing of epiphyseal ossification.
- **SAQ 2.10** Name the fontanelles and sutures in the skull and state the ages at which they ossify.
- **SAQ 2.11** The adolescent growth spurt starts at 10.3 years in girls and 12 years in boys. What factors may influence this growth?

(Answers at end of chapter.)

JOINTS

There are three major types of joint in the human body: fibrous, cartilaginous and synovial.

Each type of joint is generated as bone and connective tissue mature, but joint formation is not completed until the normal forces acting across the articulating surfaces provide the stimulus for final development (Shipman et al 1985; Fig. 2.7).

After the primary centres of ossification (in the shaft) stop their calcifying process, new bone tissue is stimulated at the interface of the metaphysis and the epiphysis; the epiphyseal plate, until the cartilage tissue is replaced by bone. Each type of joint has developed through the growth and eventual fusion of the secondary centres of ossification in the epiphysis. As the two immature bone ends

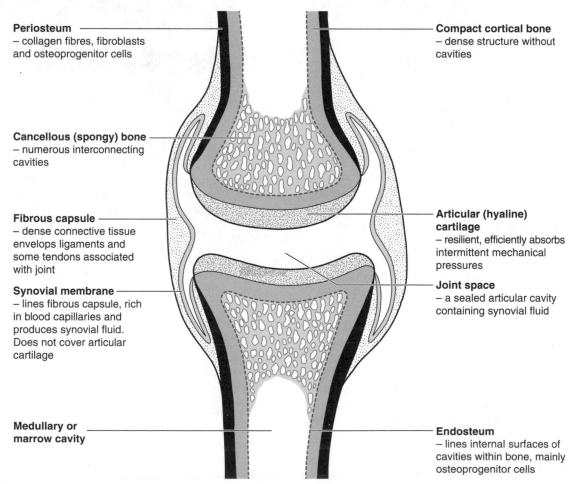

Periosteum
– collagen fibres, fibroblasts and osteoprogenitor cells

Cancellous (spongy) bone
– numerous interconnecting cavities

Fibrous capsule
– dense connective tissue envelops ligaments and some tendons associated with joint

Synovial membrane
– lines fibrous capsule, rich in blood capillaries and produces synovial fluid. Does not cover articular cartilage

Medullary or marrow cavity

Compact cortical bone
– dense structure without cavities

Articular (hyaline) cartilage
– resilient, efficiently absorbs intermittent mechanical pressures

Joint space
– a sealed articular cavity containing synovial fluid

Endosteum
– lines internal surfaces of cavities within bone, mainly osteoprogenitor cells

Figure 2.7 Anatomy of a synovial joint showing common features.

meet and start to be stressed by forces across the joint, a constant remodelling and the bone ends generate hyaline cartilage tissue at the force-bearing surfaces.

Tendons and ligaments

Three non-active components of joints are necessary to provide and maintain contact and stability: joint capsule, tendons and ligaments (Fig. 2.7).

The tendons are responsible for the attachment of muscle to bone and, as indicated earlier, they are often a continuation of the epimysium and perimysium, the fibrous covers of muscle. Ligaments, along with the joint capsule, help to control the degree of motion allowed at a joint, add stability to the joint and prevent excessive motion.

Tendons and ligaments are dense connective tissue, composed of collagen (fibrous protein) and have a meagre blood supply. Collagen gives strength and flexibility and makes up over 75% of the structure of tendons and ligaments. Tendons have more collagen than ligaments, particularly in the periphery, where the dry weight of collagen can constitute up to 99% of the total material (Amiel et al 1984). Collagen contains numerous fibrils and gains its strength from cross-linking these fibrils within the structure, giving the ability to withstand high stress levels (Carlstedt & Nordin 2001).

The collagen fibres in tendons lie in parallel so they can endure the high, uniaxial tensile loads that they have to withstand during activity. In contrast, ligaments have to bear stresses in many directions and therefore their collagen fibres are not all parallel but are interfaced with each other in a pattern relating to their functional needs (Amiel et al 1984). As the tendons and ligaments mature, the collagen fibrils increase in diameter and the number of cross-links between the fibrils increases, giving the structures greater tensile strength (Carlstedt & Nordin 2001).

Like bone, the tendons, ligaments and capsule remodel to accommodate the stresses put on them. Therefore these tissues will all respond to the stimuli of growth, increased weight bearing and increased muscle pull that accompany normal skeletal development.

Self-assessment questions

- **SAQ 2.12** Where is the secondary centre of ossification in bone?
- **SAQ 2.13** Why are epimysium and perimysium important in muscle attachment?
- **SAQ 2.14** What is the difference between the collagen in tendon and ligaments?

(Answers at end of chapter.)

Articular (hyaline) cartilage and joint lubrication

Structure of cartilage

Articular cartilage is a highly specialized tissue that is designed to withstand the stresses and strains of weight bearing and constantly altering joint mechanics. It has no vascular supply, lymph channels or nerves but has two very important roles of: 'distributing joint loads over a wide area thus decreasing the stresses sustained by contacting joint surfaces and [allowing] relative movement of the opposing joint surfaces with minimal friction and wear' (Nordin & Frankel 2001).

Cartilage is composed of two layers. The deeper layer, immediately next to the cortical bone, is constructed of long columns of chondrocytes arranged perpendicularly to the surface of the bone. These chondrocytes are fat and thickened at the end nearest the bone and at the opposing end they are thinner, healthier and still produce new cartilage (Shipman et al 1985).

The more superficial layer, the 'tangential zone', is a fibrous cover that has fingers of collagen that go vertically down between the chondrocytes to the underlying subchondral bone (Shipman et al 1985). Cartilage consists of collagen (10–30%), water and inorganic salts, including glycoproteins and lipids (60–87%), and proteoglycans (3–10%) (Nordin & Frankel 2001). Proteoglycans are large protein–polysaccharide molecules that form a concentrated solution to enmesh the collagen fibrils. Thus the cartilage is often viewed as a 'water-filled sponge' with two distinct parts: the 'fluid' or interstitial part (approximately 75% by wet weight) and the 'solid' part (approximately 25% by wet weight) (Nordin & Frankel 2001).

Synovial fluid

Articular cartilage also plays a vital role in lubrication of synovial joints, together with synovial fluid, which in turn is essential for free joint motion, chondrocyte nutrition and reduction of stresses across the joint. Synovial fluid is produced from the synovial membrane of the joint and is composed of a thick serum (the clear, watery part of blood) and two additional substances; hyaluronic acid, for viscosity and slipperiness, and a double glycoprotein.

Mechanisms of lubrication

Although many mechanisms of lubricating the synovial joints have been suggested (McCutchen 1966, Walker et al 1968, 1970), Nordin & Frankel (2001) state that a combination of mechanisms is probably involved (Fig. 2.8). Thus, as there is

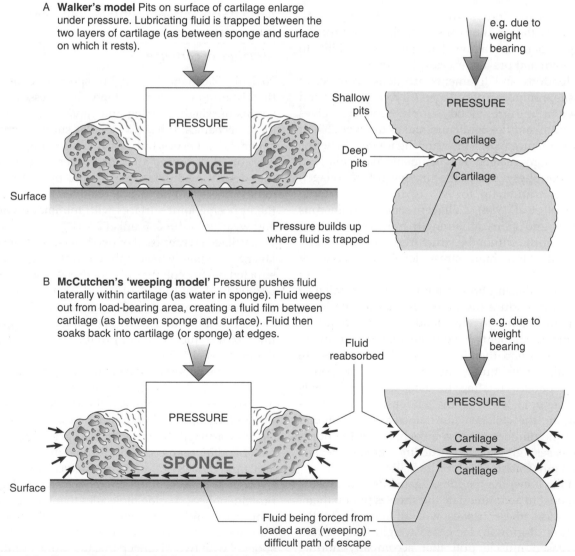

Figure 2.8 Two models of joint lubrication. A: Walker's model. B: McCutchen's 'weeping model'.

normally a cyclic function when loading a joint, lubrication will occur in two main ways.

- When a joint is subjected to a low load and is moving, a film of synovial fluid is maintained between the joint surfaces. As some load is applied to the joint, an extra supply of fluid lubricant is produced by squeezing out the fluid lying between the chondrocytes of the articular cartilage (deep pits in Fig. 2.8A). Thus a fluid film is generated in front of and beneath the articular surface, which is reabsorbed once the load bearing is reduced (Nordin & Frankel 2001).

- If loading is continued, this will cause complete expulsion of the fluid, reducing the quantity of fluid held by the articular cartilage, which will be replaced once the load is removed. A thin film of fluid will always remain but the fluid being squeezed out from the 'boundaries' will be primarily responsible for lubrication. When the load is removed the fluid can then soak back into the articular cartilage (as into a sponge) (McCutchen 1966).

Deterioration of cartilage

The mechanical response of cartilage to load is highly complex. It is regarded as a viscoelastic response, i.e. similar to that produced by a combination of a viscous fluid and an elastic solid. The main result of this combination of mechanical properties is that the cartilage can usually withstand the high forces generated by compression, stress and tension. Cartilage undergoes continual alteration of load-bearing stress, which enhances regeneration of the cartilage. However, as this is only a limited capacity, damage may then occur.

It is not until there is substantial damage to the collagen and proteoglycans and removal of the cartilage from the underlying solid bone by constant mechanical stresses (wear) that articular cartilage begins to fail. Once the cartilage starts to decrease in thickness and has small defects, it becomes softer, more permeable, starts to flake and becomes fibrillated (deep vertical clefts between chondrocytes). Therefore the lubricating fluid from between the articular surfaces then starts to leak away, allowing direct contact of the surfaces (interfacial wear) and an abrasion process is aggravated.

With alteration in the weight-bearing forces, repeated and added strain on the cartilage surfaces causes fatigue wear. This type of wear is often seen as the joints age, with increasing loss of muscle strength, and are no longer under the usual biomechanical stresses, and it can take place even if there is good lubrication of the joint (Nordin & Frankel 2001).

Articular cartilage has limited capacity for regeneration (Chubinskaya et al 2002) and is replaced by fibrous cartilage after initial injury. Fibrous cartilage does not have the same properties as articular cartilage; in particular, it cannot withstand the same loads and stress. Therefore the secondary regrowth of cartilage is not sustained for long and will break down very quickly.

Chubinskaya et al (2002) report that the articular cartilage levels of osteogenic protein-1 (protein that indicates that articular cartilage has the potential to repair) are dramatically reduced (more than fourfold; $p < 0.02$) during ageing. This suggests the possibility that osteogenic protein-1 may be critical for chondrocytes to maintain their normal homeostasis and could also serve as a repair factor during joint disease or ageing and as an indicator of joint pathology.

Research findings are coming to light in this area but, over the last decade, a number of age-related changes in cartilage have been documented, including:

- an increased denaturation of collagen type II
- a decline in synthesis of DNA, proteoglycans and link protein
- decreased responsiveness to different growth factors and many others (Chubinskaya et al 2002).

In the next few years even more advances in understanding the ageing processes of cartilage and its repair will be made, and this will help in preserving joint space width and preventing pathology.

Self-assessment questions

- SAQ 2.15 What are the functions of articular cartilage?
- SAQ 2.16 What are proteoglycans and what is their role in cartilage?

- **SAQ 2.17** Why is cartilage often described as 'a water-filled sponge'?
- **SAQ 2.18** How does a synovial joint maintain nutrition to its components?

(Answers at end of chapter.)

LIFESTYLE

The normal development of any child and the ageing process in any adult are dependent on a number of external stresses, which impinge at different times, or can remain constant, throughout life. These stresses are essentially due to lifestyle, defined as the particular attitudes, habits or behaviours associated with an individual or group (Collins 1982). But because lifestyles can be so diverse, from person to person or for the same person at different times in life, they inevitably have differing effects on the changes that occur in the body. Lifestyle, in the very wide-ranging definition given above, will obviously affect the body in a number of ways, but our main concern is how these changes influence structure, form and function during development and ageing.

Peer and family influences will dictate the environment in which a child is brought up and in which an adult lives. These influences may well be as a result of geographical, cultural and/or religious factors, together with social class, which may affect social interactions, family size and occupation (Shephard 1980). An illustration of this could be the range of dietary habits seen in our multiclass and multicultural society. The particular example of a diet with too much carbohydrate resulting in obesity or an increase in the risk of arteriosclerosis is seen in many cultures and geographical regions. Conversely, there also seems to be an increase in the number of people with vitamin deficiencies due to poor diet. Both these instances would result in characteristic but differing morphological changes in the populations involved.

To give another example, the growth and development of a fetus is directly influenced by the amount of nourishment it obtains and, if this is diminished at any time, then the internal organs undergoing cell division at that time are prone to damage (Barker 1993). Further to this, if the new-born baby is undersized, it will have an increased risk of coronary heart disease, stroke and diabetes in adult life; therefore the size of the newborn can be used as a predictor for adult health (Barker 1993). The strong implication of these points is that external influences on the womb, especially diet, can change the health and longevity of the unborn child (Barker 1993).

A strong influence on the structure and function of the body is level of activity, which can encompass occupation and hobbies. Both of these may entail varying amounts of physical exercise ranging from that of the sedentary worker to the almost continual activity of the manual labourer, postal delivery worker, professional/amateur sports person, and so on.

Motivation, either from within the individual or as a result of peer pressure, obviously plays an important part in the level of activity and the quality of physical performance achieved (Smith et al 1989). Verbal encouragement has been shown to enhance performance. Bickers (1993) demonstrated a significant increase (33.5%, $p < 0.001$) in performance of a muscle endurance task with verbal encouragement, when compared to the results attained from the same group without encouragement.

AGEING

'Stiffness, increased connective tissue, reduced muscle mass, selective atrophy of type II fibres, diminished proprioception, loss of motor neurones, decreased exercise motivation, inactivity and decreased appetite and food intake are age-related changes affecting neuromuscular function and strength' (Frontera 1989).

These natural muscular, skeletal and neural changes occurring with age are not in themselves detrimental to the capabilities of the systems but do limit the absolute control of motor performance. This limitation is characterized by a slowing down of movements, a decrease in maximum strength and a loss of fine coordination (Skinner et al 1982). These changes are only gradually noticed by individuals, especially if they have maintained a relatively high standard of health, but will present individual problems if they reach a degree of severity that causes pain, deformity and/or loss of

Figure 2.9 The 'rise and fall' of the musculoskeletal system: matching the normal physiological changes in the musculoskeletal system to the ageing process. (Adapted with permission from Govan et al 1991.)

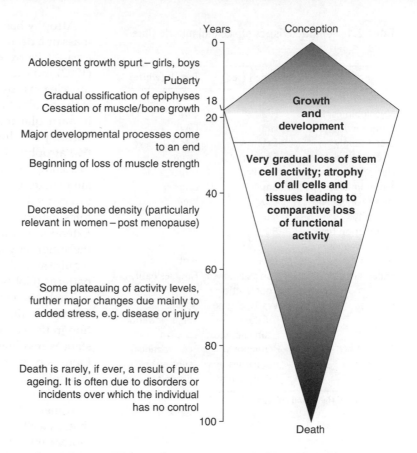

Years   Conception
0

Adolescent growth spurt – girls, boys
Puberty
Gradual ossification of epiphyses   18   **Growth**
Cessation of muscle/bone growth   20   **and**
                                             development

Major developmental processes come
to an end
Beginning of loss of muscle strength   **Very gradual loss of stem**
                                             cell activity; atrophy
                                             of all cells and
                                      40   **tissues leading to**
                                             comparative loss
Decreased bone density (particularly   **of functional**
relevant in women – post menopause)   **activity**

                                      60

Some plateauing of activity levels,
further major changes due mainly to
added stress, e.g. disease or injury

                                      80

Death is rarely, if ever, a result of pure
ageing. It is often due to disorders or
incidents over which the individual
has no control
                                      100
                                             Death

motor control, or if injury and disease predominate. The natural phenomenon of ageing, and in fact the theoretical concept also, when considered within the real environment, is accelerated and aggravated by extrinsic factors of increased pathophysiological stresses. This is amplified by the intrinsic decrease in the body's ability to respond to these stresses (Govan et al 1991). Malkia (1993) states that it is very difficult to differentiate between the natural effects of ageing on muscle and the factors causing change, which are related to environmental differences and lifestyle. This may equally be true for the other systems in the body.

Amiridis et al (2003) examined changes in posture to static balance tasks of increasing difficulty in both young (20.1 ± 2.4 years) and older (70.1 ± 4.3 years) adults. Greater centre of pressure excursions, electromyographic (EMG) activity and joint displacements were found in old compared to younger adults. Older adults displayed increased hip movement accompanied by higher hip EMG activity with increased task constraints during quiet standing.

No similar increase was noted in the younger group. Balance requires the interaction of all body systems and the differences in findings between the young and old indicate how adaptations can be made to maintain normal everyday functions. Doherty et al (1993) and Maki & McIlroy (1996) have shown that degeneration of neural, muscular and skeletal mechanisms all lead to changes in posture and balance in the elderly and increase susceptibility to falls.

Although the decline of the body systems does not truly present until the fifth decade is reached, the skeletal, muscular and neural systems start to deteriorate in the fourth decade (Lexell et al 1988) (Fig. 2.9).

Ageing and the muscular system

The first changes in the muscular system present as a result of alterations in the microscopic muscle structure leading to a loss of muscle mass (atrophy) and loss of strength and speed of contraction

Table 2.1   Characteristics of skeletal muscle fibre types

	Type I (red)	Type II (white)
Diameter (micrometres)	27	44
Myoglobin content	High	Low
Mitochondria	High	Low
Blood supply	Extensive	Less extensive
Motor end plate	Smaller	Large
Nerve fibre diameter	Smaller	Larger
Motor unit size	Small	Large
Nerve conduction velocity	Low	High
Contraction time (milliseconds)	85	25
Tension	Low	High
Endurance	Long sustained contraction	Fatigues easily
Function	Walking, long distance running, most functional activities of daily living	Rapid, high-power or sudden contractions, such as heavy lifting activities

Adapted from Harris and Watkins 1993

(Grimby & Saltin 1983, Larsson et al 1979, Vandervoort et al 1986, Young 1984, Young et al 1984, 1985). These changes also appear to arise in conjunction with impaired cardiovascular function and inactivity. Goldspink & Williams (1990) indicate 'that there is an increase in the collagen content of muscle with age with associated thickening of the endomysium and the perimysium'. This is more noticeable in slow muscle (Konanen 1989) and causes an increase in tensile stiffness and elastic efficiency (Hinderer & Hinderer 1993). Therefore the loss of the full contractile properties, in conjunction with alterations in neurotransmission (Knortz 1987), in ageing muscle also affects the performance of that muscle.

Atrophy

Prior to discussing the effects of muscle atrophy with age, some knowledge of the different muscle fibre types is needed. A brief overview is given in Table 2.1.

Atrophy has been defined as the loss of muscle mass or a decrease in whole muscle cross-sectional area (St Pierre & Gardiner 1987). Jones & Round (1992) indicate that there is a loss of up to 30% in muscle mass by 90 years of age. Atrophy in ageing is the result of loss of both muscle fibre types, but in particular reduction in the size of type II fibres (Grimby & Saltin 1983, Lexell et al 1988). The selective atrophy of type II fibres is thought to be due to accompanying inactivity and denervation. In the later stages of ageing there tends to be disuse due to a general decrease in activity levels, which constitutes a reduced demand for muscle contraction. Extended reduction in activity will mainly affect the antigravity muscles such as soleus because they require stimulation by repeated normal functional patterns (Goldspink & Williams 1990).

Thus changes occur within the tissue, which include diminished capillary density and a reduction in the amount of muscle proteins and of substances involved in energy release. Consequently there is decreased endurance, force and aerobic/anaerobic capacity, as well as a lossof elasticity due to thinning of connective tissue (St Pierre & Gardiner 1987). EMG studies have demonstrated that, as well as the reduction in muscle fibres in the motor units, there is also a reduction in the number of motor units (Campbell et al 1973). This is substantiated by Tomlinson et al (1969) and Aniansson et al (1981), who suggest that the changes in muscle are of neurological origin, rather than just originating within the muscle tissue itself.

Strength

Specific decline of muscle strength occurs after the age of 50 (Lexell et al 1988), although some decline does present after 30 years of age. Rutherford & Jones (1992) demonstrated that there is a 40% loss of strength in the quadriceps muscle alone between the third and the fourth decade, with the cross-sectional area being reduced by 23%; therefore the force generating capacity of the muscle is diminished by 20%.

This has also been shown by Young et al (1984, 1985), who found that the loss of muscle strength was proportional to the reduction in cross-sectional area in the muscle. One explanation for this could be the reduction in levels of growth hormone, which does lead to general musculoskeletal atrophy, which may be modified at particular sites by superimposed patterns of muscular activity (Rutherford & Jones 1992).

Ageing muscle strength is very often tested by using isometric contraction only, but Malkia (1993) questions this and indicates that muscle performance in ageing should only be tested in 'certain controlled movement conditions of speed, duration and load via energy pathways in movement'. The advancement of isokinetic measurement systems has assisted in this.

Fatiguability

With ageing there is greater atrophy of type II muscle fibres compared to type I. This leaves the non-fatiguable type I muscle fibres predominating, and therefore there is a greater loss of muscle strength than endurance (Stokes & Cooper 1993). It is also believed that muscle endurance declines with age more in males than in females (Lennmarken et al 1985). O'Connor et al (1993) have shown on a small sample of active elderly (63–80 years old) and young (21–33 years old), that, although the younger age group could generate higher torques (mean of 175.21 Nm compared to 102.21 Nm, $p < 0.01$), the elderly group could sustain their contraction for a longer period of time, demonstrating that elderly muscle does not fatigue as quickly as younger muscle.

This can be explained by looking at the pattern of recruitment of muscle fibres in the normal subject during maximal voluntary contraction (MVC). Initially all muscle fibre types are recruited at a high firing rate, the fast type II fibres being initiated first then the slower type I fibres coming in. The firing rate reduces as the type II fibres fatigue. The type I fibres maintain their input but, as they cannot produce the same force as the type II fibres, this will be at a reduced magnitude. Therefore in the elderly person the magnitude of the MVC is reduced but the average length of time for which it can be sustained is greater than in the younger person (O'Connor et al 1993).

Functional performance and training

Malkia (1983) demonstrated in a cross-section survey on physical performance that muscle strength is related to subjective perception of physical ability and hypothesizes that the perceived decline in physical ability in the elderly may have an effect on overall muscle strength and vice versa.

In animal and human studies (Konanen 1989) it has been shown that muscle fibre types can be changed and that with endurance training there is a change from fast to slow muscle fibres. Elderly muscle can demonstrate a similar trend in gaining strength as younger muscle (Vandervoort et al 1986) but trained athletes between the ages of 30 and 70 years can maintain greater strength than untrained people of a similar age (Sipila & Suominen 1991). Thus, lifestyle does have an effect on the ability of muscle to perform, but appropriate exercise is essential (Astrand 1986) in maintaining and retraining elderly muscle.

Nonaka et al (2002) examined the age-related changes in passive range of motion of the hip and knee joints in 77 healthy males aged between 15 and 73 years. The passive sagittal plane range of movement at the hip joint decreased with age (extension 0.27°, flexion 0.17° per year), while knee movement remained the same. There was also a reduction in the length of the biarticular muscles over the hip and knee – rectus femoris and hamstrings. The authors concluded that the changes were probably caused by shortening of the muscles and connective tissue due to reduced compliance of the joint structures and reduced muscle stretch caused by a decrease in daily physical activity with advancing age. Similar changes have been found for active range of movement (Roach & Miles 1991) but the change was smaller, 3–5°, between the groups aged 25–39, 40–59 and 60–74 years, and the variability of performance was high. As testing passive movements stresses the joint and connective tissue more, it is not surprising that a greater difference was seen by Nonaka et al (2002).

Ageing and non-contractile tissue

The maturation of collagen in the non-contractile tissues occurs around the age of 20 years and after that the magnitude of the tensile properties seems to plateau. Then, after a variable period of time, the cross-links between and within the collagen decrease in number and quality. The tensile strength and stiffness of collagen then decreases and the tissues cannot withstand deformation (Carlstedt & Nordin 2001).

Self-assessment questions

- SAQ 2.19 Outline the first ageing changes in the muscle.
- SAQ 2.20 Define atrophy.
- SAQ 2.21 During ageing the type II muscle fibres are lost to a greater extent. What is the effect of this on muscle performance?

(Answers at end of chapter.)

Cardiovascular system (total body fitness)

Capacity for whole-body exercise, particularly aerobic capability, declines first, despite the relatively normal muscle metabolism, and this decline occurs before any morphological changes in muscle are evident (Grimby & Saltin 1983).

This loss of aerobic power is thought to be due to cardiopulmonary changes, in particular to reduced maximal cardiac output and maximum heart rate (Mahler et al 1986). It should be noted that the reduced cardiovascular fitness is not completely irreversible, and useful changes can be attained through fitness training (Smith 1989), regardless of age.

It must be stressed that improvement in performance is just as feasible in the elderly as in the young, for both specific muscle function (Moritani & De Vries 1980; Frontera et al 1988) and whole body endurance exercise, which leads to an increase in maximum oxygen uptake (Makrides 1986). However, the changes associated with ageing cannot be stopped, just postponed.

Ageing of bone and joints

After bone has matured the amount of stress which it can endure slowly reduces, for a number of reasons.

During the normal ageing process, bone becomes progressively less dense, with the longitudinal trabeculae becoming thinner and the transverse trabeculae being reabsorbed (Nordin & Frankel 2001).

This reduction in bone density (osteoporosis) is greater in women than in men and is accelerated 5–10 years after the menopause (Rutherford & Jones 1992). Rutherford & Jones (1992) also note that bone mass reductions with age vary at different sites, with the mass of the distal femur decreasing after the third decade and the decrease in mass of the spinal vertebrae and the middle of the femur being delayed until the fifth or sixth decade. Therefore bones are prone to fracture or alteration from added stress, at different ages.

Thus the bone is reduced in size, strength and stiffness, as the total amount of bone tissue is diminished, particularly cancellous bone. Burstein et al (1976) demonstrated that the amount of strain older bone can withstand is only half that of younger bone, signifying brittleness and a possible loss of the energy storage capacity.

The loss of bone in the elderly is dependent on the amount of bone that was present at the point of bone maturity. Therefore as the amount of bone is extremely variable between different individuals and in the various parts of the skeletal system, the total amount of bone lost in old age is very hard to predict (Shipman et al 1985).

Yamada et al (2002), showed that the medial tibial subchondral bone (SCB) thickness was significantly lower among the elderly (age >69 years) than among the young (age <40) or the middle-aged (40–69). Lateral tibial SCB thickness also showed the same trend of decreasing thickness with increasing age but this was not statistically significant. Tibial SCB thicknesses were significantly lower in arthritic joints compared to normal. In contrast however, no significant differences were found in femoral SCB thicknesses between those in a normal and an arthritic group. The arthritic group tended to have lower SCB densities than the normal group but this was statistically significant only in the lateral femoral condyle. Although these results differ from those of others, the authors conclude that subchondral bone changes are not aetiological for osteoarthrosis but more probably secondary to loss of articular cartilage, which precedes the appearance of subchondral sclerosis.

Bone loss after maturity is also dependent on dietary factors and is enhanced by the normal reduction in the amount of calcium that can be absorbed, particularly after the age of 70 years

(Vaughan 1981). The reduction in the mineral content of bone means that the normal homeostatic balance has to be re-established; therefore, if there is an added loss of calcium due to reduced uptake of minerals, this balance will be more difficult to maintain.

As we get older, generally, less demand is made on bone, with muscle strength and weight bearing being reduced (from a reduction or loss of weight-bearing activity). Periosteal and subperiosteal bone is therefore reabsorbed, resulting in the loss of strength and stiffness mentioned earlier (Nordin & Frankel 2001). However locally, as muscle strength decreases with age, the resultant altered biomechanical alignment and stresses across bone and joints causes changes (usually an increase) in the size and shape of the joint surfaces. Thus the cartilaginous tissue at the joint surface and the underlying bone proliferates, following Wolff's law. So the joint may increase in size, with the subchondral bone appearing thicker on X-ray.

There has been some debate as to whether joint space reduces with age or just as a result of degenerative disease (Goker et al 2003). As the cartilage changes with age are different from those associated with osteoarthrosis (Hammerman 1993), any reduction in joint space width may be one of the first signs of joint pathology. The knee joint space has been shown to gradually decrease with age (Dacre et al 1991) but it is unclear if this occurs at all joints. Goker et al (2003) studied the changes in radiographic joint space width in the hip with age and concluded that there was no effect of ageing or gender but that height, femoral head diameter and leg length all were directly related to joint space width. It is unclear why the knee cartilage decreases with age while that at the hip joint does not. One explanation could be that the cartilage of the knee joint is more prone to damage as it has greater loading over flatter surface area.

The loss of muscle strength and therefore altered muscle/tendon pull, along with hormonal changes in the bone of ageing females, induce a loss of bone density (osteoporosis). Hence the bone is much more prone to fracture and/or collapse (Bland 1993). The altered muscle/tendon pull may also cause initial trauma to its bony attachment, resulting in a proliferation of new bone forming a cartilaginous or bony spur. This

usually occurs at the bony attachment of the tendons. With a reduction in muscle strength in ageing, there may be an inability to control the normal joint stresses, leading to a change in the weight-bearing forces across the joint. The weight-bearing surfaces of the joints start to fail, as a result of 'either repeated application of high loads over a relatively short period or with the repetition of low loads over an extended period, even though the magnitude of those loads may be much lower than the material's ultimate strength' (Nordin & Frankel 2001).

These changes are not necessarily noticed until further 'external stresses' such as injury, infection or inflammation occur.

Often, in fact, it is not until the additional stresses on the hyaline cartilage on the bone ends and the underlying subchondral bone progresses to eburnation (polished state) and excessive signs of 'wear and tear', with the subsequent diagnosis of osteoarthrosis, that it becomes obvious that these mechanical changes have been proceeding for some time.

Self-assessment questions

- **SAQ 2.22** What is osteoporosis and why does it occur to a greater extent after the menopause?
- **SAQ 2.23** Which type of bone is reduced most of all during the ageing process?
- **SAQ 2.24** How does Wolff's law affect ageing bone?

(Answers at end of chapter.)

Comparison of changes in the musculoskeletal system due to the ageing process and to osteoarthrosis

The results of the ageing process have been outlined in this chapter and there has been no attempt to compare them to the effects of osteoarthrosis. Meachim (1969) outlined the comparison between the two processes for bone, joint and articular cartilage. The changes in the ageing process are given in the table below. In the prerequisites for this chapter you were asked to revise the pathology of osteoarthrosis. Therefore you should be able to answer this question.

Problem-solving exercise 2.1

- From your reading, can you fill in the comparable changes that occur in articular cartilage, bone, joint and muscle in the pathology of osteoarthrosis?

Osteoarthrosis   Ageing

         Normal metabolism
         Normal enzymatic modelling
         Cartilage changes only
         No chondrocyte mitosis
         Normal rates of synthesis, collagen and proteoglycans
         No change or a reduction in the water content of cartilage
         Fibrillation of non-progressive, non-weight-bearing sites of cartilage
         No eburnation of cartilage
         Osteophytes joint edges only with excessive use
         Increased collagen cross-links
         No inflammation
         No joint effusion
         Normal pigment in cartilage
         Reduction in type II muscle fibres
         No sclerosis of subchondral bone
         Minimal loss of joint space, may occur at the periphery – should be no loss of joint congruity
         No ongoing joint/muscle pain

Modified and adapted from Bland 1993.

SUMMARY

Development and ageing involve all the components of the musculoskeletal system: muscle, bone, joint capsule, tendons, ligaments and articular cartilage. The musculoskeletal system cannot survive in isolation and is dependent on the development, maturation and ageing effects of the neural and cardiovascular systems.

All the changes that occur through the 25–30 years of development of the muscle, bone, tendon, articular cartilage and ligaments are slowly reversed at the start of the ageing process, but the time scale for ageing is much longer (from around 30 years of age until death). However, the effects of ageing are most significant after 55 years of age, especially around the time of the menopause in women.

The effects of ageing will be influenced by the lifestyle and fitness of the person throughout their active years, with the onset of the effects of ageing being less evident in the fitter and healthier individual.

The normal effects of ageing do not necessarily cause problems to the individual but may reduce their functional level, speed and performance. It is not until the effects of the stresses on the musculoskeletal structures cause failure that the ageing changes alter to pathological signs and symptoms.

ANSWERS TO QUESTIONS AND EXERCISES

Self-assessment question 2.1 (page 30)

- **SAQ 2.1** Which part(s) of a muscle constitute(s) the contractile unit?

  Answer: Myofibrils, containing the main contractile unit of the sarcomeres with filaments of actin and myosin.

Self-assessment question 2.2 (page 30)

- **SAQ 2.2** In general, which types of movement can be performed at birth?

  Answer: Reflex movements and some gross activity patterns.

Self-assessment question 2.3 (page 30)

- **SAQ 2.3** What does muscle strength directly depend upon?

Answer: Cross-sectional muscle area and the number of myofibrils.

Self-assessment question 2.4 (page 30)

- **SAQ 2.4** How does a muscle maintain the generation of force as it is lengthening, during the developmental sequence?

 Answer: By the addition of serial sarcomeres so that there is a continued overlap of actin and myosin filaments.

Self-assessment question 2.5 (page 36)

- **SAQ 2.5** Name the main functions of bone.

 Answer: Support, protection and mineral homeostasis.

Self-assessment question 2.6 (page 36)

- **SAQ 2.6** What does Wolff's law state and what does this imply?

 Answer: Bone will alter its size, shape and trabecular pattern in both the subchondral and cortical bone according to the line of physical stress. This implies that bone is constantly remodelling to accommodate for the natural stress on the body tissue.

Self-assessment question 2.7 (page 36)

- **SAQ 2.7** Name the types of ossification of bone.

 Answer: Endochondral (cartilage) ossification, intramembranous ossification.

Self-assessment question 2.8 (page 36)

- **SAQ 2.8** Name the parts of a long bone.

 Answer:
- Epiphysis – distal part.
- Metaphysis – start of the secondary centre of ossification, the site of the epiphyseal plate
- Epiphyseal plate – junction of the epiphysis and the diaphysis, the growth plate
- Diaphysis – shaft of the bone
- Medullary cavity – cavity in the centre of the shaft of the bone

- Cancellous bone – open weave, lighter and spongier bone
- Cortical bone – hard crust of bone tissue forming the exterior layers.

Self-assessment question 2.9 (page 36)

- **SAQ 2.9** Describe the pattern of timing of epiphyseal ossification.

 Answer: Elbow (13–15 years), hip (13–16 years), ankle (13–18 years), knee (14–18 years), wrist (18–20 years), shoulder (15–20 years) and medial end of the clavicle (up to 30 years of age).

Self-assessment question 2.10 (page 36)

- **SAQ 2.10** Name the fontanelles and sutures in the skull and state the ages at which they ossify.

 Answer:
- *Fontanelles*: anterior (bregmatic), sphenoidal, mastoid, posterior (lambdoid)
- *Sutures*: frontal, coronal, lambdoid, sagittal
- Fontanelles ossify between 2 months and 2 years
- Sutures ossify between 17 years and 30 years.

Self-assessment question 2.11 (page 36)

- **SAQ 2.11** The adolescent growth spurt starts at 10.3 years in girls and 12 years in boys. What factors may influence this growth?

 Answer: Alterations to the hormone level, mechanical changes and stress and pressure changes.

Self-assessment question 2.12 (page 37)

- **SAQ 2.12** Where is the secondary centre of ossification in bone?

 Answer: At the epiphysis.

Self-assessment question 2.13 (page 37)

- **SAQ 2.13** Why are epimysium and perimysium important in muscle attachment?

 Answer: They combine with the collagen of the tendon to join the muscle to the bone.

Self-assessment question 2.14 (page 37)

- **SAQ 2.14** What is the difference between the collagen in tendon and ligaments?

Answer: The collagen fibres in the tendon lie parallel but in the ligament some of the fibres are parallel but they also lie in a functional pattern, which can give multidirectional strength.

Self-assessment question 2.15 (page 39)

- **SAQ 2.15** What are the functions of articular cartilage?

Answer: To distribute joint loads over a wide area, reduce friction between opposing joint surfaces, help in the lubrication of the joint.

Self-assessment question 2.16 (page 39)

- **SAQ 2.16** What are proteoglycans and what is their role in cartilage?

Answer: Large protein polysaccharide molecules; they form a concentrated solution to enmesh the collagen fibres.

Self-assessment question 2.17 (page 40)

- **SAQ 2.17** Why is cartilage often described as 'a water-filled sponge'?

Answer: Because it is constructed of two parts – the solid part (collagen) and the fluid part (water and inorganic salts) – and acts in a similar way to a sponge in performing its functions.

Self-assessment question 2.18 (page 40)

- **SAQ 2.18** How does a synovial joint maintain nutrition to its components?

Answer: Synovial fluid is generated by the synovial membrane and it is distributed with the aid of the articular cartilage, either by pushing the fluid ahead of the motion and reabsorbing it when the pressure is reduced or by the direct pressure on the articular cartilage squeezing out the fluid from the articular cartilage.

Self-assessment question 2.19 (page 44)

- **SAQ 2.19** Outline the first ageing changes in the muscle.

Answer: Microscopic changes with resultant loss of muscle mass, strength, speed of contraction.

Self-assessment question 2.20 (page 44)

- **SAQ 2.20** Define atrophy.

Answer: Loss of muscle mass, therefore a reduction in the cross-sectional area of the muscle.

Self-assessment question 2.21 (page 44)

- **SAQ 2.21** During ageing the type II muscle fibres are lost to a greater extent. What is the effect of this on muscle performance?

Answer: A reduction in the strength that can be generated and slight loss of endurance.

Self-assessment question 2.22 (page 45)

- **SAQ 2.22** What is osteoporosis and why does it occur to a greater extent after the menopause?

Answer: Reduction in bone density, worse after the menopause because of the changes in the hormone level.

Self-assessment question 2.23 (page 45)

- **SAQ 2.23** Which type of bone is reduced most of all during the ageing process?

Answer: Cancellous bone.

Self-assessment question 2.24 (page 45)

- **SAQ 2.24** How does Wolff's law affect ageing bone?

Answer: Weight-bearing stresses across the joint change with age; therefore, where there is added pressure, the underlying cartilage and bone proliferate to accommodate the increase but when the pressure is reduced the cartilage and bone are not stimulated to remodel and there may be a loss of tissue.

Problem-solving exercise 2.1 (page 46)

- From your reading, can you fill in the comparable changes that occur in articular cartilage, bone, joint and muscle in the pathology of osteoarthrosis?

Answer:

Osteoarthrosis	Ageing
Highly anabolic and synthetic process	Normal metabolism
Enzymatic destruction of hard tissue	Normal enzymatic modelling
Remodelling all tissues about joint (articular and periarticular)	Cartilage changes only
Chondrocyte mitosis	No chondrocyte mitosis
Intense increased synthesis of collagen and proteoglycans	Normal rates of synthesis, collagen and proteoglycan
Increased water content of cartilage	No change or a reduction in the water content of cartilage
Fibrillation, focal and progressive, at weight-bearing sites	Fibrillation of non-progressive, non-weight-bearing sites of cartilage
Eburnation, ivory-like	No eburnation of cartilage
Osteophytes occur with other joint changes	Osteophytes joint edges only with excessive use
No increased collagen cross-links	Increased collagen cross-links
Inflammation	No inflammation
Joint effusion present on occasions	No joint effusion
No pigment in cartilage	Normal pigment in cartilage
Reduction in type II and type I muscle fibres	Reduction in type II muscle fibres
Sclerosis of subchondral bone	No sclerosis of subchondral bone
Narrowing of the joint space and loss of joint congruity, particularly at the greatest weight-bearing surfaces	Minimal loss of joint space, may occur at the periphery – should be no loss of joint congruity
Joint and/or muscle pain	No ongoing joint/ muscle pain

References

Amiel A, Frank C, Harwood F et al 1984 Tendons and ligaments: a morphological and biochemical comparison. Journal of Orthopaedic Research 1: 257–265

Amiridis IG, Hatzitakib V, Arabatzia F 2003 Age-induced modifications of static postural control in humans. Neuroscience Letters 350: 137–140

Aniansson A, Grimby G, Hedberg G et al 1981 Muscle morphology enzyme activity and muscle strength in elderly men and women. Clinical Physiology 1: 73

Astrand P-O 1986 Exercise physiology of the mature athlete. In: Sutton JR and Broc RM (eds) Sports medicine for the mature athlete. Benchmark Press, Indianapolis, IN, ch 3, p 3–15

Barker D 1993 What makes them grow into healthy adults? Medical Research Council News 60: 8

Bell G, Emslie-Smith D, Paterson C 1980 Textbook of physiology. Churchill Livingstone, Edinburgh

Bickers M 1993 Does verbal encouragement work? The effect of verbal encouragement on a muscular endurance task. Clinical Rehabilitation 7: 196

Bland JH 1993 Mechanisms of adaptation in the joint. In: Crosbie J, McConnell J. Key issues in musculoskeletal physiotherapy. Butterworth Heinemann, Oxford, p 88–113

Burstein A, Reilly D, Martens M 1976 Aging of bone tissue: mechanical properties. Journal of Bone and Joint Surgery 58A: 82

Campbell MJ, McComas AJ, Petito F 1973 Physiological changes in ageing muscle. Journal of Neurology, Neurosurgery and Psychiatry 36: 174

Carlstedt C, Nordin M 2001 Biomechanics of tendons and ligaments. In: Nordin M, Frankel VH (eds) Basic biomechanics of the musculoskeletal system, 3rd edn. Lippincott Williams & Wilkins, Philadelphia, ch 3, p 59–74

Chubinskaya S, Kumar B, Merrihew C et al 2002 Age-related changes in cartilage endogenous osteogenic protein-1 (OP-1). Biochimica et Biophysica Acta 1588: 126–134

Collins 1982 The new Collins concise English dictionary. Collins, London

Dacre JE, Scott DL, Da Silva JAP et al 1991 Joint space in radiologically normal knees. British Journal of Rheumatology 30: 426–428

Dandy DJ, Edwards DJ 2003 Essential orthopaedics and trauma, 3rd edn. Churchill Livingstone, Oxford

Doherty TJ, Vandervoort AA, Taylor AW, Brown WF 1993 Effects of motor units losses on strength in older men and women. Journal of Applied Physiology 74: 868–874

Espenschade A, Eckert H 1980 Motor development, 2nd edn. Charles E Merrill, Columbus, OH

Frontera WR 1989 Strength training in the elderly. In: Harris R, Harris S (eds) Physical activity, aging and sports. CSA-Albany, p 319

Frontera WR, Meredith CN, O'Reilly KP et al 1988 Strength conditioning in older men: skeletal muscle hypertrophy and improved function. Journal of Applied Physiology 64: 1038

Goker B, Sancak A, Arac M et al 2003 The radiographic joint space width in clinically normal hips: effects of age, gender and physical parameters. Osteoarthritis and Cartilage 11, 328–334

Goldspink G, Williams P 1990 Muscle fibre and connective tissue changes associated with use and disuse. In: Ada L, Canning C (eds) Key issues in neurological physiotherapy. Butterworth Heinemann, Oxford, ch 8, p 197–218

Govan A, McFarlane P, Callender R 1991 Pathology illustrated, 3rd ed. Churchill Livingstone, Edinburgh

Grimby G, Saltin B 1983 The ageing muscle. Clinical Physiology 3: 209

Hammerman D 1993 Aging and osteoarthritis: basic mechanisms. Journal of the American Geriatric Society 41: 760–770

Harris BA, Watkins MP 1993 Muscle performance: principles and general theory. In: Harms-Ringdahl K (ed) IPPT8 – muscle strength. Churchill Livingstone, Edinburgh

Hinderer KA, Hinderer SR 1993 Development and assessment in children and adolescents. In: Harms-Ringdahl K (ed) IPPT8 – muscle strength. Churchill Livingstone, Edinburgh

Jones D, Round J 1992 Skeletal muscle in health and disease. Manchester University Press, Manchester

Knortz KA 1987 Muscle physiology applied to geriatric rehabilitation. Topics in Geriatric Rehabilitation 2: 1

Konanen V 1989 Effects of ageing and physical training on rat skeletal muscle. Acta Physiologica Scandinavica 135 (Suppl.), 577

Larsson L, Grimby G, Karlsson J 1979 Muscle strength and speed of movement in relationship to age and muscle morphology. Journal of Applied Physiology 46: 451

Lennmarken C, Bergman T, Larsson J et al 1985 Skeletal muscle function in man, force relaxation rate, endurance, and contraction time – dependence on sex and age. Clinical Physiology 5: 243

Lexell J, Taylor CC, Sjostrom M 1988 What is the cause of the ageing atrophy? Journal of Neural Science 84: 275

Mahler DA, Cunningham LN, Curfman LD 1986 Ageing and exercise performance. Clinical Geriatric Medicine 2: 433

Maki BE, McIlroy WE 1996 Postural control in the older adult. Clinics in Geriatric Medicine 12: 635–658

Makrides L 1986 Physical training in young and older healthy subjects. In: Sutton JR, Brock RM (eds) Sports medicine for the mature athlete. Benchmark Press, Indianapolis, IN, p 363

Malkia E 1993 Strength and aging: patterns of change and implications for training. In: Harms-Ringdahl K (ed) IPPT8 – muscle strength. Churchill Livingstone, Edinburgh

McCutchen CW 1966 Boundary lubrication by synovial fluid: demonstration and possible osmotic explanation. Federation Proceedings 25: 1061

Meachim G 1969 Age changes in articular cartilage. Clinical Orthopaedics 64: 33

Methany E 1941 Breathing capacity and grip strength of preschool children. Child Welfare 18(2): 1

Monotoye HJ, Lamphiear DE 1977 Grip and arm strength in males and females, aged 10–69 years. Research Quarterly 48: 109

Moritani T, De Vries HW 1980 Potential for gross muscle hypertrophy in older men. Journal of Gerontology 35: 672

Nonaka H, Mita K, Watakabe M et al 2002 Age-related changes in the interactive mobility of the hip and knee joints: a geometrical analysis. Gait and Posture 15: 236–243

Nordin M, Frankel VH 2001 Basic biomechanics of the musculoskeletal system, 3rd edn. Lippincott Williams & Wilkins, Philadelphia, PA

O'Connor M, Carnell P, Manuel J, Scott OM 1993 Contractile characteristics of human quadriceps femoris muscle in active elderly and young adults. Proceedings of the Physiological Society, London

Roach KE, Miles TP 1991 Normal hip and knee active range of motion: the relationship to age. Physical Therapy 71: 656–665

Russo P 1990 Cardiovascular responses associated with activity and inactivity. In: Ada L, Canning C (eds) Key issues in neurological physiotherapy. Butterworth Heinemann, Oxford, ch 6, p 127–154

Rutherford O, Jones D 1992 Relationship of muscle and bone loss and activity levels with age in women. Age and Ageing 21: 286

Shephard RJ 1980 Population aspects of human working capacity. Annals of Human Biology 7: 1

Shipman P, Walker A, Bichell D 1985 The human skeleton. Harvard University Press, Cambridge, MA

Sipila S, Suominen H 1991 Ultrasound imaging of the quadriceps muscle in elderly athletes and untrained men. Muscle and Nerve 14: 527

Skinner J, Tipton C, Vailas A 1982 Exercise, physical training and the aging process. In: Viidik A (ed) Lectures in gerontology, vol. I: On biology of aging. Part B. Academic Press, London, p 407

Smith GA, Nelson RG, Sadoff SJ, Sadoff AM 1989 Assessing sincerity of effort in maximal grip strength tests. American Journal of Physical Medicine and Rehabilitation 2: 73

Smith WDF 1989 Fitness training in the elderly: Canadian experience. Geriatric Medicine 19: 55

St Pierre D, Gardiner P 1987 The effect of immobilisation and exercise on muscle function: a review. Physiotherapy Canada 39: 24

Stokes M, Cooper R 1993 Physiological factors influencing performance of skeletal muscle. In: Crosbie J, McConnell J (eds) Key issues in musculoskeletal physiotherapy. Butterworth Heinemann, Oxford, ch 2

Tanner JM, Whitehouse RH, Marubini E, Resele LF 1976 The adolescent growth spurt of boys and girls of the Harpenden growth study. Annals of Human Biology 3: 109

Thelen E 1985 The developmental origins of motor coordination: leg movements in human infants. Developmental Psychobiology 18: 1

Tomlinson BE, Irving D 1977 The numbers of limb motor neurones in the human lumbosacral cord throughout life. Journal of the Neurological Sciences 34: 213–219

Tomlinson BE, Walton JN, Rebeiz JJ 1969 The effects of ageing in and cachexia upon skeletal muscle. A histopathological study. Journal of the Neurological Sciences 9: 321

Vandervoort AA, Hayes KC, Belanger AY 1986 Strength and endurance of skeletal muscle in the elderly. Physiotherapy Canada 38: 167

Vaughan J 1981 The physiology of bone. Clarendon Press, Oxford

Walker PS, Dowson D, Longfield MD, Wright V 1968 'Boosted lubrication' in synovial joints by fluid entrapment and enrichment. Annals Rheumatology Disease 27: 512–520

Walker PS, Unsworth A, Dowson D et al 1970 Mode of aggregation of hyaluronic acid protein complex on the surface of articular cartilage. Annals Rheumatology Disease 29: 591–602

Yamada K, Healey R, Amiel D et al 2002 Subchondral bone of the human knee joint in aging and osteoarthritis. Osteoarthritis and Cartilage 10: 360–369

Young A 1984 The relative isometric strength of type I and type II muscle fibres in the human quadriceps. Clinical Physiology 4: 23

Young A, Stokes M, Crowe M 1984 Size and strength of quadriceps muscle of old and young women. European Journal of Clinical Investigation 14: 282

Young A, Stokes M, Crowe M 1985 Size and strength of quadriceps muscle of old and young men. Clinical Physiology 5: 145

Chapter 3

Recognition of change in the musculoskeletal system: assessment

Anne-Marie Hassenkamp

CHAPTER CONTENTS

OBJECTIVES

By the end of this chapter you should:

- Have an awareness of how different philosophies can drive assessment
- Have an understanding of the different changes measured by different assessments and be aware of the suitability of certain kind of assessments for different kinds of situations
- Have an insight into factors possibly indicating serious pathology and which should not be dealt with by physiotherapy as a first line approach (red flags)
- Have an appreciation of psychosocial factors which might be indicative of a slower pace of recovery (yellow flags)

KEY WORDS

Assessment, change and measurement of it, physiotherapy management, health models, red and yellow flags.

Prerequisites

Before continuing with this chapter you should revise the different assessment techniques and schedules you have used up to now for assessing musculoskeletal changes.

INTRODUCTION

The Chartered Society of Physiotherapy's Code of Conduct (1990) charges its members with the absolute need to assess each patient before treating him or her.

The assessment acts as the baseline for the decisions we take after that point in time. It is therefore of ultimate importance for our patient as his or her future management will depend on it. By looking at its different facets in detail and developing a good rationale based on a sound theory base, the physiotherapist will become flexible in using only those aspects of the very detailed assessment apparatus that are meaningful and relevant for the particular patient about to be assessed. This is true for the subjective as well as the objective assessment. Time spent on requiring good and flexible assessment skills always pays off in terms of treatment outcome. A poor assessment cannot be compensated for by a technically excellent treatment, as one would not be able to ascertain the extent of the possible change.

The first question we need to ask is 'assessment of what'? Do we assess change or do we assess needs? Is the assessment aimed at, for example, a change in range of movement, or is it geared towards establishing what would be necessary to enable the patient to be as independent as possible?

Physiotherapists are experts in recognizing when change has taken place. We understand the wide variety of what is normal but also have an understanding of what changes are beyond the realm of normal. This specialized discernment is something our particular training/education can bring to the assessment procedure. The movement continuum theory of physical therapy (Cott et al 1995) has already been mentioned in the Introduction. It gives an excellent structure to the ever-expanding field of our practice. This model can further offer a real understanding of the interconnectedness of the structures and the factors that drive these (anatomy and physiology as well as the wish/necessity to move at a certain level). In order to grasp this quite complex theory, why not try and identify where you operate on that continuum: is your preferred movement capability the same as your current movement capability? If not, why do you think that is? What would you need to investigate to get to the bottom of this?

Demonstrating and measuring this change is the underlying core of assessment. The recognition and validation of change has been at the centre of physiotherapists becoming recognized as independent and autonomous practitioners. This identification and measurement of change is becoming authenticated by a slowly expanding area of research (Parry 1985). Since Anne Parry's work there has of course been a very active debate within our profession on the pros and cons of evidence-based physiotherapy. For an interesting discussion that puts practice on the horns of the dilemma, read Bithell (2000), Bury (1996) and Sackett et al (1996).

HEALTH MODELS

Before this discussion goes any further we need to consider different models of health and the resultant roles of physiotherapist and patient within these. As will be seen, the model the practitioner works in has a defining influence on the patient. These different paradigms feed the assessment philosophy and hence are directly related to outcome.

In a strict biomedical model the patient's referring problem is defined in terms of system breakdown. His/her body is seen as a biological entity, which has developed a fault. The role of the practitioner is therefore to identify the area of breakdown while the role of the patient is to co-operate with the treatment and to get better. Years of 'the fracture in bed 5' or 'the total hip replacement in the side ward' give evidence of the ultimate starkness of this approach. It is believed that the body is governed by certain natural laws, which can be predicted and which assume a vaguely linear pattern. The implication for assessments within this model is clearly that of identifying the pathological or mechanical change rather than trying to understand the impact of the current happening on the patient's life. Questions about the patient's personal life, his hobbies, profession and general belief about his problem, etc. seem to be less important, if not irrelevant, within this model, as they will not influence the treatment avenue.

As long as physiotherapists saw themselves more as doctors' assistants than autonomous practitioners, working in this model was appropriate and congruent with our treatment approaches. In strict terms, though, this model suggested that, as we all shared bodies that reacted along similar physiological lines, we would react similarly to therapeutic advances. This is clearly not so as all of us will be able to recall situations that demonstrated how differently we all respond to the same stimulus. Even though the noxious insult may be the same, the level of pain it causes is likely to be quite different in different people. The experience and perception of pain were possibly quite different. The biomedical model found it hard to generate acceptable explanations for these happenings and it has been felt not to be altogether congruent with the different therapies. However, it is difficult to fully explore other models as long as we work within a referral system that is still steeped for the most part in the biomedical approach. I do not want to be too critical about this model, however, as there are clear situations in which this is the most appropriate structure to assess and work in.

Over the past years, therefore, health professionals in general and physiotherapists in particular have moved away from this very powerful mind set and have shifted more towards a model that incorporates the patient as a partner and does not just look at him/her as a biological system that has broken down. This biopsychosocial model (Engel 1977) was first reported as a counterbalance to the biomedical model and tried to challenge its assumptions of only anatomical–physiological system failure.

It views the patient as presenting with a problem, which could lie in the spheres of the patient's body, psyche or social environment. Here the role of the health professional is to empower the patient to deal with the existing problem in an individual way. Cott and colleagues' movement continuum theory model (1995) again helps with integrating into this different mind set and its implied assumptions. This automatically assumes that the patient and the therapist have to negotiate goals (rather than the therapist informing the patient of his/her objectives). The treatment outcome, as well as the assessment does not merely

deal with the identification of a biological breakdown but also with the meaning this has for the patient and the influence this has on his/her life style.

This model takes into account the fact that all of us are different and that we are affected quite differently by happenings. Remember how some patients do not want to know anything about their clinical diagnosis and just want to leave it up to the professional to get on with it and 'cure' them while others ask a lot of very detailed questions and wish to be in a situation where they can take an informed choice about their future. This might include the decision not to avail themselves of our treatment.

Another driver for the assessment process and its interpretation is of course the thought behind what we are looking for. Mostly we are determined to discover the impairment, disability and handicap dimension. This division has served the WHO for many years (WHO 1980). The recent re-interpretation of these dimensions is classified into:

- impairment (a loss or abnormality of body structure or of a physiological or psychological functioning)
- activity (the nature and extent of functioning at the level of the person – activities may be limited in nature, duration and quality)
- participation (the extent of a person's involvement in life situations in relation to impairment, activities, health conditions and contextual factors – participation may be restricted in nature, duration and quality)
- context (includes the features, aspects, attributes of, or objects, structures, human-made organizations, service provisions, and agencies in, the physical, social and attitudinal environment in which people live and conduct their lives (WHO 2001)).

Going back to the beginning of this discussion, you can see how different the assessments of these two patients would need to be in order to get the best result for them. It is therefore vital that you search your physiotherapist soul and become aware of how you tick within certain physiotherapy situations. Do you lean more towards a biomedical or biopsychosocial approach in your patient assessments? Are your assessments geared to elicit 'hard' measures only (measurable signs) or do you include 'soft' measures, which are more focused on the individual? This will clearly be different according to the setting you most work in. Imagine assessing a patient in a community setting in contrast to an Intensive Therapy Unit. It is essential that we consider these points before the assessment is planned and executed.

ASSESSMENT IN GENERAL

The physiotherapy assessment usually consists of two or even three components (Parry 1985):

- a subjective examination, meaning an interview, the listening to the patient's story
- the objective examination, the measuring of hard findings
- the interpretations.

Physiotherapists are spending a lot of time becoming accomplished in the cohesiveness of these three subsections of assessment and have developed a certain thoroughness in this. Thoughts that come to mind include the fact that, although the patient shares a disorder with others (i.e. his/her biological system has failed in a predictable way), the patient's needs are individual and therefore the priorities that are set have to be individual priorities, incorporating an individual potential for response (Watts 1985). This process is done with scientific rigour and follows predictable and strictly ordered thought processes. As mentioned earlier, we set a lot of store by this approach and base the right to be autonomous practitioners on this element of our practice and education.

Watts (1985) links the decision-making process, which is the consequence of assessment really, to having a vision that is clearly related to the physiotherapist's understanding of her role and responsibility in this interaction. Is she meant to be the powerful healer or does she see herself more as the patient's partner, who is able to empower him? Watts refers further to the possible danger of a narrowness of vision if the choices in assessment/decision making are made in an unconscious way. How can we make these choices explicit and hence conscious? Self-awareness, as

previously mentioned, can be a considerable step in this direction. Another suggestion would be the implementation of regular peer supervision amongst physiotherapists as a routine avenue to ensuring good practice. Are there some assessment – and hence management – options we never consider and, if so, why is that? The disadvantage of having a predictable and well-structured route through the information-gathering process is the possible lack of safeguards for recognizing something different as relevant. The quickly expanding area of clinical reasoning might help us with the making explicit of our thought processes and hence might allow us to develop more breadth rather than just more depth.

Self-assessment question

- **SAQ 3.1** Do we use all the information gained in an assessment? Is our assessment aimed to only pick out the useful information for this patient? Is it ethical to collect data that will/might not be used in treatment planning?

Watts (1985) stresses the importance of exploring what our assessments are based on. Are they based on theory or on professional anecdotes? Are we aware of where this theory comes from? Is it borrowed from the fields of medicine and sociology or is it based on physiotherapy observations? What markers do we use in our assessments? Do we use the concepts of normal/abnormal or stability/mobility or disorder pathways (e.g. osteoarthritis versus rheumatoid arthritis, etc.)? How do we report change? Do we report it in terms of judgemental statements or descriptions of state or in any other way? How do we ensure the relevance of this information that we collect? Hislop (1985) states that evaluation/assessment by the physiotherapist must display a concept for the uniqueness of the relationship of the patient as a person and a disorder of the social context of society or community in which the person or the patient lives. This is a very taxing standard and can only be achieved by clinicians who are dealing with quick, high-level decision-making processes at all times. This Hislop (1985) says cannot be taught but can only be achieved through continuous practice, and of course reflection on these processes. Every individual clinician seems to attain this along pathways but it seems clear that a critical stance and self-awareness are vital ingredients, rather than conformity.

Four ingredients for the achievement of clinical excellence have been stated to be memory, knowledge, competence and performance (Hislop 1986). As stated earlier, change can only be evaluated if one has an accurate knowledge of the normal variations in people, which then allows clinicians to decide when something is beyond normal. The same is true, of course, of the predictability of treatment effects. Another call, therefore, for a sound knowledge base. As you can see from the age of these references, the debate about assessment paradigms is not current.

Elsa Ramsden (1985) looked at the different stages influencing the decision-making process in an assessment.

Self-assessment question

- **SAQ 3.2** Which of these categories are you aware of as a physiotherapist? Do you put them into the same order?

Her model takes it for granted that people process data, decode the information, which comes via the eyes, and encode the messages they send. She proposes the following four strategies for change resulting from this assessment.

1. Identify the need for change
2. Establish goals for change
3. Select means for the attainment of change (= a goal)
4. Evaluate the results of change.

These four stages are at the heart of each and every assessment but they do not occur automatically. For this to happen, Ramsden says, three things have to happen in the change process. First, there has to be a need for change; second, the necessary relationship between patient and therapist needs to be established; last, an appropriate course of action working towards the desired change or goal needs to be established. This mirrors the influential Kolb Learning Cycle (1984), which also speaks about four stages:

- Experiencing or immersing oneself in the doing of the task
- Reflection, which involves reviewing what has been done and experienced
- Conceptualization, which involves interpreting the events and understanding the relationships among them
- Planning looks at predictions about what is likely to happen next or what actions should be taken.

Self-assessment question

- **SAQ 3.3** Does this sound familiar to you? Can you try and verbalize and identify your own implicit structure of assessments?

It is the working on this relationship between patient and therapist that needs to be the focus for the assessment or treatment if progress or co-operation is to be achieved.

The quality of this relationship is of paramount importance if we want to achieve the very best results in our assessment and hence needs working on and must be included in our scrutiny of our practice.

In sympathy with Kolb, Ramsden (1985) again argues that a model for change must be put within the context of a problem-solving analysis. Again, she identifies several stages, first recognizing the problem, then identifying and locating resources, and finally making out alternative courses. Only then does Ramsden embark on selecting the course of action, initiating it and starting to collect data. These are followed by the evaluation process.

Stanley Paris (1986) approaches thoughts about assessments from a different angle. Rather than being immersed in the process of assessment as Ramsden is, his concerns are more focused on outcome and hence on our understanding of the underlying causes of the patient's distress and the course our assessments will take.

He challenges our understanding of pathology, which leads to pain, which in turn leads to spasm. This cycle would keep our assessments firmly within the realms of the biomedical model, hence leaving us with the problem of how we would identify the need for change in terms of disease process. Paris's own thinking had led him to identify a triad consisting of *dysfunction*, which in turn creates or contributes to a *noxious stimulus*, which then leads to an *involuntary muscle holding*. Should the involuntary muscle holding not resolve, it will automatically cause a *circulatory problem* (stasis) which needs to lead to the *retention of metabolites* hence again *pain*. Paris's point (1986) is that an assessment therefore should not try to identify a syndrome but rather symptoms, which when treated will relieve the syndrome and hence the pain.

The need for change in this concept is couched in terms of function and this by definition must result in an individually differing goal.

Paris (1986) reminds us that, while most physicians will wait for laboratory results to confirm the suspected diagnosis, physiotherapists tend to feel that they need to be able to come to an instant opinion on which to base judgements about treatment and further management. Needless to say, this often leads to premature decisions and incorrect information handed to the patient. It is at times necessary to postpone the first treatment of the patient until after that assessment has been evaluated properly.

Should you use examination sheets or not?

There are obviously clear advantages for using examination sheets (e.g. neatness, speed, consistency, easy transferability). The disadvantages are not to be minimized either. Are all the patients going to need the same kind of questioning/approach? Or would it be possible to branch off much earlier into a more acute or chronic part of the interview and assessment? This will depend largely on the experience or lack of it of the examiner.

It seems important that the use of examination sheets is assessed for each assessment setting. They should therefore be used in a flexible way and the motives for using them must be clear to the user. In any team setting they can surely be regarded as a standardized way of documenting a baseline and subsequent change and therefore might be regarded by the team members as a useful and necessary tool. These assessment sheets are surely less helpful if they act purely as a prompter for the assessor. In that case a standardized approach might automatically mean a non-individualized approach to the patient's problem. Clearly, then, a patient-centred problem-solving approach will be impossible and this could therefore be regarded as poor practice.

We must, however, at all times be aware of the limitations of what we record. The validity and especially specificity of our tests (and those of the medical practitioners, for that matter) are often poor and nebulous.

How should you go about assessing a patient?

Paris (1985), committed to symptoms rather than syndromes, divides his evaluation into the following 15 points:

1. Interview with receptionist
2. Pain assessment
3. Initial observation
4. History and interview with physio
5. Structural observation
6. Active movements
7. Upper/lower extremity evaluation
8. Neurological assessment
9. Palpation for condition
10. Palpation for position
11. Palpation for mobility
12. X-rays and other medical findings
13. Summary of objective findings
14. Plan of treatment for objective findings
15. Prognosis

Self-assessment question

- SAQ 3.4 Reflecting on the Ramsden and the Paris approaches to assessment, where does your own thinking fit in? In order to be/become a good assessor, it is important that you become aware of your own thinking patterns in this.

The physiotherapy assessment has so far been firmly linked to problem solving. Is it therefore possible to predict who is going to be a good problem solver and who is not? Newble et al (1995) suggest that the problem-solving skill is not a stand-alone skill and that it is therefore impossible to predict someone's problem-solving skill in one area by having observed them problem-solve in another. It appears, therefore, that this skill is very context-specific. A marvellous illumination of this was published by De Groot (1965), who observed chess grand masters problem solving. This group of subjects was unable to transfer their exceptionally highly developed skill from chess to another area. Problem solving in assessments therefore needs to be linked to the very specific knowledge of the theories underpinning the area of muscular skeletal problems and recognition of the specificity of that particular context.

What is needed for a good assessment?

The function of the assessment is to make sense of the examination findings. Grieve (1981) defines the role of the examination as 'to understand fully how the patient is troubled and then to seek a physical basis for these symptoms in terms of objective signs'. He goes on to say that assessment is 'the judgement that is necessary to make sense of these findings; hence to identify a relationship between the symptoms reported and the signs of disturbed function'.

This makes it very clear that the assessor needs very specific knowledge, but s/he also needs specific skills, and it seems that the interdependence of these two ingredients, knowledge and skills, is the vital ingredient. This interdependence is not an abstract thing but a continually changing entity fed by our attitudes (Newble et al 1995). Self-awareness, which has already been mentioned several times, is an essential part of being a physiotherapist and this needs as much training and continual development as the more technical side of our profession. Participation in experiential learning (i.e. in or through clinical practice) is essential. More on this aspect can be read in the literature on clinical reasoning in physiotherapy (Carr et al 1995, Higgs & Jones 2000).

Remember the patient with whom you just were unable to forge any relationship and who seemed to bring out the most impatient side of you? Have you any idea why that was? Do the patients whom you cannot help have anything in common? Are you aware what or who they remind you of? Or are you aware that the very angry patient who seems unable to co-operate with you has projected his feelings on to you although they really belong to a totally different setting, and retaliation on your part is therefore going to be the most damaging reaction? This is clearly not only true for negative happenings but also for really successful encounters. What was it in your patient that made it so easy for you to get on to the same wavelength as them?

Unless these issues are clearly understood their impact on the assessment might be harmful and unhelpful. Skills and knowledge are enhanced by experience. The less experience the assessor has, i.e. the less the patient mileage s/he has, the more the therapist will have to stick to clearly signposted routes. Feltovich & Barrows (1984) refer to this as 'illness scripts'. At the other end of the continuum is the experienced clinician who has in his/her mind a vast bank of previous experiences or memories on which s/he can draw quickly and efficiently. It is therefore much easier for the experienced clinician to recognize patterns and to extrapolate information about these (Brooks et al 1991). They are able to perceive relations between different bits of information. The expert therefore seems to do less problem solving than the novice as the former has already stored solutions to a lot of everyday problems s/he may be confronted with in clinical practice (Kahney 1993).

Having reviewed the background to assessment per se it is now important to consider assessment in a more specific way as it relates to orthopaedics.

What is the role of the physiotherapist in an assessment?

Hertling & Kessler (1990) believe this to be to 'clarify the nature and extent of the lesion, to assess the extent of resulting disability and to recover significant data in order to establish a basis against which to judge progress'.

Self-assessment question

- SAQ 3.5 Do you agree with this statement or would you like to add to it or qualify it more?

As mentioned earlier, physiotherapists have to come to their opinion by evaluating, first, purely subjective data offered by the patient plus, second, objective data elicited by a clinical examination. In this they are quite different from, for example, doctors, who on the whole have the benefit of laboratory results.

Many well-known orthopaedic surgeons (e.g. Dandy 1993) and physicians (e.g. Cyriax 1982) as well as physiotherapists (e.g. Grieve 1981) have suggested assessment schedules.

The actual sequence of your assessment plan will depend a lot on the setting you work in. Do you work in an outpatients' department with independent patients coming for a well-defined problem or do you work on a ward with bed-bound patients who have undergone surgery or experienced the diagnosis of a progressive disease? Or perhaps you work in the community with patients in their own home coping with a chronic and perhaps disabling disease.

Self-assessment question

- SAQ 3.6 How do you think the assessment might change with the setting you work in? Why?

The aim of the assessment – whichever way you elicit the information – is to establish what the patient's problem is, what it means to the patient (i.e. which aspect of it is the most disturbing to the patient) and what clinical objective findings can be found to narrow down the possible clinical diagnosis.

ASSESSMENT OF ORTHOPAEDIC PATIENTS

After having looked at assessment per se, it is time now to look at how the assessment can be addressed for an orthopaedic patient. How should we and how can we elicit the information needed for the professional judgement (assessment) that we discussed earlier? Jones et al (1994, 2000) remind us of the need to use open-ended questions rather than just yes/no questions, using the patient's words as much as possible when investigating the problem and repeating part of the patient's story for clarification. How many times though do we put words into the patient's mouth in order to clarify a point our way or hurry him/her towards a solution that we anticipate?

What is your favourite way of structuring the initial interview? Do you allow patients to tell their own story in a semi-structured way or do you lead them along a very strictly controlled path?

For a more detailed discussion of the skills needed for the subjective assessment, refer to Thomson (1992).

Certain information has to be elicited and the sorts of thing that you would need to find out are discussed below.

Why is the patient here?

Was the patient referred by a general practitioner, consultant or another health professional, or did he refer himself to you? This might give you an insight into how the patient thinks about his health. Does he feel responsible for it and able to influence it; does he indicate that he would be quite prepared and happy to work towards the solution of his problem? Or does he give the impression that he expects you to be the solver of all his problems? Perhaps he already hints to you that he has no faith in medicine in general and physiotherapy in particular. As you know, past experiences influence the cognition of the present. If the patient, therefore, has had a good or unsatisfactory experience with physiotherapists in the past this will influence his present expectations of you and of himself.

What is the problem?

Self-assessment question

- SAQ 3.7 What sort of physiotherapy problems do you know or have you dealt with?

On the whole patients get referred to physiotherapists for pain, loss of function and associated signs, e.g. swelling. If the patient is able to describe a very clear incident (e.g. trauma, disease onset) it will be important to discover as much as possible about this incident and to get a feel for the patient's own assessment of the situation. What is the meaning for him of all that has happened? Make sure to be open to all the innuendoes and not only to listen to the obvious. A lot of very pertinent but hidden meaning is conveyed in this part of the patient interview.

How does the patient's life style contribute to or detract from his problem? Are you dealing with a very fit and independent person who has a good understanding of how his body works or are you treating a person whose life style is such that he is under continual mental stress without the necessary time to relax or even to feel what his body is telling him.

What else would you want to know under this heading? You have established how the problem arose and the meaning of it to the patient and you now need to find out if this was the first occurrence of this particular trouble or not. This is important when you are trying to make sense of the patient's words and non-verbal cues, as it will again link in with his and your expectations.

Where and what is the problem and how does it impinge on the patient's life?

It is important now to ascertain if the patient is able to be precise about the problem or not. The physiotherapist tries to understand the location of the pain. For instance, is it a large area or a very specific, narrow area? Can the extent of the pain perimeter be identified as a recognizable anatomical or neurological segment? If not, does it remind you of a description of disease (e.g. diabetes can mirror musculoskeletal problems) and if so which one?

Self-assessment questions

- **SAQ 3.8** You will remember from your previous reading and experience that some anatomical entities have a very precise pain distribution. Where do muscles, ligaments, bones, nerves,

blood vessels and capsules refer pain to? Do not forget the viscera in this. Many a person with low back pain has been offered an operation when the real origin of his/her symptoms was a duodenal ulcer (Weiss et al 1998).
- **SAQ 3.9** Can you remind yourself of the mechanism they use for referral?
- **SAQ 3.10** Are you clear why some of them refer pain in keeping with their geographical situation while others are able to refer pain to locations distant from their anatomical position? Kellgren (1938, 1939) did some of the pioneering work in this field. He managed to map pain referral by irritating pain-sensitive structures (e.g. ligaments) and recording the subject's pain distribution once he had manipulated these structures.

Once you have established whether the pain is limited to a specific area or not you now want to find out if it ever changes in its geography or extent when it is relieved or exacerbated.

How does it behave?

In many ways, this may be the linchpin of this part of your examination. As physiotherapists we deal mainly with problems that incorporate a mechanical element rather than being purely cases of disease. This means that we are looking for a behaviour pattern that is indicative of this aspect.

Self-assessment questions

- **SAQ 3.11** How would you expect the behaviour of symptoms to vary in someone who had a mechanical problem and someone who was suffering from a disease process?
- **SAQ 3.12** What cues would you be hoping for from the patient?

The first thing to establish, therefore, is whether this problem changes with movement or rest. Most pain problems that we can treat have an element of 'being helped by rest'. It is rare that someone with unremitting pain will be helped by physiotherapeutic, hence mechanical or electrical, techniques.

Once you have established that there is a movement element to it you need to find out as much as possible about this relationship: what exact movement increases or decreases the pain?

How quickly does the pain come on once the exacerbating movement has occurred, how severe is it in comparison to the 'normal' level and how long does it stay for once the aggravating movement has been stopped? These three points will help you to identify the irritability of the problem, which will then guide you when you are thinking about the objective examination, which is to follow. This helpful concept of irritability has been around for a long time and has been explored in physiotherapy by Maitland (1964).

Contraindications

Clearly, as in all aspects of physiotherapy there are clues to look or listen for when examining a patient with an apparent orthopaedic or musculoskeletal problem. As discussed at the beginning of this chapter, you will have scanned your memory (often in an unconscious manner) for possible theories underpinning the patient's story while you were listening to him. By now, therefore, you might already have some ideas as to the nature of the problem (i.e. which structure is responsible).

What alternatives to your vague and not yet fully developed hypothesis do you need to exclude?

We said earlier that a hallmark of a musculoskeletal problem is its reaction to movement and rest. Hence, in someone complaining of unremitting pain that was unchanged by either rest or movement we would suspect a serious disease process that would need to be explored.

The following questions might be asked:

- Have you had any significant weight loss? Patients with malignant disease often exhibit marked weight loss.

- What sort of tablets are you on? While it is important to chart the rhythm of pain killers and anti-inflammatory drugs when assessing the patient's pain levels, it is also essential that you investigate the long-term use of systemic steroids or anticoagulants. These medications can be associated with osteoporosis.

- Has any member in your family suffered from rheumatoid arthritis? Remind yourself of the possible hereditary nature of this disease.

- Have you noticed any change in your bladder or bowels? Naturally, the lack of exercise resulting from pain or injury and the use of painkillers interfere with these functions but you need to explore whether either retention or incontinence might be present, as this could be a sign of cord or cauda equina involvement. This would clearly not be a problem primarily for a physiotherapist but for investigation by an orthopaedic surgeon or neurosurgeon.

Results of the subjective examination

At the end of this first part of the assessment you should now have gained a thorough insight into:

- the patient's problem and how he views it
- the patient's expectations of you and himself
- the history, nature and behaviour of the problem
- its degree of irritability
- possible contraindications to treatment (red flags = signs and symptoms that might be indicative of a serious pathology)
- a working hypothesis of which structures might be involved
- a sound theoretical reason for planning certain investigations
- a list of factors (yellow flags) that might indicate a slower progression to treatment avenues. Kendall et al (1997) described them as:
  A ttitudes and beliefs (e.g. pain is harmful and an indication of harm and damage)
  B ehaviours (avoidance of 'normal' activities and roles)
  C ompensation
  D iagnosis and treatment issues (is there any test that has not yet been done?)
  E motions (fear of increased pain with activity)
  F amily (overprotective spouse/partner)
  W ork (history of manual labour; repetitive, boring work).

The message of the yellow flags is on the one hand a signal for slower than anticipated progress and on the other an indication that other (more psychologically trained) professionals should be involved with this patient's care.

Summary of the subjective examination

1. Why is the patient here?
2. What is the problem?
3. Where is the problem?
4. How does it behave?
5. Are there any contraindications to treatment by a physiotherapist (red flags)?
6. Are there any factors that might indicate a slower rate of improvement?

Before moving on you now need to ask yourself: what is the relevant information gained so far? What particular working hypothesis (or hypotheses) have you arrived at? The answers might be, for example, 'Young woman with very specific problem relating to right ankle after inversion injury' or 'Middle-aged man complaining of repeated bouts of mild aches and general stiffness'.

The objective examination

You are now set to start the second and equally important aspect of the assessment process: you need to identify the extent of the disturbed function.

Objective findings will help you to establish a firmer relationship between the patient's symptoms and your own hypothesis. While physiotherapists usually do not diagnose a condition in the medical sense, we continually check our memory banks for recognition of previous groupings of symptoms that might help us in the planning of the tests to be done on and with the patient's problem. An assessment has to be carefully prepared and will depend totally on the findings of the subjective assessment. Part of the preparation might include the revision of basic facts from the fields of anatomy, physiology, kinesiology and pathology and the way in which these are influenced by psychosocial considerations.

For example, in the case of the young woman with the ankle injury: What is the anatomy of the ankle joint? What are the biomechanical issues relating to the ankle joint? Does the patient's life style contribute to the problem experienced at the moment? Are there any yellow flags that might slow down her progress?

It becomes clear that, without a good knowledge base, it will be difficult to make sense of the clinical presentation, a management plan will be extremely shaky and it will be virtually impossible to make a good prediction of the outcome.

Hence the questions to ask yourself now are:

- What are the essential findings of the assessment so far?
- What tests or investigations are needed to 'firm them up' and harden my hypothesis?
- Which findings are red herrings, or 'tombstones' of previous incidences, as Grieve (1981) called them; in other words, which findings do not directly or immediately contribute to the current problem?
- What do you know about the problem so far and what do you need to look up?

An extensive objective examination will include aspects of:

1. observation
2. active movements
3. passive movements
4. resisted or repeated movements
5. palpation of the area
6. neural tension testing
7. neurological testing (if indicated)
8. muscle patterning.

Clearly, only the most potent tests are going to be employed and only those that are going to shed most light on the problem. For a more detailed discussion of the various tests to be considered, refer to other orthopaedic texts (e.g. Hertling & Kessler 1990).

Novice examiners tend to employ an 'overkill' strategy. They will do every test in the book in order to find objective data to confirm the very vague hypothesis. This is because they are new at the game and therefore have not yet collected the multitude of information and knowledge that allows for speedy pattern recognition. With growing experience you will be able to tailor your investigations more specifically to your needs.

Self-assessment question

- **SAQ 3.13** Would you want to employ the same objective examination on these two patients, both complaining of low back pain?
  1. A 25-year-old woman has been referred with a 2-week history of intense left-sided low back pain radiating into her left calf after lifting shopping out of the boot of her car. Remember that all root pain is referred pain but that not all referred pain is root pain. Are you happy with the difference?
  2. A 56-year-old man has been referred with a history of several years of repeated bouts of general backache and stiffness without a specific onset.

  They clearly both have back pain, but what is different in these two scenarios?

  If you need to, refer back to Chapter 2.
  After you have worked out your answers to this question, read the next section.

Differences between the two scenarios

Some differences are:

- age of patient
- time since onset of problem
- description of onset
- location/specificity of pain
- intensity of pain.

Age of patient.   What might be the diagnostic relevance of the patient's age? It is generally less likely that there would be degenerative processes causing the problem (hence more generalized) in a 25-year-old than in a 56-year-old. That might lead you to a very localized testing procedure for the woman while you might want to test the male patient's movements more generally. What do you know about the mechanisms of degeneration of joints?

Time since onset of problem.   On the one hand there is a very short time span with a 'fresh' injury and on the other hand a long-standing problem appearing in repeated bouts of pain. You would expect to find the previously discussed 'tombstones' of old pain events in the older patient but would not anticipate them in the younger one. Hence your investigations would need to be much more far-ranging in the man than in the woman when it came to movement tests. Are you happy with your knowledge of the difference between acute and chronic pain and their associated effects on mood and motivation?

Description of onset.   The big difference here is the exact mechanical nature of the one (lifting) in contrast to the unknown one of the other. The anatomical and neurological entities that are stressed by hyperflexion and perhaps twisting need to be concentrated on fully in the young woman while others might be excluded. Clearly, the man with his more generalized and vague history needs a more general movement examination in order to narrow down the multitude of possibilities. A close look in this patient at the kinetic chain functioning versus general muscle patterning will bring in important data.

Localization of pain.   What anatomical entity do you know to refer pain to the calf? You need to remind yourself of the different patterns of referral and their relevance. For example, a specific pattern below the knee often suggests nerve root involvement while more general referred pain can be a symptom of, for example, muscle or ligament involvement, although these rarely refer pain below the knee. This differentiation clearly narrows down the options in our two patients: the woman's examination needs to be focused on possible nerve root involvement while, because of the non-specific nature of his problem, examination of the man should cover joints, muscles and ligaments. General aching is rarely a symptom of nerve root involvement and hence this does not have to be given a priority in the initial assessment.

Intensity of pain.   Again, authors like Grieve (1981) will be able to help you with the differentiation of certain pain descriptors that hint at their anatomical source. We mentioned earlier the importance of irritability and the role that intensity of pain plays in its definition. Clearly, the more irritable a patient's problem seems to be, the less aggressive the objective examination has to be.

So, at the end of your preparation for the objective examination, what are you left with in terms of necessary tests and investigations? Which procedures do you need to employ to get to the bottom of these patients' back pain?

For the 25-year-old woman:

1. *Observation*
   Is there evidence of the patient avoiding flexion?
2. *Active movements*
   - Gentle testing of extension (is this pain-free?) and then flexion (is this painful?)
   - Testing of side flexion and rotation most probably have little extra to offer, so can be left out initially, but try a side glide to right or left.
3. *Passive movements*
   Muscles and ligaments are not suspected as a cause for the patient's pain, so passive movements will not add anything to test the provisional hypothesis (nerve root involvement).
4. *Resisted movements*
   Again these would not add anything to our provisional knowledge about this lady's problem.
5. *Repeated movements* could clearly be indicative of a joint or ligamentous problem (not our hypothesis for this patient) but could also add a decisive bit of information if one remembers McKenzie's thinking about nerve root involvement (McKenzie 1981). Hence there might be an increase of pain when repeating flexion (the patient's hypothesized mode of injury) and a possible decrease when repeating extension (the opposite of her hypothesized mode of injury).
6. *Palpation* will be useful to get an insight into the degree of soft tissue agitation but passive intervertebral joint movement would have nothing to offer as this is not part of the hypothesis so far.
7. *Neural tension*
   Clearly, in someone with suspected nerve root involvement the neural tension needs to be tested as a positive test will really help to firm up the hypothesis.
8. *Neurological testing*
   In anyone with pain radiating away from the midline, muscle strength, sensation and reflexes need to be checked, as they are directly related to nerve root involvement

- Look for areas of classic wasting (e.g. wasted extensor digitorum brevis is a good indicator of a L5 lesion)
- Into this category, of course, falls the whole area of adverse mechanical (neural tension/Ant) tension
- Calf tenderness is an indicator of denervation tenderness (medial calf S1/lateral L5).

What would this examination involve for the 56-year-old man with generalized back pain? Because he has a general and repetitive problem it is more difficult to come up with a working hypothesis for him. This means that the examination needs to include more tests rather than being able to focus on a particular anatomical apparatus. Revision of pain referral patterns (e.g. Grieve 1981) and bearing in mind his age will indicate, however, that he is less likely to have a nerve root problem caused by an intervertebral disc; hence tests particularly aimed at that diagnosis can be left out (at first) of the battery of intended tests as they will not be able to help the investigator's quest to confirm the working hypothesis.

At the moment one would have to say that the cause of his problem might be a degenerative process. This will lead to tests that stress spinal joints, the intervertebral discs, the surrounding muscles and ligaments.

1. *Observation*
   - Is there any movement, position, etc. that the patient seems to dislike? This will help you to narrow down the vast range of possibilities for his back pain
   - Are you able to discern that, perhaps, a particular movement direction seems to be worse than others?
2. *Active movements*
   Unless a clearer picture has emerged by observing the patient undress or get on/off a chair or plinth, you need to test all movements in the hope that you will be able to discern a particular movement pattern that is more troublesome than the others (e.g. are you able to identify a compression or stretch pattern?). This is still in line with the hypothesis of joints, muscles or ligaments being involved in the cause of the patient's problem, as active movements test all of these.

3. *Passive movements*

   These might add a little bit of insight with regard to joint involvement (the patient will not be able muscularly to protect a possibly painful range) but it will add a lot to your knowledge of his muscle and ligament length and tightness.

4. *Resisted movements*

   This will have little to offer unless suspicion has arisen that the patient's muscles are the prime reason for the problem; the other anatomical entities do not really respond to this kind of testing in a clear way.

5. *Palpation*

   This is necessary to localize the problem as much as possible; the soft tissue condition (swelling, fibrosis, spasm, etc.) has to be identified but the palpation findings of the individual spinal joints are going to add the most potent objective data to your finding as they will help to narrow down the anatomical possibilities as well as the actual location. The biggest danger here is the identification of 'tombstones' (remnants of previous episodes that have burnt themselves out but resulted in stiff or painful joints); it is important, therefore, to link your findings to the patient's present problem rather than just identifying a painful spot unrelated to the patient's current pain (which one would be able to find in most of the asymptomatic population).

6. *Neural tension*

   Nerve root involvement has been excluded earlier on and hence we do not need more

information along this line, but we are dealing with a repetitive problem that might quite reasonably have affected the nervous structures (by inflammatory processes?), e.g. as they travelled through the layers of effected soft tissues or past joints that were inflamed and swollen; a steadily increasing body of literature (Butler 1991) makes it imperative to test the length of the neural tissues.

7. *Neurological testing*

   We decided earlier that the patient's problem was unlikely to be caused by nerve root involvement and hence data collected under this heading would be unhelpful and confusing.

INTERPRETING THE ASSESSMENT RESULTS

Now you have finished the initial data collection, you need to come up with a reasoned hypothesis that can result in a management plan. It is here that a lot of problems occur. You have ended up with an enormous amount of information, not all of it meaningful, and you are left needing to identify certain patterns of findings that you must recognize as belonging to together in a relevant way. It is obvious that you will not be able to recognize these patterns unless you have actually come across them before. This point has elaborated in more detail and depth by Cox (1988).

Here, at the end of the chapter, you might want to test yourself on how far you have travelled on the road to pattern recognition. This test has been researched by Case et al (1988):

Self-assessment questions

What are the various options you might want to consider as the cause of back pain? Remember to include referred visceral pain, which could mimic back pain. Some possible options are listed below:

A Intervertebral disc prolapse
B Muscular sprain
C Ligamentous sprain
D Postural strain
E Spondylosis
F Arthrosis of spinal joints

G Fracture of a vertebra
H Kidney problem
I Spondylolisthesis
J Hypermobility syndrome
K Spinal tumour
L Scheuermann's disease
M Dysfunction
N Osteoporosis.

For each of the following patients with back pain, select the most likely diagnosis and make sure that you have a rationale for it (otherwise testing for the diagnosis can be difficult).

- SAQ 3.14 A 35-year-old computer analyst has back pain after a severe bout of gardening; he developed leg pain after about 2 days; flexion is most painful.
- SAQ 3.15 An 18-year-old student developed back pain after falling 10 metres through a snow bridge; all movements are equally painful; rest relieves pain somewhat.
- SAQ 3.16 A 25-year-old ballet dancer complains of severe back pain; it is aggravated by end-range positions; more than seven joints (!) seem to have excess movement.
- SAQ 3.17 A 15-year-old boy noticed a dull central back ache that is aggravated by loading his spine and is mostly relieved by rest.
- SAQ 3.18 A 48-year-old mother of five has had a long history of episodic back pain, which for the first time has travelled down her leg and into her foot; she presents with a hyperlordosis in her spine.
- SAQ 3.19 A 39-year-old man complains of a dull central backache on prolonged sitting that is on the whole relieved by walking around and getting up from a chair; flexion is limited and painful but repeated flexion eases his pain and range increases.
- SAQ 3.20 A 58-year-old bus driver complains of central sharp back pain that is worse at the end of the day and helped by rest; no particular movement makes his pain worse.
- SAQ 3.21 A 30-year-old woman felt a sharp twinge on the left side of her back while playing tennis; she was able to continue to play but felt totally 'seized up' after she had stopped playing.
- SAQ 3.22 A 40-year-old machine operator, after years of repetitive bending to the left, noticed a sharp and very localized pain on the left side of her back; extension and left side bending increase her pain.
- SAQ 3.23 A 70-year-old woman has started to notice a generalized and sharp pain around the centre of her back; extension seems to make it worse.
- SAQ 3.24 A 28-year-old accountant experienced sharp general pain in his back after pulling a surprisingly heavy weight; passive movements are pain-free but active extension is very painful.
- SAQ 3.25 A 20-year-old student complains of general back pain after sitting in front of his computer for more than 1 hour; pain is relieved once he gets up; all movements are pain-free.
- SAQ 3.26 A 25-year-old man complains of severe central back pain that is unrelieved or aggravated by any movement or position; night pain is persistent; general malaise was noticed.
- SAQ 3.27 A 57-year-old woman has started to complain of severe colic-like pain in her central back which is unrelieved or aggravated by any movement; certain unpredictable positions seemed to affect it, as well as going to the toilet.

SUMMARY

This chapter has introduced you to the various thoughts of assessment, the skills needed for it and how to acquire them, and finally has offered you the opportunity to work through an example of testing hypotheses.

The examples have focused very much on pathology. Fleming (1991), in her 'three track mind model', focuses on the three different strands of reasoning going on in the therapist's mind:

- *Procedural reasoning*: this focuses on the disease or pathology (e.g. the examples above)

- *Interactive reasoning*: the face to face encounters and the ensuing relationship is at the centre here; the experience the particular problem has engendered is looked at
- *Conditional reasoning*: this takes into consideration both the patient as a social being and the condition s/he complains of and hence is a much more involved multidimensional thinking process.

Clinical reasoning is obviously one of the hallmarks of an autonomous health worker and the assessment is an early opportunity to put this into practice.

ANSWERS TO SELF-ASSESSMENT QUESTIONS 3.14–3.27 (PAGE 67)

- **SAQ 3.14** A 35-year-old computer analyst has back pain after a severe bout of gardening; he developed leg pain after about 2 days; flexion is most painful.

  Answer: A – intervertebral disc prolapse.

- **SAQ 3.15** An 18-year-old student developed back pain after falling 10 metres through a snow bridge; all movements are equally painful; rest relieves pain somewhat.

  Answer: G – fracture of a vertebra.

- **SAQ 3.16** A 25-year-old ballet dancer complains of severe back pain; it is aggravated by end-range positions; more than seven joints (!) seem to have excess movement.

  Answer: J – hypermobility syndrome.

- **SAQ 3.17** A 15-year-old boy noticed a dull central back ache that is aggravated by loading his spine and is mostly relieved by rest.

  Answer: L – Scheuermann's disease.

- **SAQ 3.18** A 48-year-old mother of five has had a long history of episodic back pain, which for the first time has travelled down her leg and into her foot; she presents with a hyperlordosis in her spine.

  Answer: I – spondylolisthesis.

- **SAQ 3.19** A 39-year-old man complains of a dull central backache on prolonged sitting that is on the whole relieved by walking around and getting up from a chair; flexion is limited and painful but repeated flexion eases his pain and range increases.

  Answer: M – dysfunction.

- **SAQ 3.20** A 58-year-old bus driver complains of central sharp back pain that is worse at the end of the day and helped by rest; no particular movement makes his pain worse.

  Answer: E – spondylosis.

- **SAQ 3.21** A 30-year-old woman felt a sharp twinge on the left side of her back while playing tennis; she was able to continue to play but felt totally 'seized up' after she had stopped playing.

  Answer: C – ligamentous sprain.

- **SAQ 3.22** A 40-year-old machine operator, after years of repetitive bending to the left, noticed a sharp and very localized pain on the left side of her back; extension and left side bending increase her pain.

  Answer: F – arthrosis of spinal joints.

- **SAQ 3.23** A 70-year-old woman has started to notice a generalized and sharp pain around the centre of her back; extension seems to make it worse.

  Answer: N – osteoporosis.

- **SAQ 3.24** A 28-year-old accountant experienced sharp general pain in his back after pulling a surprisingly heavy weight; passive movements are pain-free but active extension is very painful.

  Answer: B – muscular sprain.

- **SAQ 3.25** A 20-year-old student complains of general back pain after sitting in front of his computer for more than 1 hour; pain is relieved once he gets up; all movements are pain-free.

  Answer: D – postural strain.

- **SAQ 3.26** A 25-year-old man complains of severe central back pain that is unrelieved or aggravated by any movement or position; night pain is persistent; general malaise was noticed.

  Answer: H – kidney problem.

- **SAQ 3.27** A 57-year-old woman has started to complain of severe colic-like pain in her central back which is unrelieved or aggravated by any movement; certain unpredictable positions seemed to affect it, as well as going to the toilet.

  Answer: K – spinal tumour.

References

Bithell C 2000 Evidence-based physiotherapy. Physiotherapy 86: 58–61

Brooks LR, Norman GR, Allen SW 1991 The role of specific similarity in a medical diagnostic task. Journal of Experimental Psychology: General 120: 278–287

Bury T 1996 Evidence-based practice: survival of the fittest. Physiotherapy 82: 75–76

Butler D 1991 Mobilization of the nervous system. Churchill Livingstone, Edinburgh

Carr J, Jones M, Higgs HJ 1995 Teaching towards clinical reasoning expertise in physiotherapy practice. In: Higgs HJ, Jones M (eds) Clinical reasoning in the health professions. Butterworth Heinemann, Oxford

Case SM, Swanson DB, Stillman PS 1988 Evaluating diagnostic pattern recognition: the psychometric characteristics of a new item format. In: Proceedings of the 27th Conference on Research in Medical Education. Association of American Medical Colleges, Washington, DC

Cott C, Finch E, Gasner D et al 1995 The movement continuum theory of physical therapy. Physiotherapy Canada 47: 87–95

Cox K 1988 How to teach clinical reasoning. In: Cox K, Ewan CE (eds) The medical teacher, 2nd edn. Churchill Livingstone, Edinburgh

Cyriax J 1982 Textbook of orthopaedic medicine, vol 1: The diagnosis of soft tissue lesions, 8th edn. Baillière Tindall, London

Dandy D 1993 Essential orthopaedics and trauma, 2nd edn. Churchill Livingstone, Edinburgh

De Groot A 1965 Thought and choice in chess. Monton, The Hague

Engel GL 1977 The need for a new medical model: a challenge for biomedicine. Science 196: 129–136

Feltovich PJ, Barrows HS 1984 Issues in generality in medical problem solving. In: Schmidt HG, De Volder ML (eds) Tutorials in problem-based teaching. Van Gorcum, Assen

Fleming M 1991 The therapist with the three-track mind. American Journal of Occupational Therapy 45: 1007–1014

Grieve G 1981 Common vertebral joint problems. Churchill Livingstone, Edinburgh

Hertling D, Kessler R 1990 Management of common musculoskeletal disorders. In: Physical therapy principles and methods, 2nd edn. JB Lippincott, Philadelphia, PA

Higgs J, Jones M 2000 Clinical reasoning in the health professions, 2nd edn. Butterworth Heinemann, Oxford

Hislop HJ 1985 Clinical decision making: educational, data and risk factors. In: Wolf SL (ed) Clinical decision making in physical therapy. FA Davis, Philadelphia, PA

Jones M, Christensen N, Carr J 1994 Clinical reasoning in orthopaedic manual therapy. In: Grant R (ed) Clinics in physical therapy. Physical therapy of the cervical and thoracic spine, 2nd edn. Churchill Livingstone, New York

Kahney H 1993 Problem solving: current issues, 2nd edn. Open University Press, Buckingham

Kellgren JH 1938 Observations on referred pain arising from muscle. Clinical Science 3: 175

Kellgren JH 1939 On the distribution of pain from deep somatic structures with charts of segmental areas. Clinical Science 4: 303

Kendall NAS, Linton SJ, Main CJ 1997 Guide to assessing psychosocial Yellow Flags in acute low back pain: risk factors for long-term disability and work loss. Accident Rehabilitation & Compensation Insurance Corporation of New Zealand, and the National Health Committee, Ministry of Health, Wellington

Kolb D 1984 Experiential learning: experience as a source of learning and development. Prentice Hall, Englewood Cliffs, NJ

Maitland G 1964 Vertebral manipulations. Butterworths, London

McKenzie R 1981 The lumbar spine. Mechanical diagnosis and therapy. Spinal therapy. Waikanae, New Zealand

Newble D, van der Vlenten C, Norman G 1995 Assessing clinical reasoning. In: Higgs HJ, Jones M (eds) Clinical reasoning in the health professions. Butterworth Heinemann, Oxford

Paris SV 1985 Clinical decision making: orthopaedic physical therapy. In: Wolf SL (ed) Clinical decision making in physical therapy. FA Davis, Philadelphia, PA

Parry A 1985 Physiotherapy assessment, 2nd edn. Croom Helm, London

Ramsden EL 1985 Bases for clinical decision making: perception of the patient, the clinician's role and responsibility. In: Wolf SL (ed) Clinical decision making in physical therapy. FA Davis, Philadelphia, PA

Sackett DL, Rosenberg WM, Muir Gray JA et al 1996 Evidence-based medicine: 'what it is and what it isn't'. British Medical Journal 312: 71–72

Thomson DJ 1992 Counselling. In: French S (ed) Physiotherapy: a psychosocial approach. Butterworth Heinemann: Oxford

Watts NT 1985 Decision analysis: a tool for improving physical therapy practice and education. In: Wolf SL (ed) Clinical decision making in physical therapy. FA Davis, Philadelphia, PA

Weiss DJ, Concliffe T, Tat N 1998 Low back pain caused by a duodenal ulcer. Archives of Physical Medicine and Rehabilitation 79: 1137–1139

WHO 1980 International Classification of Impairment, Disability and Handicap (ICIDH). World Health Organization, Geneva

WHO 2001 International Classification of Functioning, Disability and Health (ICF). WHA 54.21 (22 May). World Health Organization, Geneva

Chapter **4**

Decision making and clinical reasoning in orthopaedics

Karen Atkinson

CHAPTER CONTENTS

OBJECTIVES

By the end of this chapter you should:

- Have an overview of the areas of orthopaedics covered in this book
- Have a basic understanding of problem solving within the clinical situation
- Understand the elements involved in successful clinical reasoning
- Be able to relate this to the process of clinical reasoning in the orthopaedic setting
- Understand the reasons for the differences in novice and expert clinical reasoning processes
- Have some ideas about your own reasoning processes and the strategies that may help to develop these
- Start to appreciate how you can use problem solving and clinical reasoning in your decision making in orthopaedic practice.

KEY WORDS

Orthopaedics, clinical reasoning, knowledge base, novice–expert differences, patient focus, hypothetico-deductive model, backward reasoning, pattern recognition, forward reasoning, knowledge–reasoning integration.

Prerequisites

In order to obtain most benefit from this chapter, you should have read Chapters 1–3.

INTRODUCTION

This chapter, along with the previous three, is introductory. Here, you will be considering the elements involved in clinical reasoning in a general sense and links will be made to the issues raised in Chapter 1. Later on in the book you will be looking at specific areas of orthopaedics, so continuing the process of developing your own problem-solving and reasoning skills by applying them to particular scenarios.

By now you should understand something of the changes that occur naturally in the body during ageing, and how in some cases these changes can become severe enough to cause problems for the individual, often manifesting as pain and loss of function. There are also situations where the body is affected by disease or injury, which can themselves cause problems and/or emphasize the changes due to ageing. In terms of the movement continuum theory of physical therapy (Cott et al 1995), this is the point at which people note differences between their preferred movement capacity (PMC) and their current movement capacity (CMC), i.e. they are at present unable to carry out all the movements and functions they would wish to. Remember that these changes in movement potential go on at all levels of the movement continuum, from the microscopic level, where pathological processes may be occurring in the tissues, through to the macroscopic level of the person not being able to function at the expected level in society, e.g. having a reduced ability to carry out work, leisure and/or daily living activities. It is most likely to be at this point, where 'changes' turn into 'problems' and people note reductions in their functional abilities that they seek out some form of help from health professionals. Physiotherapists may however, be involved before this stage if part of their role is in the education of individuals or groups regarding healthy living, fitness and the avoidance and prevention of injury.

We cannot stop the normal changes of ageing but the effects of these changes can be minimized by keeping the body as healthy and active as possible. It is also impossible to stop people succumbing to disease or injury but it is possible, by education, to reduce the risk of accident or exacerbation. This type of intervention attempts to influence everyday activities such as lifting techniques or habitual postures adopted for work situations; and, in some cases, certain elements of lifestyle, e.g. levels of exercise.

In both educational and treatment situations, it is important for the physiotherapist to have knowledge of normal and pathological change. According to Higgs & Titchen (2000), knowledge is an essential element for reasoning and decision making, both of which are considered central to professional practice. When taking a patient through an educational process, it is important for the physiotherapist to be able to explain the reasons behind recommendations to carry out exercise or to change daily activities. In the treatment setting, the physiotherapist must be aware of the underlying changes in the tissues and how these may affect the patient physically, psychologically and socially, as discussed in Chapters 2 and 3. If the physiotherapist has a well organized and easily accessible knowledge base this will facilitate the clinical reasoning processes that are necessary for the formulation of problem lists, goals and treatment plans.

According to Patel & Kaufman (2000) 'well-organized, coherent information is easier to remember than disjointed collections of facts'. If you can put information into context and explain something clearly to yourself so that you can understand it, this will make it much easier for you to communicate the information effectively. This process also means that you will be able to retain it in memory for future use. Our experience in talking to many teachers is that the time they really learn a subject thoroughly is when they have to teach it to someone else!

These processes are closely related to the issues discussed in Chapter 3, where knowledge about the recognition of change in the musculoskeletal system could be used to facilitate the subjective and objective assessment.

If you are able to remember these points when interacting with patients, they will contribute to your ability to problem solve. As you will recall from Chapter 1, the best way to become skilled in problem solving is to actually do it and, as stated earlier, the case studies in this book have been designed to start you off. The more you practise and reflect on your performance, both with the case studies and when you deal with real patients, the more quickly you will enhance your ability to make effective clinical decisions.

THE RANGE OF ORTHOPAEDICS

Physiotherapists come into contact with patients who have orthopaedic problems in virtually all areas of healthcare. These problems are usually of primary importance when working on orthopaedic wards or in the outpatient setting. The incidence of patients with orthopaedic problems is, however, much higher than this. You will come into contact with these patients even if you are a specialist in another area, such as intensive care, neurology or care of the elderly. Orthopaedic problems span the whole spectrum, cutting across all ages and specialities. In some cases these problems may be secondary issues but they can still have an impact upon patients' overall outcomes if they are not addressed. This is why it is important for you to have a good grounding in the subject. It is perhaps also true to say that orthopaedics is one of the fundamental fields for the physiotherapist. It is often seen as being rather more straightforward and easier to understand than other areas, and so is covered early on in the syllabi of most courses. This, unfortunately, can cause underestimation of its importance.

Fractures

Fracture, i.e. loss in the continuity of a bone, may be what most people would think of if they were asked to explain the term orthopaedics. This loss of bony continuity can be due to many causes such as trauma, repeated small stresses or pathological change, e.g. neoplasia.

In this area, the physiotherapist is usually involved once the fracture has been reduced and immobilized.

Soft tissue injury

This area of orthopaedics covers damage to tissues such as ligament, tendon or muscle. As with fracture, there can be various causes of this damage. It could be due to a single traumatic event such as a fall or sports injury, or perhaps to longer-term stress on a structure, e.g. inflammation of the synovial lining of a tendon sheath after many repetitions of the same movement.

Here the physiotherapist may be the first-line contact for the treatment of the patient.

Rheumatology

This area of healthcare is concerned with patients with rheumatic diseases, also known as the connective tissue diseases. They are commonly thought of as only affecting the joints but in fact they can affect connective tissues in any area of the body. This means that patients with rheumatic conditions often have widespread and sometimes systemic symptoms, which can cause significant problems that are superimposed over the dysfunction due to the articular manifestations. Generally these diseases are incurable, chronic diseases of unknown causation. We are including rheumatic conditions with orthopaedics as patients often present with similar problems, e.g. pain, swelling and loss of function. The approach of the physiotherapist may need to be modified, however, because of the long-term nature of rheumatic diseases and the reliance on pharmacological management.

In this instance the physiotherapist is more often part of a team of healthcare workers who are involved with the management of each patient.

Bone disease

The diseases that can affect the skeleton are many and varied. Some, such as osteomyelitis (infection of bone following fracture), can be acquired as a result of previous trauma, some such as neoplasms (e.g. osteosarcoma) are of unknown causation and some, such as osteoporosis, may have a connection with the changes of ageing.

Here again, the physiotherapist is often part of a healthcare team involved in the management of the patient. Some signs and symptoms will be different depending on the specific disease but many of the problems experienced by patients, such as pain, swelling, muscle weakness and loss of function, mirror those mentioned earlier in relation to other areas of orthopaedics. The overall approach to each patient may therefore differ to an extent, depending on the disease, but because of the similarity in the symptoms the basic skills and techniques used by the physiotherapist will be the same.

Congenital and paediatric orthopaedic problems

This area of orthopaedics deals with particular orthopaedic problems and deformities in children. These can occur for a range of reasons such as trauma (e.g. a fracture through the epiphyseal growth plate, which affects the development of the bone), congenital conditions (e.g. congenital dislocation of the hips) or some diseases (e.g. idiopathic juvenile arthritis).

Once more the approach of the physiotherapist will be similar to that in the previously mentioned areas, working with other members of the healthcare team but with special consideration given to the age of the patient. It is extremely important to address these problems as early as possible in the child's life in order to avoid further complications later on. You will find information in the appropriate chapters about how physiotherapists address orthopaedic problems with children as the client group.

Joint replacement

A number of the above-mentioned injuries and diseases can lead to patients needing joint replacements. For example, many patients with rheumatic disorders, which can seriously damage the joints, may eventually require a replacement. This will enable more effective function, helping patients to reach their preferred movement capacity or at least to reach their maximum achievable movement potential. Joint replacement may also be necessary after certain fractures, such as those that divide the neck of the femur. In this injury the blood supply to the head of the femur can be compromised, resulting in avascular necrosis (death of the bone). If this is the case the decision may be taken to replace the femoral head with a metal implant.

Some centres specialize in replacements of large areas of bone that have been affected by neoplasia. These carefully designed and custom-made prostheses are produced for individual patients.

Joint replacement can therefore span a wide variety of patients with problems due to injury or disease. Here again the physiotherapist will be part of a team dealing with the patient. Orthopaedic surgeons often have very specific postoperative regimens that physiotherapists are required to use in their patient interventions. In the ideal situation, physiotherapists should have been involved in the design of these regimens.

ORTHOPAEDIC PROBLEMS: GENERAL POINTS

The areas of orthopaedics discussed above are covered in the following chapters. There are also two more general chapters, one on gait and one on hydrotherapy. In all the areas mentioned above you will come across patients with gait problems and we felt that this was an essential area for you to consider. Hydrotherapy is a treatment modality that can be effectively used in the management of patients with a wide range of conditions but particularly those with orthopaedic problems. It is a non-weight-bearing or reduced-weight-bearing environment, meaning that patients can be treated in the pool much earlier than on dry land. This chapter brings all areas of the book together by requiring you to return to each of the other chapters to consider how you would use hydrotherapy for the patients in the case studies.

It is useful to remember that any of the conditions mentioned in the various chapters may be complicated by damage to other structures, such as blood vessels or nerves. As the physiotherapist involved, it is essential that you take all the necessary points into consideration during your clinical reasoning process, i.e. physical, psychological and social factors. You must remember that the patient and any carers involved are part of the team, and their opinions and needs should be central in the rehabilitation process.

Now you have a clear picture of the content of the following chapters it is hoped that it will be easier for you to transfer the earlier information on problem solving into that setting. The remainder of this chapter will focus on the issues of clinical reasoning in the clinical, and particularly the orthopaedic, situation.

CLINICAL REASONING IN ORTHOPAEDICS

In Chapter 1 you thought about problem solving in very general terms, beginning in childhood and continuing throughout life on a daily basis. This now needs to be put into the context of physiotherapy and related to the decisions you make and the clinical reasoning that occurs in order to reach those decisions.

Clinical reasoning can be defined as 'a process attempting to structure meaning from a mass of confusing data and experiences occurring within a specific clinical context and then making decisions based on this understanding' (Higgs 1996). Hassenkamp (1998) also describes clinical reasoning as a way of safeguarding against adopting the most fashionable technique without evaluation. Both these descriptions underline the importance of the individual therapist in the process. Jones (1997) describes clinical reasoning as being influenced by a number of factors: the therapist (his/her needs, goals, values, beliefs, knowledge and cognitive, interpersonal and technical skills), the patient (his/her values and beliefs along with psychological, physical, social and cultural factors) and the environment (resources, time, funding and externally imposed requirements). This brings in a wide range of elements that are of importance in the overall 'real' clinical context.

Richardson (1999) also discusses the importance of the physiotherapy 'culture' in which students and newly qualified practitioners find themselves when in the clinical environment, and how much this can influence the development of an individual's clinical reasoning skills. Sometimes this influence can be positive and sometimes rather negative, depending on the approach of the experienced clinicians. Are you there to learn the knowledge and behaviour of the more experienced practitioners, which could be seen as an apprenticeship, or are you there to develop your own knowledge and skills base through guided practice and critical reflection, so becoming an autonomous and independently thinking practitioner? Inevitably you will gather information from the knowledge and practice of others but it is essential that you also have the opportunities to build up confidence in your own perspectives. Teachers in the academic setting can facilitate this process, extending learning into the clinic by the use of videos, tape recordings and transcripts of practice to stimulate debate and analysis (Richardson 1999). Case studies can also be used to do this, particularly where context- and domain-specific knowledge remain constant but the details of the cases vary. This can help you to develop your own representation of a particular field of practice as well as an understanding of the usual problems, outcomes and treatments appropriate for a patient group (Robertson 1996).

Basic skilled clinical reasoning, for the individual practitioner, involves three main elements: knowledge, the act of cognition (thinking) and the process of metacognition (awareness and monitoring of thinking; Jones 1997). This last is seen as an essential part of clinical reasoning. It suggests that it is not sufficient to have a sound knowledge base, to think analytically and to synthesize data; it is also necessary to be able to critically self-evaluate and to reflect on observations while interacting with patients (Thomson 1998). The process is therefore not purely logical because it deals with unpredictable human data. This means that it is not possible to use an algorithm (see Chapter 1) to reach a conclusion.

Reasoning and problem solving in making clinical decisions is not like attempting a maths problem but more like arranging a wedding (Higgs 1996). It is a situation where you need to be flexible and use creative approaches in your thinking. In the wedding scenario some logistics are involved (e.g. Look at the size of the church – how many guests can be fitted in? or What menu shall we choose for 82 guests and how much will it cost?) but there are also the social and psychological issues such as who will be offended if they are not invited – and does it matter? The seating plan for the reception might also cause some headaches! So a mixture of problem solving and reasoning methods must be applied to deal with both the logic and the more unpredictable elements of the situation.

> ## Review points
>
> You need to have a sound knowledge base, to be able to think analytically and to synthesize data in your clinical reasoning skill development. What other factors must you consider and why are these important?

To be an effective practitioner you must develop your problem-solving skills. It is essential that you are able to look at the large amount of information you obtain from an assessment and then organize it and identify specific patient problems. From this point it is possible to formulate goals and treatment plans. If the goals and treatments are appropriate, then in order to get to this stage you must have used clinical reasoning to come to these decisions.

Clinical reasoning involves thinking about what you do and why you do it, talking to others about the way you work and giving reasons for your thoughts and actions. Practical experience underpinned by reflective practice is fundamental to professional learning (Richardson 1999). As discussed in Chapter 1, some of the processes that lead to problem solving go on at an unconscious level because everyone starts to use them very early in life. But in the clinical setting where you are a novice, it is unlikely that this will be the case. The reasoning of a new practitioner is recognized as requiring conscious effort while that of an expert practitioner is more tacit or unconscious (Unsworth 2001).

Research has shown that, when a person is less practised in a particular task s/he tends to use slower, more labour-intensive analytical processing methods that put a strain on short-term memory. When someone is more practised at a task and the information is familiar, e.g. an expert clinician working in his/her specialist area, intuitive strategies are often used. These strategies are rapid and automatic and as such are difficult to map, i.e. the clinician is probably largely unaware of the

factors influencing the decision-making process and would find it hard to verbalize them. 'It appears that the more experienced we are, the less able we are to tell what we know' (Harries & Harries 2001). Just because it is difficult, however, this should not stop us from trying to reflect upon these processes in an attempt to understand how reasoning occurs. It is not until you consciously acknowledge these processes that you can start to think about them and work to improve your skills.

> ## Self-assessment question
>
> - SAQ 4.1 What are the three main elements of basic, skilled clinical reasoning?
>
> (Answer at end of chapter.)

KNOWLEDGE BASE AND NOVICE/EXPERT DIFFERENCES

As discussed in Chapter 1 it is important to remember that what you already know influences the decisions you make. A well-organized knowledge base gleaned both from background theoretical work and from experience will, therefore, help you to make decisions more efficiently. It is interesting to note, however, that students often see theory and practice as separate events and it is impossible to predict how well they will be able to make links with theory once an area of practice has been experienced (Robertson 1996).

When assessing a patient, students and novice practitioners have access to the same information as the expert clinicians but may not come to the same conclusions. This seems to be a result of what they do with the available data. Novices tend to note all the information and find it difficult to recognize what is relevant and what is not, thus slowing the process down (Jones 1997, Stewart 2001). Experts still consider the whole picture but are able to pick out the salient points. They can make sense of the patient's condition and how it might impact upon his/her life while taking into account the uniqueness and individuality of that patient. As mentioned earlier, this is done smoothly and rapidly in a rather automatic or intuitive way. You may not be able to do this effectively until you have had more experience and this is seen as part of the natural development process of your clinical reasoning skills (Stewart 2001).

So what is different between the expert and the novice? Box 4.1 shows the seven key characteristics of experts that have been identified across a range of domains. It might be interesting for you to note these as you read through this section of the chapter.

Experts have differences in the organization of their knowledge base and in their use of cognitive strategies. According to Case et al (2000), experts have:

- highly organized knowledge bases
- integrated their theoretical knowledge with their experiential knowledge as a result of having more clinical experience.

Previously acquired knowledge has been structured into schemata or 'chunks' and stored in this way and is, therefore, much more accessible. The information is domain-specific, it is meaningful and already interconnected, and so this, along with the previous factor, increases the overall speed and efficiency of the reasoning process. Information is more organized and clearly defined and linked to well-developed schemata that experienced clinicians can draw on as required (Robertson 1996).

Patient focus

One difference that seems to be identified regularly in work on clinical reasoning is how much attention is directed to patient issues. Experienced clinicians consider interaction with the patients to be a very significant aspect in defining the specific problems and in identifying the relationship between those problems and the goals of intervention (Robertson 1996). Jensen et al (2000) carried out a piece of work looking at clinical expertise with experienced physiotherapists from a range of specialist areas. It was found that they all shared a relatively common understanding of their role regardless of the area in which they worked and this was that 'practice begins and ends with patients'. The focus rested on the knowledge gained in learning from patients in their practice and collaboration between the patient and the therapist was seen as central to the clinical reasoning process.

This is not necessarily the case with novice practitioners, who tend to be question-centred and are only able to begin to change this focus with more experience. Initially they can note the patient's concerns but appear to have no in-depth understanding of the issues raised. Thomson (1998) alludes to some health professionals who complained that they 'could not stop their patients talking' as though the problem lay with the patient rather than being anything to do with the way they were conducting the assessment. The key aim seemed to be to obtain responses to specific questions rather than to listening to the patient's story and focusing on the patient 'first as a person' (Jensen et al 2000).

This question-centred approach often appears to be used by insecure novice practitioners (Thomson 1998). Doody & McAteer (2002) note that expert practitioners allocated approximately equal time to carrying out the subjective and objective assessments whereas novice therapists spent twice as much time on the physical examination as on the subjective part of the assessment. The shorter physical examination performed by the experts was found to be the result of better focus on patient issues that had arisen in the subjective assessment, thus enabling the practitioner to carry out a more effective objective assessment. Experts tailor the examination to suit the patient's clinical presentation and are more flexible and open to unexpected issues arising. Robertson (1996) states that, as practitioners move from being novices to the level of 'advanced beginners', there is a shift from question-centred to patient-centred assessment.

It seems clear that experience is essential in the development of clinical reasoning skills. Novice practitioners do, however, need to have a basic mastery of skills, techniques and domain-specific knowledge before it is possible for them to have an increased awareness of the patient.

A number of strategies have been suggested that may enable faster development of clinical reasoning processes in students/novices. Some of these can be actioned by academic staff, some by clinical educators and some by the student/novice.

- Case scenarios
- Analysis of problem solving during placements
- Earlier clinical placements
- Role plays and simulations
- Observation of and interaction with experienced clinicians – witness them thinking out loud as they identify and solve patient problems
- Recent, frequent and intensive patient contact
- Being aware that it is necessary to develop cognitive skills and to have the ability to observe and skilfully use your hands and bodies to facilitate patients' functional movement
- Teaching students to value the patient as well as the clinical educator as a source of knowledge
- Carefully listening to patients (active listening) and understanding the meanings patients attach to health and illness
- Placing more emphasis on the subjective assessment and the planning of the physical examination

- Developing self monitoring skills and practising reflection-in-action (Robertson 1996, Jensen et al 2000, Stewart 2001, Doody & McAteer 2002).

Review points

Think about the last time you assessed a patient.

How much time and attention did you give to listening to the patient's story? How important do you feel this information was?

How often have you felt overwhelmed by the amount of information you have obtained during an assessment? Can you think of anything that might help you to focus more?

Look at and consider the list of suggested strategies above. Which of these have you tried? Which do you think might be helpful to try or to suggest to your clinical educator?

Self-assessment questions

- **SAQ 4.3** Why is it not possible to use algorithms to solve problems in the clinical setting?
- **SAQ 4.4** When you know you are about to see a new patient, you will need information about that person. List as many sources of this information as you can.

(Answers at end of chapter.)

MODELS OF CLINICAL REASONING

A large amount of work has been carried out on clinical reasoning by a number of the health professions, particularly medical practitioners and occupational therapists. In physiotherapy, the study of clinical reasoning is a developing area of interest and the research that has been produced has served to raise awareness and to facilitate the development of improved reasoning skills across the profession (King & Bithell 1998). The use of clinical reasoning models is an attempt to logically guide clinicians through assessment and treatment planning and evaluation of outcomes. As stated earlier, the process of clinical reasoning is now considered to be an integral component of clinical practice and the term is used interchangeably with others such as clinical decision making, clinical problem solving, clinical judgement and clinical rationale (Case et al 2000). A number of models have emerged from the work on clinical reasoning but as yet there is no unifying framework that incorporates all theories and concepts.

Hypothetico–deductive model

The hypothetico-deductive model of clinical reasoning originated from research in the medical field. This method of reasoning is often used in scientific work, where hypotheses are generated from observations; the hypotheses are tested through the collection of more data and then modified accordingly. This method tends to focus on diagnosis and so has some limitations for physiotherapy practice in that it gives little attention to issues that we consider to be important, such as treatment selection and management (Doody & McAteer 2002). It is also a relatively inefficient method in that it places a large demand on clinicians' working memory (Noll et al 2001). This said, however, many studies have found evidence of hypothetico-deductive reasoning taking place in both experts and novices (King & Bithell 1998, Case et al 2000, Noll et al 2001, Doody & McAteer 2002).

In the clinical setting this approach involves a physiotherapist generating hypotheses based on clinical data about a particular patient from the initial assessment and then testing these hypotheses through further inquiry and investigation in order to support or reject them (Higgs & Jones 2000). This model has been commonly used for a number of years, either alone or as one of a number of strategies, in medicine, physiotherapy, occupational therapy and nursing.

Jones et al (2000) describe an initial hypothesis, which the physiotherapist develops on first coming into contact with the patient. In the outpatient setting, for example, this would occur through the process of greeting the patient, listening to any comments made and observing general points such as posture, build, movement, facial expression, age and so on. Information might also be obtained from a referral or from the case notes if these had been requested. This collection of information in different ways is also referred to by some

authors as cue acquisition (Doody & McAteer 2002). This is preliminary information, i.e. it is obtained prior to the actual assessment beginning, but it still provides an initial impression and the physiotherapist will already be interpreting and sorting these data into broad categories.

This initial hypothesis (or more than one) may be physical, psychological and/or social in nature and not necessarily diagnostic (Jones et al 2000). If we take a patient with rheumatoid arthritis, for example, the physiotherapist observes her as she gets up from the chair, walks to the cubicle, gets undressed ready for examination (with permission) and sits on the plinth. There would also normally be some verbal interaction with the patient regarding the activities she is performing. During this early cue acquisition period the physiotherapist will be formulating the initial hypotheses regarding the source of any problems with these activities, e.g. which joints are affected and their degree of involvement. Although most physiotherapists have some routine factors in their assessment process, these initial hypotheses should help focus the interview and examination procedures on to the particular issues of importance for the individual patient. These hypotheses will then be tested as the assessment goes on and additional data are collected. The thinking (cognitive) process that goes on during this time will include a search for evidence that either supports or refutes the hypotheses and so the physiotherapist has an evolving understanding of the patient and her problems.

This idea can be focused further by considering the example of a patient who is referred for physiotherapy because of a shoulder problem. After formulation of the initial hypotheses, the physiotherapist goes on to ask specific questions and to examine the patient physically. The data gathered here, however, do not support the hypothesis of a damaged shoulder; in fact the evidence from the physical examination and from talking to the patient points to the symptoms coming from an injury to the neck. The hypothesis would, therefore, need to be modified and the line of enquiry refocused to collect data referring to the new problem area identified.

This hypothesis generation and testing continues until enough data are obtained to make a diagnostic decision (Jones et al 2000). The speed and efficiency with which this process proceeds with any patient will depend on a number of factors. The knowledge base of the physiotherapist, the cognitive skills to analyse and synthesize data or cues (i.e. cue evaluation) and the person's level of awareness and monitoring of these thinking processes (metacognitive skills) were mentioned earlier. If the physiotherapist has a lot of experience with a particular type of patient, the process of hypothesis modification should be completed more quickly than with someone who is a novice in the field. Doody & McAteer (2002) identify a number of errors in cue evaluation in novice practitioners that may hinder the clinical reasoning process:

- Not able to perform tests properly
- Not able to correctly interpret results of correctly performed test, possibly due to deficits in knowledge base. The novices did not recognize patterns and so could not decide if the test results were positive or negative
- Omitted tests
- Disregarded the results of tests in that they did not recognize the significance of test results.

There are many other possible reasoning errors and generally less-experienced clinicians tend to make more of them. Examples of these are: making assumptions, prematurely limiting the number of hypotheses, making a decision based on limited or biased data and the physiotherapist only attending to data that support his/her hypothesis while ignoring (probably unconsciously) negating factors. It has been shown, however, that experts may also be biased in their use of information obtained from the assessment of patients.

In the hypothetico-deductive model as originally postulated, the point at which the diagnosis is made might be where the process stops, i.e. the diagnosis is the outcome from the clinical reasoning process. This is why we may need to be cautious in our use of this essentially medical model in its application to allied health professions in which diagnostic issues are not as central to practice. This has been a very useful model in initiating understanding of the clinical reasoning process but in physiotherapy, as in other similar professions, we have a greater emphasis on psychosocial issues, which may not sit so comfortably in the hypothetico-deductive mould (Case et al 2000).

Generally the hypothetico-deductive model is a reliable method, being both safe and solid. It involves backward reasoning, whereby hypotheses are generated from an exhaustive collection of subjective and objective data, and is used when no familiar patterns are noted (Noll et al 2001). It seems to be particularly useful when domain knowledge is inadequate (Doody & McAteer 2002). Overall it tends to be rather slow and related very much to physical disorders. Novices are more likely to use this method but they will gradually move on from this stage with more experience. If an expert is dealing with an unfamiliar scenario, however, there is a tendency to fall back on this model of reasoning.

Pattern recognition

As you already know, expert practitioners have greater, better organized and more easily accessible stores of knowledge in memory than novices. This enables the use of different types of clinical reasoning methods although, as noted above, there may still be a degree of use of the hypothetico-deductive model in conjunction with these, particularly in unfamiliar situations.

Pattern recognition can be defined as 'direct, automatic retrieval of information from a well structured knowledge base' (Higgs & Jones 2000). As discussed earlier, clinicians gradually gather experience and begin to integrate their biomedical knowledge with their clinical knowledge, creating clusters of organized and accessible schemata. This allows them to filter through patient information to look for and recognize familiar patterns (Noll 2001).

Pattern recognition can also be described in terms of inductive reasoning – 'a method of reasoning by which a general law or principle is inferred from observed particular instances' (Flew 1984). In very basic terms this means that if, on observation: A1 is x, A2 is x, A3 is x and so on, then all As are (probably) x. In clinical parlance, if a physiotherapist observes that the A-type gait of patient 1 is due to OA hip, the A-type gait of patient 2 is due to OA hip, the A-type gait of patient 3 is due to OA hip and so on, s/he may deduce that all patients with A-type gait (probably) have it because of the same condition – OA of the hip joint. Hopefully, however, you can see that there are weaknesses in this argument, which appears rather simplistic, especially taking into account the unpredictable nature of human data. There is also a danger in that the clinician could make assumptions about the patient as soon as certain signs/symptoms are discovered and a misdiagnosis could be made if all the evidence is not considered. Conversely, while it lacks certainty, there are strengths to this method, as it enables conclusions to be reached in the face of imprecise data and limited premises (Higgs & Jones 2000).

The recognition of patterns of patient presentation in order to come to a diagnosis is a form of forward reasoning. This is the process of hypothesis formation based on the physiotherapist's organization of knowledge and subjective information from patients seen in the past (Noll et al 2001). In contrast to backward reasoning, forward reasoning requires good domain knowledge (Doody & McAteer 2002) and is most likely to occur in familiar cases with experienced clinicians. Having said that this method is useful, it is important to remember that the same sorts of possible errors in reasoning can occur here as with the previous model.

Self-assessment question

- **SAQ 4.5** Try to remember as many possible errors in the reasoning process as you can. Think back to your clinical experience – have you made any of these errors in the past?

(Answer at end of chapter.)

There is no doubt that an expert in a particular area does recognize patterns in patient presentation, especially if the type of patient has been seen many times before. Higgs & Jones (2000) also describe this as pattern interpretation – it is a fast and efficient method and, as we discussed earlier, leads to descriptions of this type of reasoning as automatic or intuitive. It is considered to be a characteristic of expertise (Case et al 2000).

As the expert physiotherapist gains more data during the examination of a patient there are probably repeated instances of pattern recognition going on throughout, not just for the initial

diagnosis of the condition. Decisions are then made based on the perceived connections between the current case and those previous experiences stored in memory. The new case is placed in the same category and the past case and given the same label or diagnosis (Higgs & Jones 2000). It has been found that therapists who are more experienced automatically consider a range of options before making their decisions, whereas novices on the whole are not able to do this. Students and newly qualified physiotherapists tend to have a narrower approach, being less able to think more widely because of their rather limited knowledge/ experience base. Alsop & Ryan (1996) stress the importance of developing the skill of thinking widely and inductively as this leads on to the ability to generate and actively seek new ideas, and so find possible solutions to problems (Fig. 4.1).

Whereas the hypothetico-deductive model depends on both inductive and deductive reasoning, the pattern recognition model relies on inductive reasoning as the new information is compared against existing patterns of knowledge.

This method is not generally used by novices as they do not have such a well-organized knowledge base or the automatic ability to categorize data. Some of these skills can be developed to a degree in a number of ways, one of which is the consideration of case studies of typical patients in a particular area. Prion (2000) describes the use of case studies as an instructional method when teaching clinical reasoning and, in the training of student nurses, this was shown to be a positive step. This method provides opportunities for students and novice practitioners to try out clinical reasoning and decision making and, more importantly, to be able to make and correct mistakes in a safe situation. It also encourages students to bring in the range of aspects that impinge on the patient in the clinical setting, i.e. psychological, social and physical aspects, so looking at the patient as a whole. We mentioned earlier that it is more difficult for novice practitioners to be patient-focused until all the basic skills and knowledge have been acquired. That does not mean, however, that you should not be encouraged to consider these issues from the beginning. The use of case studies also enables the essential processes of self monitoring and reflection to be initiated.

Figure 4.1   Inductive reasoning.

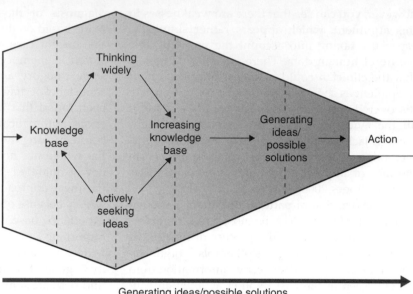

Generating ideas/possible solutions

Students have reported that case studies make the information more 'real' and tutors have found that the students learned and remembered more than ever before. One of the comments that came up quite often was that it was very useful to talk ideas through and to see how the instructors were thinking about the particular cases. This would seem to support the idea that novices can improve their clinical reasoning skills by observing and interacting with experienced clinicians and by listening to them thinking out loud when working through a clinical problem.

When you are using this book to consider case studies, perhaps you might have the opportunity to discuss your ideas with another reader or a colleague. If this is not possible, at least you can compare your thinking with that offered by the authors. When you are working in the clinical situation, try to take every opportunity to discuss cases, both with physiotherapists who are at the same level as you and with those you consider to be 'experts'. This will help you to develop your knowledge base and clinical reasoning skills.

It would seem, however, that there is no real substitute for experience. Without this experience it is possible to get sidetracked during assessment or to attend too much to irrelevant data. Dealing with patients is never straightforward, because of the unpredictability of human data and the immense range of individual differences.

It is important to note, however, that the pattern recognition approach to clinical reasoning is not particularly useful even to experts when they find themselves in a different situation. If a senior physiotherapist who has specialized in treating patients with sports injuries is suddenly placed in the intensive care situation, s/he will probably fall back on the hypothetico-deductive model.

Knowledge–reasoning integration

Much of the research into clinical reasoning in the allied health professions suggests that clinical reasoning skills cannot be developed independently of other skills (e.g. clinical and investigative skills) and professional knowledge. Higgs & Jones (2000) propose the idea of knowledge–reasoning integration, where knowledge acquisition and clinical reasoning skills develop in parallel. Most researchers looking at novice–expert differences emphasize the development of the experts' highly structured, easily accessible and organized knowledge base and seem to attribute much of the development of their clinical reasoning ability to this change. Knowledge is restructured as it is used in clinical reasoning and it ultimately becomes a store of specific detailed case studies with all the associated information and biomedical knowledge that has been used in past instances. It also allows for intuitive and interpretative approaches in the use of that knowledge and in clinical reasoning.

Some researchers in the occupational therapy field have looked at these more integrated ways of clinical reasoning. Schell & Cervero (1993) discuss different methods of reasoning:

- *Scientific reasoning*, where effective use is made of research-based theory and technique. This is felt to have helped with the 'professionalization' of the field. This professionalization is still an ongoing process in physiotherapy. The emphasis is on evidence-based practice, setting of guidelines and standards of practice, looking at outcome measures and audit of these outcomes. These activities are being used extensively in the hope that they will establish physiotherapy more firmly as based on available research. Much of this work is occurring in response to changes in the healthcare system in the UK, where purchasers and users of the system are asking for evidence that physiotherapy is effective.

  On its own, however, this scientific reasoning approach is not adequate to explain the complexity of clinical practice.

- *Narrative reasoning* (Mattingly 1991), in which clinical reasoning is considered to be 'an imagistic and phenomenological mode of thinking'. Here the unpredictability of human data is again considered and most clinical reasoning is thought to occur during treatment rather than during assessment. There are two main ways in which narrative reasoning occurs while considering the whole patient: 'through the therapists sharing stories and through therapists creating therapeutic stories with current patients'. These stories can help the physiotherapist to reason through and understand a little of the patients' experience of the biomedical conditions affecting them. It is possible to examine issues around the meaning the disability has for the patient and the motivation that will affect patient performance.

  This model takes contextual issues into account. One way to think of this is that the physiotherapist considers the patient as the main character in a book, which then allows him/her to form a story or narrative about that person's life. This includes looking at what has gone on in the past, where that person is now and what might occur in the future. This tends to personalize the approach of practice, with the physiotherapy input at least attempting to mirror aspects of the person's lifestyle. This can in turn increase levels of participation and the treatment may become more meaningful to the patient. In order for this to occur, however, it is essential that the narratives of the patient and the therapist are the same (Alsop & Ryan 1996).

  This is an area where good communication and interpersonal skills are essential on the part of the physiotherapist. The patient and/or carers must be consulted and considered to be an integral part of the healthcare team. If this does not occur then the patient's progress could be hindered as s/he may not see the relevance of the treatment. As we have discussed earlier, consideration of what the patient perceives to be the main problems or issues is an essential element for the physiotherapist to address. If a patient is most worried about whether she will be able to return to her own house or not after her hip replacement, it is essential that the physiotherapist addresses this and does not skirt around the issue or avoid the subject altogether.

- *Pragmatic reasoning* takes wider issues, such as organizational, political and economic realities, into account. These may well have an effect on practice. This aspect is related to contextual issues but this time not the patient's context but rather institutional issues that could either inhibit or facilitate therapy.

  This is a great driving force for therapists working within the health service in the UK. Physiotherapists, although autonomous practitioners, may find they have less control over who they treat, when they treat them and how, because of financial or policy constraints. This could have a major influence on clinical reasoning processes whatever the beliefs or attitudes of the individual therapist.

These issues emphasize the multifaceted nature of clinical reasoning. Inevitably it is not just about the physiotherapist–patient interaction but also involves a large range of other aspects.

Fleming (1991) who is also from an occupational therapy background, talks about this multifaceted approach to clinical reasoning in her theory regarding the therapist with the 'three-track mind'. Again three types of reasoning are postulated:

- *Procedural reasoning*, which guides the therapist when thinking about the physical performance of the patient. This involves knowledge about the condition, pathophysiology, course, prognosis, how long the patient has had the condition, the effects, possible interventions, possible problems, assessment techniques, possible findings and so on. In the physiotherapy setting much of this occurs before the patient is even seen, with an image being formed of what might be expected in each particular case.

- *Interactive reasoning* is used to help with understanding the patient as a person and how s/he is managing within the environment. This will tend to occur more as the physiotherapist interacts with the patient during assessment and treatment.

- *Conditional reasoning*, which integrates the previous two but also helps the physiotherapist to 'project an imagined future condition or situation for the patient'. It is therefore the imaginative and integrative part of the reasoning. How might that patient progress in the next few weeks/months? – depending on all of the factors in the previous categories. This is a very dynamic process.

Problem–solving exercise 4.1

Imagine you are about to see a new patient with rheumatoid arthritis. Try to work through the three tracks of reasoning described above, considering how you might use your clinical reasoning skills in your contact with her. (*Procedural reasoning*: consider your knowledge of the condition and possible consequences, i.e. signs and symptoms/disability – problems you might expect, how you could identify them and what you might find out; *Interactive reasoning*: forming an image of the person in your mind,

how is she performing within her particular setting?; *Conditional reasoning*: synthesizing from the previous two – what to do? This is how she is now, how might she progress in the next few weeks?)

These are the three tracks of reasoning and experienced clinicians are apparently able to shift rapidly from one to the other, as well as being able to analyse different aspects of the patient's problem simultaneously. It is important to point out that not all of these processes are easy even for a very experienced physiotherapist, particularly seeing a picture of the patient in the future. It is, however, a good level to aim for as it is much more complete, putting the patient in context and not focusing on the medical model, which tends to miss so much.

Many of these issues begin to be addressed in the following chapters during consideration of the case studies. It is only when in contact with 'real' patients, however, that the physiotherapist can begin to fully develop these skills.

CONCLUSIONS

As mentioned earlier in this chapter, a great deal of work is being carried out with regard to clinical reasoning and the steps that occur during the process. It is the foundation of successful problem identification and thus, in turn, treatment decisions. It is not simple; this would not be possible given the complexity and unpredictability of humans and their health problems. The solution is to do as much as possible to acquire the knowledge base and the skills for physiotherapy practice, and along with this to develop the ability to think widely and creatively and to actively seek out new ideas.

It would seem that there is no substitute for experience. All the research seems to point to a natural development process that occurs as physiotherapists move through their career. This experience can, however, be guided rather than being a matter of trial and error. Without a helping hand a student or newly qualified clinician could be making mistakes in reasoning without being aware of it.

This is where reflection and critical appraisal of performance becomes essential, i.e. the metacognitive processes mentioned earlier, where the physiotherapist actively thinks about his/her thinking and reasoning methods.

The models of clinical reasoning presented here are examples of many different ones available in the literature – however, they seem to encompass the essential factors involved. Novices are said to use the hypothetico-deductive model as it is the one based on the actual condition of the patient and seems most grounded in the medical model of healthcare. It is perhaps the easiest one to grasp. This is not, however, a stepwise process with the physiotherapist being 'promoted' through the ranks of clinical reasoning levels. Rather, it is a flexible scenario where new skills and knowledge are added as experience increases. The novice practitioner may indeed use some elements of the reasoning methods mentioned in the other models at an early stage – but perhaps not as intuitively as an experienced physiotherapist.

The learning process continues throughout life and this is no less true of clinical reasoning. Practice and experience are needed to achieve and maintain competence in this area. Clinical reasoning is a complex and multifaceted process that takes a long time to master. But it is essential to develop a self-awareness and self-monitoring approach to attaining knowledge and to the thinking processes that are necessary for sound, clinical problem-solving skills (knowledge, cognition and metacognition).

SUMMARY

This chapter has outlined the areas of orthopaedics dealt with in the later chapters of the book to help the reader to think about clinical reasoning and problem solving within the specific clinical setting.

A brief outline of clinical reasoning was given, along with examples of some models – the hypothetico-deductive model, the pattern recognition model and the knowledge–reasoning integration model. These have been described in outline and related where possible to the orthopaedic situation.

If you are particularly interested in the subject of clinical reasoning, please refer to the texts and journal articles in the reference list.

ANSWERS TO QUESTIONS

Self-assessment question 4.1 (page 76)

- **SAQ 4.1** What are the three main elements of basic, skilled clinical reasoning?

Answer: Basic skilled clinical reasoning, for the individual practitioner, involves three main elements: knowledge, the act of cognition (thinking) and the process of metacognition (awareness and monitoring of thinking; Jones 1997).

Self-assessment question 4.2 (page 77)

- **SAQ 4.2** What is the process of metacognition? Why is it important in the development of your clinical reasoning skills?

Answer: Metacognition is the awareness and monitoring of thinking. It is seen as an essential part of clinical reasoning, in that, in order for your clinical reasoning to be effective, it is not sufficient to have a sound knowledge base, to think analytically and to synthesize data: it is also necessary to be able to critically self-evaluate and to reflect on observations whilst interacting with patients (Thomson 1998). Development of this skill takes time and practice.

Self-assessment question 4.3 (page 78)

- **SAQ 4.3** Why is it not possible to use algorithms to solve problems in the clinical setting?

Answer: Reasoning and problem solving in the clinical setting are not purely logical processes because they deal with unpredictable human data. This means that it is not possible to use an algorithm to reach a conclusion. Reasoning and problem solving in making clinical decisions is not like attempting a maths problem but more like arranging a wedding (Higgs 1996). There are social and psychological issues to consider. It is a situation where you need to be flexible and to use creative approaches in your thinking.

Self-assessment question 4.4 (page 78)

- **SAQ 4.4** When you know you are about to see a new patient, you will need information about that person. List as many sources of this information as you can.

Answer: We suggest a number of possibilities in the following list. You may, however, come up with other suggestions:

- The patient
- Medical notes
- X-rays and/or results of other imaging techniques
- Referral
- GP
- Records of previous physiotherapy interventions
- Colleagues in the healthcare team, e.g. other physiotherapists, nurses, doctors, occupational therapists, social workers and so on
- Family/carers
- Possibly books, journals, the Internet, lecture notes and other sources to improve your background knowledge about the patient's particular condition.

Self-assessment question 4.5 (page 81)

- **SAQ 4.5** Try to remember as many possible errors in the reasoning process as you can. Think back to your clinical experience – have you made any of these errors in the past?

Answer:

- Not able to perform tests properly
- Not able to correctly interpret results of correctly performed test, possibly because of deficits in knowledge base – did not recognize patterns and so could not decide if the test results were positive or negative
- Omitted tests
- Disregarded the results of tests not recognizing their significance.

References

Alsop A, Ryan S 1996 Making the most of fieldwork education – a practical approach. Chapman & Hall, London, ch 14

Case K, Harrison K, Roskell C 2000 Differences in the clinical reasoning process of expert and novice cardiorespiratory physiotherapists. Physiotherapy 86: 14–21

Cott CA, Finch E, Gasner D et al 1995 The movement continuum theory of physical therapy. Physiotherapy Canada 47: 87–95

Doody C, McAteer M 2002 Clinical reasoning of expert and novice physiotherapists in an outpatient orthopaedic setting. Physiotherapy 88: 258–268

Fleming MH 1991 The therapist with the three track mind. American Journal of Occupational Therapy 45: 1007–1014

Flew A 1984 A dictionary of philosophy. Pan Books, London

Harries PA, Harries C 2001 Studying clinical reasoning, Part 1: Have we been taking the wrong 'track'? British Journal of Occupational Therapy 64: 164–168

Hassenkamp AM 1998 Clinical reasoning: a student's nightmare. British Journal of Therapy and Rehabilitation 5: 75–77

Higgs J 1996 Personal communication

Higgs J, Jones M 2000 Clinical reasoning in the health professions. In: Higgs J, Jones M (eds) Clinical reasoning in the health professions, 2nd edn. Butterworth Heinemann, Oxford, ch 1

Higgs J, Titchen A 2000 Knowledge and reasoning. In: Higgs J, Jones M (eds) Clinical reasoning in the health professions, 2nd edn. Butterworth Heinemann, Oxford, ch 3

Jensen GM, Gwyer J, Shepard KF, Hack LM 2000 Expert practice in physical therapy. Physical Therapy 80: 28–43

Jones M 1997 Clinical reasoning: the foundation of clinical practice. Part 1. Australian Journal of Physiotherapy 43: 167–170

Jones M, Jensen G, Edwards I 2000 Clinical reasoning in physiotherapy. In: Higgs J, Jones M (eds) Clinical reasoning in the health professions, 2nd edn. Butterworth Heinemann, Oxford, ch 12

King CA, Bithell C 1998 Expertise in diagnostic reasoning: a comparative study. British Journal of Therapy and Rehabilitation 5: 78–88

Mattingly C 1991 What is clinical reasoning? American Journal of Occupational Therapy 45: 979–986

Noll E, Key A, Jensen G 2001 Clinical reasoning of an experienced physiotherapist: insight into clinician decision-making regarding low back pain. Physiotherapy Research International 6: 40–51

Patel VL, Kaufman DR 2000 Clinical reasoning and biomedical knowledge: Implications for teaching. In: Higgs J, Jones M (eds) Clinical reasoning in the health professions, 2nd edn. Butterworth Heinemann, Oxford, ch 4

Prion S 2000 The case study as an instructional method to teach clinical reasoning. In: Higgs J, Jones M (eds) Clinical reasoning in the health professions, 2nd edn. Butterworth Heinemann, Oxford, ch 18

Richardson B 1999 Professional development. 2. Professional knowledge and situated learning in the workplace. Physiotherapy 85: 467–474

Robertson LJ 1996 Clinical reasoning, Part 2: Novice/expert differences. British Journal of Occupational Therapy 59: 212–222

Schell BA, Cervero RM 1993 Clinical reasoning in occupational therapy: an integrative review. American Journal of Occupational Therapy 47: 605–610

Stewart LSP 2001 The role of computer simulation in the development of clinical reasoning skills. British Journal of Occupational Therapy 64: 2–8

Thomson D 1998 Counselling and clinical reasoning: the meaning of practice. British Journal of Therapy and Rehabilitation 5: 88–94

Unsworth CA 2001 The clinical reasoning of novice and expert occupational therapists. Scandinavian Journal of Occupational Therapy 8: 163–173

Chapter **5**

Management of fractures

Fiona Coutts

OBJECTIVES

By end of this chapter you should:

- Have an overview of the classification, management, normal healing times and complications of fractures
- Understand the assessment of a patient post-fracture, in both the in- and outpatient situation
- Recognize how to problem solve in patient treatment and assessment, irrespective of the fracture site, extent or medical management.

KEY WORDS

Fracture, classification, management, complications, physiotherapy management, stability.

Prerequisites

Read the section in Chapter 2 on bone and joint changes during development. Familiarize yourself with fracture healing and medical management.
   Recommended reading:

- Dandy DJ, Edwards DJ 2003 Essential orthopaedics and trauma, 3rd edn. Churchill Livingstone, Edinburgh
- McRae R, Esser M 2002 Practical fracture treatment, 4th edn. Churchill Livingstone, Edinburgh
- Crawford Adams J, Hamblen D 1999 Outline of fractures. Churchill Livingstone, Edinburgh.

INTRODUCTION

Fractures or loss of continuity in the substance of a bone (McRae & Esser 2002) are a common occurrence and represent considerable treatment time and financial costs in the accident and emergency (A&E) department, inpatient wards through to physiotherapy outpatient departments and then to community care (Audit Commission 1995, Dinah 2002). The healthcare system of today has to manage a much greater number of elderly people with fractures because of the extended life expectancy of the population (Gomberg et al 1999, Swiontkowski & Chapman 1995). This brings added costs of care in the hospital environment, with a growing demand for early discharge and 'hospital at home' schemes (Coast et al 1998). There is also a greater interest in the management of falls prevention as a pre-empted attempt to reduce the number of people admitted with fractures, under the government-led initiatives through the National Service Framework for Older People (Department of Health 2002). Falls prevention uses a multidisciplinary team approach to the management of a complex problem and, because of the extent of this practice, will not be covered in this chapter, but the management of fractures as a result of falling will be covered.

Although the human skeletal system demonstrates both strength and a degree of flexibility, unfortunately we subject it to some very difficult trials and mishaps, testing its strength and endurance. When the forces become too great, exceeding the normal stress or strain load of bone, a fracture will occur. The forces required for a fracture are far less in an older person because of the normal changes that take place with ageing (Chapter 2). This is particularly so in women in the post-menopause years (De Laet & Pols 2002, Dinah 2002).

The skeletal system forms a frame to which muscles, tendons, ligaments and connective tissue are affixed, allowing a firm attachment so that they can perform their movement functions. Without this 'solid' frame the soft tissue could not exert the forces needed to perform the functions of motion – a fundamental requirement of human life. Further to this, the skeletal system offers protection to the more vulnerable viscera: lungs, heart, digestive system, bladder, etc., which would otherwise be extremely prone to injury.

In Chapter 2 we have already addressed the role and function of bone as we develop and age. If you have not already re-read this chapter, go back there now and refresh your memory.

This chapter does not cover all aspects and types of fractures but will outline the general management of fractures and then, through case studies, explore physiotherapy rehabilitation of specific fractures, which may be extrapolated to other skeletal areas. Rehabilitation starts at the point of fracture fixation from advice to the patient through to the restoration of function to as full capacity as possible. It is well documented that muscle weakness in particular may either take a long time to be restored or be decreased permanently (Marks et al 2003, Sato et al 2002), so that in most cases the physiotherapist will not see the patient through to full recovery. Rehabilitation should not stop with the cessation of visits to the outpatient physiotherapy department.

(Note: '#', which is the sign for fractures, is sometimes used in this chapter.)

CLASSIFICATION OF FRACTURES

Fracture classification is undertaken according to several factors:

1. **Skin damage**
   - *Open (compound)*: the skin is broken either from an external source or as a result of the bone fracturing then piercing the skin (compound from within)
   - *Closed (simple)*: skin remains intact.
2. **Shape or line of fracture** (Fig. 5.1) – the name describes the shape
   - *Transverse* or *horizontal*
   - *Oblique/spiral*
   - *Comminuted*: in many small parts
   - *Crush*
   - *Greenstick*: a bend in an immature bone, with a break in one of the bone cortices.
3. **Displacement**
   - *Undisplaced*: bone ends are still in apposition although there is a clear break; there is usually no need for reduction
   - *Displaced*: bone ends do not meet and reduction is necessary to achieve good anatomical

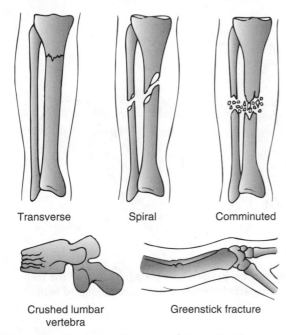

Transverse   Spiral   Comminuted

Crushed lumbar vertebra   Greenstick fracture

Figure 5.1   Patterns of fractures. (Adapted with permission from Dandy & Edwards 2003.)

Self-assessment question

- **SAQ 5.1** Outline and/or draw what you understand by the two fracture descriptions given above.

Answer

a. *Open spiral fracture of the tibia*: the tibia has a fracture in the shape of a spiral, which has broken the skin at the fracture site. This needs manipulation back to the anatomical position prior to stabilization.
b. *Closed impacted fracture of the neck of the femur*: the neck of the femur has been pushed into the head of the femur resulting in a stable fracture which does not need reduction by manipulation but will need some protection from weight bearing. No skin damage (Fig. 5.2).

position prior to stabilization, which is always needed. Soft tissue between the bone ends or muscle spasm may be causing the displacement and this has to be corrected by surgical removal prior to reduction
- *Impacted*: bone ends have been firmly shunted together so forming a stable but shortened bone. Often minimal external support is needed except for reduced weight bearing in lower limb fractures
- *Stable*: fracture where the bone ends are held firmly, either by position or by the surrounding tissues. Thus reduction is often unnecessary and minimal support is needed – e.g. an impacted fracture or a fracture of the metacarpals where the surrounding muscle tissue is holding the bone ends in place.

Therefore a fracture can be described, for example, as:

a. an open spiral fracture of the tibia
b. a closed impacted fracture of the neck of the femur.

A fracture can also be classified by its position, using the *Arbeitsgemeinschaft für Osteosynthesefragen* (AO) classification of proximal (1), central diaphyseal (2) and distal (3) segments (McRae & Esser 2002; Fig. 5.3).

Both segments 1 and 3 can include either epiphyseal or intra-articular fractures, where the break traverses either the epiphyseal (bone growth) plate of a child or the joint surface. Further details of AO classification and the Harris & Salter epiphyseal fracture classification (Fig. 5.4) can be found in McRae & Esser (2002).

Both epiphyseal and intra-articular fractures can cause major secondary problems and are regarded as complex. Epiphyseal fractures may cause a total lack of growth stimulation at the plate, if it has been crushed; thus the bone will be shorter than the contralateral side. If the fracture involves only one side of the plate, the bone will grow with an anteroposterior or valgus/varus deformity, if not corrected.

The term intra-articular fracture describes any fracture that includes the articular surface of a joint (Fig. 5.5). When this occurs it is very important that joint congruity is restored so that no roughened or misaligned surfaces remain, predisposing the joint to excessive secondary wear and tear.

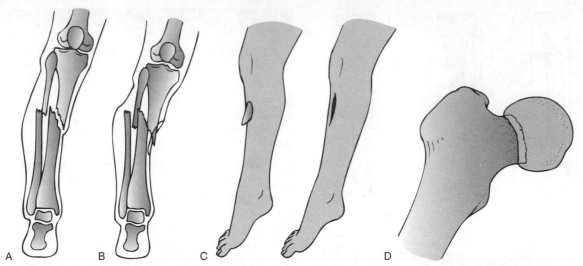

Figure 5.2   A: Spiral fracture of the tibia and fibula with no skin damage. B: Open (compound) fracture of the tibia and fibula. C: External view of open fracture of the tibia. D: Closed impacted fracture of the femur. (Adapted with permission from McRae & Esser 2002.)

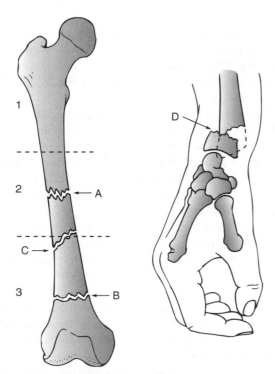

Figure 5.3   *Arbeitsgemeinschaft für Osteosynthesefragen* (AO) classification of fracture position. A: Transverse fracture of the middle third of the femur. B: Transverse fracture of the distal third of the femur. C: Spiral fracture of the distal third of the femur. D: Epiphyseal fracture of the distal third of the radius. (Adapted with permission from McRae & Esser 2002.)

CAUSES OF FRACTURES

Whatever the classification of fractures there will also be some soft tissue damage and possible nerve or vascular involvement, although not necessarily all at the same time, except in severe injuries.

Direct trauma

Here fractures have been caused by a direct blow such as:

- a kick on the shin in football
- a car hitting a pedestrian
- a person falling and landing on both feet from a great height.

In these situations the force of the blow is more likely to cause a transverse or crush fracture, and the layers of tissue from superficial to deep may be affected, i.e. skin, fascia, connective tissue, muscle, nerves and blood vessels.

Indirect trauma

Examples of indirect trauma include:

- a fall on to the outstretched hand resulting in a rotatory force with a spiral/oblique fracture of the humerus
- football boot studs placed firmly on the ground with the body weight of the person still moving

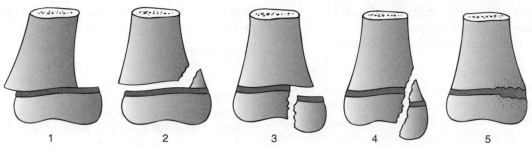

Figure 5.4   Harris & Salter epiphyseal classification of epiphyseal injuries. 1: Epiphyseal slip only. 2: Fracture through the epiphyseal plate with a triangular fragment of shaft attached to the epiphysis. 3: Fracture through the epiphysis to the epiphyseal plate. 4: Fracture through the epiphysis and shaft crossing the epiphyseal plate. 5: Obliteration of the epiphyseal plate. (Adapted with permission from Dandy & Edwards 2003.)

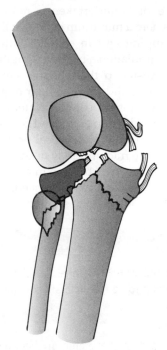

Figure 5.5   Intra-articular fracture. (Adapted with permission from McRae & Esser 2002.)

over the foot, leading to a spiral/oblique fracture of the tibia.

These events therefore result in less soft tissue damage but often more displacement of the bone ends. The greater the indirect force the more extreme the break, which can lead to greater soft tissue damage.

Pathological causes

Pathological fractures occur where there is already a weakened area or diseased portion present, e.g.

osteoporosis, tumours, cysts, metabolic disorders. The bone fractures from within because its internal structure is weakened or engorged with tissue other than bone. Damage can occur to the soft tissue and muscle attachments surrounding the fracture, either through pressure from the growing tumour/cyst or from the collapse of the bone.

Stress or fatigue fractures

These fractures are caused by repeated excessive loading of a bone. This results in mechanical bending of the bone, of small magnitude, which eventually summates to cause a fracture. Therefore, anyone who repeatedly places high forces across a bone is prone to this injury. For example:

- Fracture of the second metatarsal (MT) in anyone repeatedly walking for excessive distances
- Fracture of the upper third of the tibia in long-distance runners
- Pars interarticularis fractures in fast bowlers.

Avulsion

These fractures arise when either a sudden muscular action of high force 'pulls off' a segment of bone to which it is attached or a high traction force occurs across a joint and the ligament or joint capsule remains intact but a small piece of bone attachment is 'pulled off'. For example, the medial collateral ligament of the knee may pull off the medial epicondyle of the femur.

Common sites for avulsion fractures through muscle pulls are:

- Base of the fifth metatarsal (peroneus brevis)
- Tibial tuberosity (quadriceps)

- Upper pole of the patella (quadriceps)
- Lesser trochanter (iliopsoas)
- Anterior superior iliac spine (iliopsoas).

Severe avulsion fractures are one cause of joint instability resulting in a fracture dislocation, where the joint surfaces become displaced but there is no ligamentous damage. The fracture usually occurs near to or into the joint surface, thus allowing excessive joint movement to take place with only a slight additional force. Intra-articular fractures may also cause a fracture dislocation, where a larger piece of bone, with ligamentous or joint capsule attachment, becomes detached from the main part of the bone. Fracture dislocations are usually managed as for a fracture and, with good bone healing, normal joint laxity is restored.

Subluxation and dislocation

Joint surface displacement without a fracture is always accompanied by severe stretching of ligamentous and capsular tissue, resulting in a partial malalignment (subluxation) or, if the soft tissue becomes torn, a total malalignment or dislocation takes place.

Both subluxation and dislocation will be discussed in Chapter 6, on soft tissue injury, as no fracture is involved.

MANAGEMENT OF FRACTURES

There are three stages in the management of fractures:

- *Reduction*: manipulation of the bone to its correct anatomical position
- *Immobilization*: a means of holding the bone in the correct reduced position
- *Rehabilitation*: returning the person to as full function as possible after the trauma or disease.

REDUCTION

It could be argued that bone can heal whatever position it is left in so there is no need to reduce the fracture. Unfortunately, poor position of bone ends can lead to malunion (union in a poor position) and thus severe deformity or loss of bone

length can occur. With either of these primary problems, secondary changes may ensue:

- Shortening or lengthening of muscle length, with resultant alteration in muscle force
- Altered biomechanics and weight bearing across joints both ipsi- and contralaterally
- Alteration in range of motion at all joints in the limb (Dandy & Edwards 2003, McRae & Esser 2002).

Both primary and secondary factors predispose the joints above and below the fracture site, and possibly all joints in that limb, to osteoarthrosis (Tetsworth & Paley 1994). Therefore, manipulation of the bone ends is undertaken to reduce them to a position where a minimum of 50% of the bone ends are overlapping and in contact with each other. During manipulation a traction (longitudinal) force is exerted distal to the fracture site to pull the shortened bone ends back to their required length, and then an anteroposterior, lateral or rotatory force may be added to gain good correction. This is usually done under either local or general anaesthetic but some fractures may need to be surgically reduced. Too much distraction may cause a disturbance of bone healing, as there needs to be contact between the bone ends to stimulate bone growth.

Self-assessment question

- **SAQ 5.2** Which fractures by classification do not need to be reduced, and why not?

Answer

Those that are:

- *Impacted*: the bone ends are held together and usually motionless. The fracture may become loose prior to union, especially if weight bearing begins too soon, so it may need to be reduced if the position of the bone ends changes.
- *Stable*: the bone ends have to be in good apposition for a fracture to be stable, with at least 50% overlap, and they are held in place by the surrounding soft tissues.
- *Undisplaced*: there is already a good anatomical position, with a minimum of 50% overlap of bone ends, for the fracture to be termed 'undisplaced'.

Healing times

Before going on to discuss immobilization and rehabilitation we should consider how long it takes for fractures to heal.

In general the healing time of a fracture depends on its position in the body. For full details of fracture healing please consult any of the books mentioned in the Prerequisites box.

The two most important stages of fracture healing to consider are:

- *Union*: the partial repair of the bone, when the initial callus forms around the bone ends so that there is minimal movement. The bone under pressure will still give a little and will be painful. On X-ray the fracture line will still be visible. Full bone maturity has not been reached, so full weight bearing cannot be undertaken and some external support is still needed. This can be moderated as the healing moves from union to consolidation.
- *Consolidation*: full repair of the bone, where no movement takes place at the fracture site. On X-ray no fracture lines are seen and the bone trabeculae now cross the site where the fracture used to be. Full function can now commence without damaging the fracture. The bone has full maturity and is back to its original strength.

Although most references to fracture healing will, rightly, not give exact time scales for fracture healing, there are some basic guidelines (Crawford Adams & Hamblen 1999, Dandy & Edwards 2003, McRae & Esser 2002). Table 5.1 lists the approximate times for union and consolidation in normal bone.

Union will usually take place at any time between 3 and 10 weeks after the fracture occurred.

Consolidation will take approximately double the union time, and full remodelling double the consolidation time. At the consolidation stage the excess bone stabilizing the fracture site is fully mature but it is not until the final stage of remodelling that the bone returns to its prefracture shape.

In children all the stages are reached more quickly and callus can occur in the first 2 weeks post-fracture; therefore all the times must be adjusted accordingly.

In the older adult both the union and consolidation times may be extended if there is evidence of poor bone stock (e.g. osteoporosis), but this is highly variable.

The trauma of the fracture to the bone and surrounding tissues will inevitably give rise to a number of complaints, including:

- pain
- inability to move the joints above and below the fracture site
- muscle weakness
- alteration in proprioception
- slowing down of the circulation
- altered sensation.

Bleeding into the tissue and the formation of inflammatory exudate will result in tissue engorgement and resultant adhesions. Therefore, as a result of the trauma of fracture and the normal healing process, as well as immobilization, the surrounding muscle, soft tissue and joint structures will become shortened, fibrosed and weakened, leading to some

Table 5.1 Approximate union and consolidation times in normal adult bone

Fracture position	Union time (weeks)	Consolidation time (weeks)
Proximal third of humerus	7–10 days	3–4
Distal third of radius/ulna	4–6	8–10
Scaphoid	3–4	6–8
Proximal third of femur	4–6	8–12
Distal third of femur	6	12
Proximal third of tibia	6–8	12–16
Distal third of tibia	8–10	16–20

degree of post-fracture joint stiffness. The main issue for the rehabilitation phase is therefore to reduce the extent of post-fracture joint stiffness and muscle weakness (Marks et al 2003, Sato et al 2002) once the fracture is healed.

IMMOBILIZATION

Once reduction has been achieved the bone segments must be held in place by immobilization. This is achieved by one of three means:

- conservative, with an external fixation device (plaster of Paris – POP, splints, etc.)
- external fixators
- internal fixation.

It is quite common for more than one form of immobilization to be used in the management of the patient before the fracture has united.

The type of immobilization used depends on a number of factors such as the type and extent of the fracture and the health and age of the patient. These will not be discussed here as, on the whole, the medical staff make this decision.

The type of immobilization is important to the physiotherapist as it dictates when therapy commences (O'Connor et al 2003) and the extent of the physiotherapy allowed. All forms of immobilization, to a greater or lesser degree, inevitably predispose the affected part to post-immobilization joint stiffness, muscle weakness, alteration in proprioception, slowing down of the circulation and altered sensation through disuse. These therefore become the main issues for the rehabilitation phase.

Conservative: external fixation

Immobilization in slings, collar and cuff (c&c), Tubigrip, splints (e.g. Futuro wrist splint) splinting materials (Plastazote, Orthoplast, etc.), POP, polymer resin casts and other such methods all fall into this category. Skin or skeletal traction is also included but this obviously requires hospitalization and is therefore dealt with at the end of the section. All other forms of conservative immobilization either need only 1–2 days hospitalization or, as in most cases, none at all.

In this category non-surgical means are used to support the fracture and a sling, c&c or POP cast are

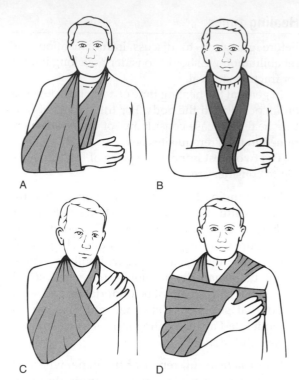

Figure 5.6   Support for upper limb fractures. A: A simple triangular bandage. B: Collar and cuff. C: High sling. D: Swathe and body bandage. (Adapted with permission from Dandy & Edwards 2003.)

the commonest appliances used. These are cheap and easy to apply but it is mainly the anatomical area of the fracture that dictates the choice of appliance within this category.

Slings and collar and cuff

Obviously, slings and c&c are used only in upper limb fractures and there are four types of immobilization (Dandy & Edwards 2003; Fig. 5.6):

- *A simple triangular bandage or broad arm sling* is used to support the weight of the forearm and hand, thus relieving the weight on the upper arm. It can therefore be used for fractures or injuries around the shoulder, humerus or elbow.

- *A collar and cuff (c & c).* Although this can be used to support the whole forearm/arm, as with the triangular bandage, the main advantage offered by using collar and cuff is support from the wrist only. Thus the c&c takes the weight of the forearm but the humerus is left unsupported so that a gravitational traction force is exerted on it, allowing longitudinal correction of shaft fractures.

- *A high sling* supports the whole arm, keeping the hand/wrist in elevation so reducing the risk of swelling in the hand. Thus it does not act directly to support the fracture but to eliminate one complication. This type of sling is therefore used in hand, wrist and forearm fractures treated either with or without POP or external splint. It should be remembered that the patient should be encouraged to remove the sling to exercise the limb through as full range as possible, and then to return the limb to the elevated support on completion.

- *A body bandage* is a sling that supports the arm, as with the triangular bandage, but the arm is then bandaged to the side, so it can only be worn under the clothes. A body bandage is used predominantly to prevent movement of the upper arm, especially in the very early stages (1–10 days) after fracture of the neck/head of humerus or after shoulder surgery. The body bandage offers extreme support but does loosen in time and needs to be reapplied regularly.

With any form of sling or c&c, the patient must keep the non-painful joints moving and, when possible contract all muscles isometrically to maintain minimal tone. It is also very important that the patient notes any changes in sensation (numbness or paraesthesia), colour (bluish), severe increase in swelling or loss of motor function in the hand/wrist. All these are signs of complications and will be discussed in the section on POP.

Self-assessment question

- SAQ 5.3 A patient has been issued with a collar and cuff immediately after a fracture of the upper third of the humeral shaft. Which joints would you advise him/her to move?

(Answer at end of chapter.)

Plaster of Paris casts

Plaster of Paris (POP) is the term used to describe Gypsona-impregnated bandages, which have been used for many years to maintain bone and joint position. The bandages, after being soaked in cold water, produce a semi-liquid POP and are then moulded to the part, encompassing the joints above and below the fracture. After 20–30 minutes the POP starts to dry and hold its shape, but full drying takes up to 24 hours, so weightbearing must be delayed at least until after this time.

The advantages of POP are that it is cheap, easy to apply, useful in immobilizing most fracture sites, can be easily reinforced or replaced and can be placed over small wounds or scars after they have been dressed. The disadvantages include potential vascular occlusion, pressure sores, undiagnosed infection and joint stiffness after POP use. The main disadvantages to the patient are the weight of the cast, especially in the lower limb, and the facts that it is quite warm and itchy, that if wet it will disintegrate and that children especially can get items caught between the skin and the cast, which may cause undetected pressure sores and/or infection.

When they dry, POP bandages become rigid and brittle and are therefore prone to cracking, particularly with overuse; skin irritation or rubbing can ensue.

The advantages far outweigh the disadvantages, however, and POP would be the first choice of immobilization for most simple fractures. If the patient is elderly or frail and would benefit from a lighter support, if the fracture is in a young patient who continues to lead an active life or if a patient has more than one fracture, a synthetic cast (fibreglass, polypropylene, polyurethane or polymer resin) may be applied. Trade names include Dynacast Extra (a rigid fibreglass bandage), Dynacast Optima (a high-performance polypropylene casting tape; both from Smith & Nephew plc, London UK), 3M Primacast Splint and 3M Soft Cast Tape (3M, Berkshire, UK).

To make the cast lighter and more durable and to stop disintegration when wet, a normal Gypsona POP is applied with a synthetic bandage overcoat. The main disadvantage of using synthetic bandages is that they are more than twice as expensive as Gypsona POP bandages. The synthetic material

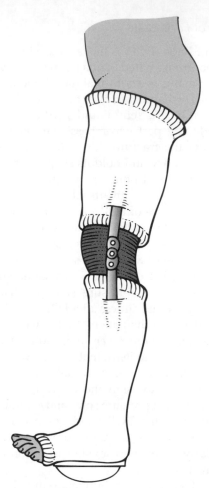

Figure 5.7 A cast brace.

occur without causing additional pressure on the vascular tissues.

A dynamic brace can also be applied using POP/polymer resin or a plastic such as Orthoplast (Pesco & Altner 1993). The dynamic (cast) brace has the benefit of allowing controlled movement at a joint while maintaining the position and stability of the fracture (Fig. 5.7). Fractures of the shaft of femur are very often treated with POP or synthetic braces, after either traction or internal fixation, when extra fracture support is needed. Thus patient hospitalization time is reduced and function and joint mobility can start earlier. Dynamic braces can also be used for fractures of the tibia, radius and ulna and lower humerus. Plastic materials can be used to brace these fractures but as they are very expensive should be used sparingly.

Self-assessment question

- SAQ 5.4 How would the patient know if the POP was causing too much pressure and what advice would be given to them?

(Answer at end of chapter.)

Case study 5.1: Mrs Andrews, immediately post injury (1)

Mrs Andrews, a 67-year-old lady, arrives at the A&E department at her local hospital following a fall on to her outstretched (right) hand. After X-ray and orthopaedic assessment she has been diagnosed as having a (R) Colles fracture. Following manipulation and reduction under local anaesthesia, a dorsal POP back slab has been applied and she is to return in 5 days time to attend the fracture clinic.

Self-assessment questions

- SAQ 5.5 What is a Colles fracture?
- SAQ 5.6 How long will this fracture take to reach union and consolidation? What do these terms mean?

---

is also much more brittle than POP when dry and again can cause skin rubbing or cuts, but it does come in a variety of colours, which is very attractive to all ages! POP or synthetic bandages need to be applied carefully and instruction on how this is done can be found in McRae & Esser (2002).

Both these types of bandage will shrink as they set and, given also the natural tendency for the soft tissue around the fracture site to swell 24–48 hours after the injury, this means that the bandage should not be applied too tightly. A cotton sleeve and then wool covering must be placed over the limb prior to application of the POP.

The cast may also be split after setting, or the POP may only be applied to one side of the limb (a back slab) to ensure adequate room for swelling to

Answer

A Colles fracture is a fracture of the distal radius within 2.5 cm of the wrist. The classic 'dinner fork' deformity that results is due to the dorsal and radial displacement of the distal fragment of bone.

Colles fractures occur predominantly in older people following a fall on to the outstretched hand. Similar mechanics in a younger person would be more likely to cause fractures of the forearm or humerus. There is a common belief that there is an association between this fracture and osteoporosis as it is much more common in post-menopausal women.

Problem-solving exercise 5.1

What type of support will be given for the arm, and what instructions should be given to the patient prior to review in 5 days time? (See end of chapter to check your answer, or if you have problems, and also see below.)

There are now a number of different treatments for the acute Colles fracture, including external fixation, splint or semi-rigid cast as well as the normal rigid POP or fibreglass casts. O'Connor et al (2003) have shown that minimally displaced Colles fractures can be treated with a simple Futuro splint (Smith & Nephew plc) instead of a rigid POP. The results compared favourably with the patients in the splint group having better subjective and objective functional assessment and movement 6 and 12 weeks post-injury. Likewise White et al (2003) compared the functional outcome of Colles and tibial fractures treated with either semi-rigid or rigid glass fibre casting materials and found that the semi-rigid cast provided slightly better immobilization and functional movement. Thus the traditional POP cast for the management of Colles fractures may be replaced in the near future, particularly for minimally displaced fractures.

Skin or skeletal traction

The changing management of patients with fractures means that long-term traction is not often used

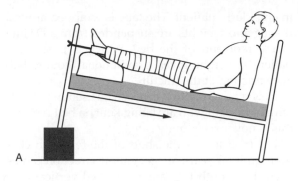

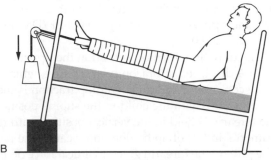

Figure 5.8   Skin traction. A: Fixed traction: the weight of the patient provides traction. B: Sliding traction: the weight of the patient still applies traction but his own weight is counterbalanced by a weight attached to a cord running over a pulley. (Adapted with permission from Dandy & Edwards 2003.)

as an individual treatment. It is more routinely used as a temporary holding immobilization until:

- skin wounds are healed
- muscle spasm has reduced so that correct limb length can be achieved
- other injuries are treated
- the patient is fit enough for surgery or operation time becomes available and in young children (who heal more quickly anyway).

There are two basic types of traction: skin and skeletal.

Skin traction (Fig. 5.8)

Tape or elastic adhesive bandages are placed around the limb distal to the fracture and weight is suspended from the end to apply traction. The commonest form of this is sliding skin traction before internal fixation of a fractured neck of femur in an elderly patient. The tape is wrapped around the leg and weights are suspended from a D sling at the foot end of the bed, which is raised; the patient's weight gives gravitational counterbalance traction at the fracture.

This type of traction can also be used in patients with back pain who are being kept on bed rest, but this is now exceedingly rare.

For fractures of the shaft of the femur in children under 3 years of age, gallows traction can be used. Here both legs are suspended vertically by strong tapes, thereby lifting the buttocks off the bed and applying traction to the femur (Dandy & Edwards 2003).

The only time traction is used in the upper limb is for a displaced supracondylar fracture, which is more common in children. Dunlop traction is then used, where, with the child in the supine position, the forearm is held in the vertical position with the humerus in 90° of abduction and clear of the bed. The pull on the forearm gives a vertical force on the radius and ulna, elbow joint and the distal third of the humerus, which pulls the bone ends into place.

Skeletal traction

The commonest form of skeletal traction is that used to manage fractures of the femoral or tibial shaft but it is also used to provide stabilization for unstable cervical spine fractures.

In fractures of the cervical spine, two screws are inserted into the skull and weights (1–5 kg depending on the location of the fracture) are attached to the callipers to distract and re-align the cervical segments, reducing pressure on the spinal cord (Grundy et al 1996).

(This chapter will not explore spinal fractures and their consequences in detail. If you want to find out more on this area try reading Bromley (1998), Grundy et al (1996) or McRae & Esser (2002).)

In femoral shaft fractures the leg is placed in a Thomas splint for support and then either a Steinmann or Denham pin is surgically inserted behind the tibial tubercle so that an appropriate weight can be attached to it. A longitudinal force is exerted through the tibia on to the quadriceps, hamstrings and knee joint. Thus the lower end of the femur is pulled into correct alignment. If too much weight is applied the femoral length will be over-corrected and a gap will be created between the bone ends. Canvas straps and pads are placed around the leg and attached to the Thomas splint to ensure correction of the fracture in the anteroposterior and lateral planes. X-rays of the femur in traction will ensure correct alignment. Finally, the Thomas splint is then suspended from an overhead 'Balkan' beam, with counterbalance weights, to allow free movement of the leg (Fig. 5.9).

A similar set-up can be used to supply traction to the calcaneus when severe tibial fractures are present.

General points concerning traction

Traction allows the free joints to be mobilized and the free muscles to be contracted much earlier than POP or other external splints. The main disadvantage is that the patient is kept on bed rest, although only for a few days in most cases using skin traction. Thus, as with anyone on bed rest, care must be taken to ensure good bed mobility, skin care and respiratory function.

With either skin or skeletal traction, during exercise or general body movements, rubbing can occur under the tapes or canvas supports, particularly during muscle contraction as this causes localized movement. Therefore the underlying skin must be inspected with great care if the patient complains of either soreness or rubbing. Pressure areas should be checked by all staff, especially the area of the Achilles tendon at the end of the tape or the canvas of the Thomas splint, the patella and the ring top of the Thomas splint.

Self-assessment question

- SAQ 5.7 What are the specific disadvantages of bed rest and which groups are most at risk?

Answer

Loss of motion, either of the specific limb or generally, which predisposes to a number of other problems:

- Slowing down of circulation, which may predispose to vascular problems (deep vein thrombosis, pulmonary embolism)

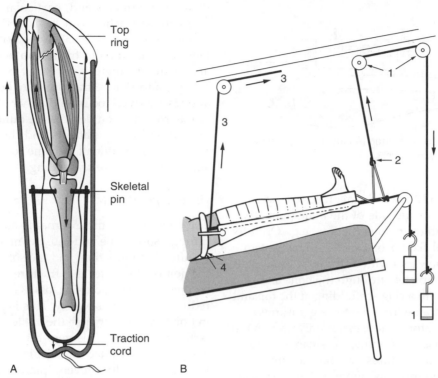

Figure 5.9 Skeletal traction provided by a Thomas splint. A: The top ring provides one point of traction. The traction cord is attached to the skeletal pin and to the end of the Thomas splint. B: A 'lively' system may be preferred, which may be achieved in various ways, e.g. by weights and a system of pulleys (1). The suspension cord may be arranged in a Y-fashion to straddle both irons of the Thomas splint (2). Although it is often attempted, support for the proximal end of the splint (3) is less clearly of benefit as it may cause extra pressure beneath the ring (4). (Adapted with permission from McRae & Esser 2002.)

- Loss of ability to maintain full respiratory function because of lack of mobility and compression of the bases and posterior lobes of the lungs, therefore more risk of chest infections
- Increased risk of pressure sores through extra pressure being exerted over greater trochanters, ischial tuberosities, sacrum, calcanei, Achilles tendons, elbows, scapulae and the back of the head
- Loss of generalized muscle tone
- Loss of independence
- Poor posture, as patient tends to be in half lying or slumped lying, so over time back pain or stiffness can ensue.

The groups most at risk are the elderly; those with a previous medical history, which would make them more prone to the complications above, and those with multiple injuries.

All these complications can occur even if patients are not in traction but, because traction grossly limits movement and patients are already in shock from the trauma, they are even more at risk of these occurring. A report on the incidence of pressure sores in a single NHS Trust hospital showed that 10.3 patients per 100 admitted to orthopaedic wards developed pressure sores, this was 6% higher than on other wards (Clark & Watts 1994). Although this rate was for all patients and not just those on traction, it is still important to note that there is a very high incidence of patients with pressure sores on orthopaedic wards, and many of these will be elderly patients who will inevitably spend some time in skin traction following a fracture of the neck of the femur.

External fixators

With this type of immobilization, the bone fragments are held by an external scaffolding attached

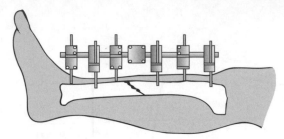

Figure 5.10   External fixator. (Adapted with permission from Dandy & Edwards 2003.)

to pins (Fig. 5.10), which are inserted percutaneously, either to one side of the bone (monofixator using cantilever construction, e.g. Orthofix Dynamic Axial fixator or Distal Radius System – Smith & Nephew plc) with a strong external rigid support, or completely through the bone and skin at both sides with a ring scaffolding at the top and bottom of the frame (ring fixator, e.g. Ilisarow).

The monofixator is more commonly used in the management of acute trauma, Hessman et al (1994) report that tibial fractures are the fractures most commonly fixed this way (Emami et al 1995), particularly for severe fractures (Weiner et al 1995). Pelvic (Rieger et al 1996), forearm (Helber & Ulrich 2000), humeral (Lavini et al 2001), ankle (El-Shazly et al 2001), fingers (Syed et al 2003) and Colles (Fischer et al 1999, Pesco & Altner 1993) fractures are also reported to have been treated using external fixators.

Halopelvic traction was one of the first forms of external ring fixator to be used in the management of spinal correction or after operation (Calliet 1975). Here a ring is placed around the skull and two or four screws are inserted, rods are surgically implanted through the pelvis and two or four strong external uprights support the upper and lower fixation points. Both this device (Cheung et al 2003) and a modification of this device (halopelvic jacket, where a POP or polymer resin jacket replaces the pelvic rods) are still used in the stabilization of cervical fractures after skeletal traction.

The advantage of external fixation in the management of long bone fractures is that it can be used in patients with severe skin loss or infection (Dandy & Edwards 2003) or soft tissue or vascular injury (Salihefendic et al 1997). It also allows easy alteration, under X-ray control, of the alignment of the bone fragments and, particularly, either compression or traction can be added as necessary (Dandy & Edwards 2003). The greatest disadvantages are that the pin tracks can become infected and therefore there is a risk of osteomyelitis or osteitis, and that re-fracture may occur if the fixation is removed too soon (Palmer et al 1997).

External fixation devices are quite unsightly to look at and many patients and their relatives or friends find it difficult to come to terms with the sight of the fracture scaffolding.

General points

The bone pins of the external fixator are inserted through soft tissue and muscle, making the latter painful on contraction, and the soft tissue around the joints distal to the fracture may therefore become shortened, causing loss of motion and often reducing function severely. This is particularly so in tibial fractures, where the ankle is held in plantarflexion because it is very difficult to dorsiflex. Some surgeons attach a footplate to the external fixator to try to prevent plantarflexion taking place. Even if plantarflexion is present, dorsiflexion exercise (active and passive) must take place, to maintain and restore movement and strength.

Thus the role of the physiotherapist must be to:

- maintain the soft tissue length of the plantar flexors by passive or active assisted movement, i.e. place a sling around the distal part of the foot and gently pull the sling towards the body. This will stretch the posterior calf muscles – gastrocnemius with the knee straight and soleus with the knee bent; the spring ligament and the plantar aspect of the foot will also be stretched
- mobilize the subtalar joint (inversion and eversion), distal joints (pronation and supination) and long and transverse arches of the foot
- maintain full knee extension as the tight plantar flexors will tend to pull the knee into flexion
- maintain isometric contraction of the dorsiflexors as much as the patient is able
- keep the skin from sticking to the pin sites by encouraging gentle oscillatory joint movements
- maintain venous return to prevent swelling and vascular problems, by gentle ankle movements with good strong contraction of the long toe flexors/extensors while in elevation

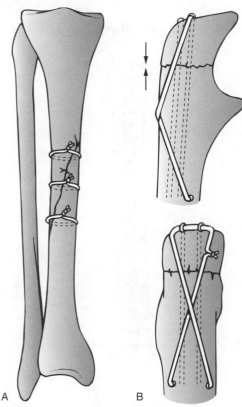

Figure 5.11   Internal fixation: wire. A: Cerclage wiring of the tibia. B, C: Tension band wiring of the olecranon. (Adapted with permission from Dandy & Edwards 2003.)

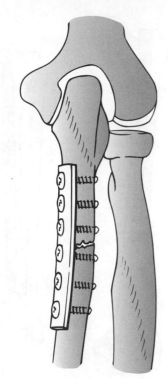

Figure 5.12   Internal fixation: plates. (Adapted with permission from McRae & Esser 2002.)

• encourage the patient to check the skin distal to the fracture daily to keep it hydrated with moisturizer.

External fixation that does not pierce large muscle groups, such as halopelvic traction, halobody jacket, or pelvic fracture fixation, is much easier to maintain and produces far fewer problems from muscle involvement. Pelvic external fixation does however bring problems of its own as the pins can damage the internal organs within the pelvis such as the urethra or bladder. Hip flexion can become limited because of the size of the frame (Palmer et al 1997) and this needs to be assessed regularly. All other types of external fixation, e.g. of the humerus and radius, will incur similar muscle or joint problems.

Operative internal fixation

In the patient's operation notes you will often see the abbreviation 'ORIF'. This stands for 'open reduction internal fixation' and describes the act of reducing the fracture at the time of fixing it internally. Thus you will know that the patient has had some form of internal fixation but not the specific details.

The type of internal fixation will again depend on the position and extent of the fracture and the size, texture and strength of the bone (McRae & Esser 2002). Therefore there has to be a huge variety of internal fixation devices that the surgeon can insert to stabilize the reduced fracture. These include screws, plates, intramedullary nails, locking nails, wires or nail-plates (sliding or compression) (Figs 5.11–5.15). They can be used either singly or in combination in severe fractures (Fig. 5.16).

Further information about the various kinds of internal fixation can be obtained from Dandy & Edwards (2003), McRae & Esser (2002).

Internal fixation is indicated when:

• fractures cannot be controlled in any other way, i.e. other methods of immobilization have failed
• patients have fractures of more than one bone

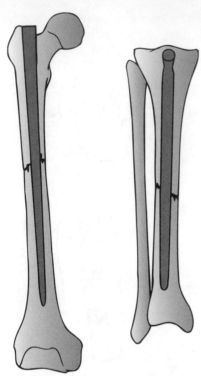

Figure 5.13   Internal fixation: intramedullary nails. (Adapted with permission from Dandy & Edwards 2003.)

- the blood supply to the limb is jeopardized by the fracture and the vessels must be protected (Dandy & Edwards 2003)
- bone ends cannot be reduced without opening the fracture site to remove muscle and soft tissue debris.

Internal fixation is very often used with multiple fractures, providing the patient is suitable for a general anaesthetic. The internal fixation provides the quickest form of stability to the fractures, stopping the blood loss that automatically occurs when a bone is broken. Severe loss of blood can increase the shock experienced by the patient and, left uncontrolled, can be fatal. Internal fixation will also provide early stability for the multiple fractures, thus reducing pain and increasing function for the patient.

The advantages include:

- better chances of obtaining good reduction and union (McRae & Esser 2002)
- early mobilization both generally and specifically.

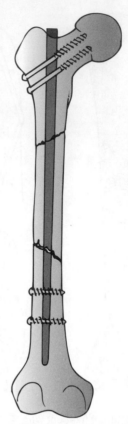

Figure 5.14   Internal fixation: locking nails. Screws are passed into the fragments above and below the fracture to hold the bone out to length. (Adapted with permission from Dandy & Edwards 2003.)

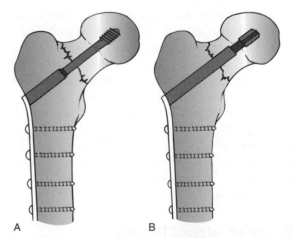

A   B

Figure 5.15   Internal fixation: nail-plates. A: Compression. B: Sliding. (Adapted with permission from Dandy & Edwards 2003.)

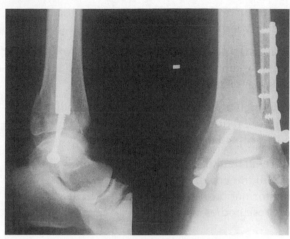

Figure 5.16   Internal fixation: combination of screws and plates. (Adapted with permission from Dandy & Edwards 2003.)

The disadvantages are:

- risk of infection
- additional trauma of surgery to bone and surrounding tissue.

Internal fixation, like splints/casts and external fixators, acts as an immobilization device until fracture healing takes place but, unlike the other devices, internal fixation is not visible. Thus there is often a misunderstanding among patients and junior staff alike that the internal fixation device is strong enough to support the normal stress or strain loads of bone. This is not the case and extra support with reduced loading must be given to the internal scaffolding until initial callus formation occurs. Thus a patient with an internally fixed fracture of the humerus should have a broad sling or collar and cuff supplied in the early stages to help support the weight of the arm and reduce function. Similarly, the patient with an internally fixed femur or tibia should remain non-weight-bearing until initial callus forms, to ensure that no excess loading occurs across the fracture site.

Normally after internal fixation, only limited joint movement will take place, in the initial stages because of pain, swelling, bruising and apprehension. When these reduce after 10–14 days the patient may be tempted to use the limb normally. It is important that at this time the patient is seen again by either medical or therapy staff to remind them of the basic 'do's and don'ts'.

Postoperative care

As the patient has had a general anaesthetic then alongside the physiotherapy aims of treatment for the fracture site, are those for postoperative care. The physiotherapist must assess the respiratory and vascular performance and general mobility. These will be discussed in the rehabilitation section.

REHABILITATION

Initial rehabilitation instructions after the injury

Rehabilitation starts as soon as the fracture has been reduced. From the first contact with the patient, the physiotherapist must ensure that the patient fully understands the rehabilitation process to aid full recovery.

It has been well documented that complications can commence immediately after the fracture if the patient or care staff are not aware of potential problems. Thus suitable care instructions must be clear to all concerned. All members of staff are still involved at this stage and any of the medical, nursing or therapy staff may contribute this information depending on the policy at specific hospitals.

Basic instructions

The instructions to Mrs Andrews described earlier (Problem-solving exercise 5.1, Answer) should be given to all patients with upper limb fractures. Therefore to refresh your memory revise Problem-solving exercise 5.1.

> #### Self-assessment question
>
> - SAQ 5.8 What instructions should be given to a patient with a fracture of the lower third of tibia and fibula who is being sent home non-weight-bearing in a long leg POP cast from thigh to toes?
>
> (Answer at end of chapter.)

These basic instructions underpin the process of rehabilitation. The overall objective of post-fracture rehabilitation is to aid fracture healing in the appropriate timescale, returning the patient to his/her functional norm with as few complications as possible.

Longer-term complications of fracture

Some of the complications of fractures have been mentioned before but need to be highlighted again before addressing rehabilitation.

Alteration to the healing rate

Delayed union.   The fracture takes a longer time to heal than usual, accompanied by abnormal bone changes. This is usually managed by having a longer immobilization time.

Non-union.   The fracture does not unite in the recognized time frame. Bone infection and excessive movement at the bone ends are two of the causes of non-union. Non-union is usually managed initially by a longer time of immobilization, then, if it persists, surgical management by internal fixation with excision of bone ends and bone grafting is used. In very severe cases of non-union, with long-standing pain and/or infection, amputation of the limb may be necessary. Osteoporosis can result from delayed weight bearing, particularly when there is an issue with the length of time of healing, and in some cases of non-union external fixators are used to assist healing and also to enhance weight bearing (Lavini et al 2001).

Malunion.   The fracture unites but with an unacceptable degree of angulation or rotation. If severe, the bone can be re-aligned by manipulation if ununited, or if union or consolidation has occurred then an osteotomy may be performed to correct the malalignment.

Shortening

As a result of malunion the bone ends may heal in an overlapped position, thus shortening the bone length. This is particularly important in the lower limb, where a resultant leg length imbalance of greater than 1.25 cm may cause secondary low back pain and greater loading across the hip joint, possibly leading to secondary osteoarthrosis.

Joint stiffness.   There may be loss of full joint range of motion from either periarticular or intra-articular causes.

Periarticular causes.   Include pain, swelling, haemorrhage, reduced muscle function or muscle tethering, capsular or ligamentous damage.

Intra-articular causes.   Include joint adhesions, malalignment of joint surfaces and excessive callus formation if there are intra-articular fractures or loose bodies.

Avascular necrosis

The blood supply to the bone has been interrupted and therefore the bone dies and crumbles, and the joint involving that bone becomes painful and stiff. This commonly occurs with fractures of the neck of femur, scaphoid, talus or lunate, or in segments of a comminuted fracture where the blood supply has been totally severed.

Autonomic problems – Sudeck's atrophy or reflex sympathetic dystrophy

Sudeck's atrophy refers to hand symptoms that may occur after a Colles or other wrist fracture and reflex sympathetic dystrophy is a term used when symptoms occur in the foot after ankle fractures. In Sudeck's atrophy the Colles fracture is fully united but on X-ray there is patchy osteoporosis. There is severe post-traumatic pain with autonomic changes, including swelling of the hand and fingers. The skin is warm, pink and has a polished, shiny appearance. Excessive pain along with the swelling inhibits movement of the fingers and wrist. The symptoms slowly subside as movement returns and pain reduces, but this takes a considerable length of time.

Myositis ossificans

This is usually seen at the elbow, after a supracondylar fracture but can occur at any joint, especially the hip, shoulder or knee. It is especially seen in patients with a paraplegia or head injury, where passive movements or stretching are carried out regularly, often against tight muscles or increased tone. A calcified mass develops in the soft tissues of a joint after severe trauma and may be associated with intense haematoma. As there is a strong belief that passive movement or stretching predisposes the tissue to myositis, many physiotherapists will not use passive stretching of the elbow joint. Limited passive motion may be carried out, or the practitioner may err on the side of caution and only do active assisted motion.

Infection (osteitis)

This often presents following an open fracture or through the pin tracks of an external fixator. The normal signs of infection appear (pain, raised temperature, swollen area with local tenderness) and there may be a foul-smelling discharge or staining of POP. Bone death (necrosis) will occur in severe, long-term cases.

Postcallus complications

These can include either nerve damage or tendon rupture. Following the normal development of callus, the soft tissue in the surrounding area may become compressed or frayed by movement over the extra bone. Thus any soft tissue near the fracture can become involved. (Note: the extensor pollicis longus tendon is very prone to rupture after a Colles fracture.)

Osteoarthrosis

Alteration in the joint articular surface, biomechanical stress changes or alteration in the bone length post-fracture all predispose the adjacent joints to increased wear and tear and early osteoarthrosis (OA). OA may occur at any joint associated with the altered mechanics, not just the joint involving the fracture (e.g. the contralateral knee joint following a fractured neck of femur).

Muscle weakness

This has been mentioned previously but because of the trauma associated with the fracture and the subsequent immobilization there is evidence of muscle weakness even from 6 hours post fracture and

that muscle strength loss increases exponentially (Heslinga et al 1995, Williams & Goldspink 1978).

Physiotherapy cannot prevent these complications but, if you are aware of them, then you will be able to recognize and treat them accordingly during the rehabilitation period.

PHYSIOTHERAPY ASSESSMENT AND TREATMENT

Much more caution must be exercised when assessing for the first time an inpatient with an acute fracture. By the time the patient comes to outpatient therapy, usually after bone union, a much fuller examination of the part can take place, without causing damage.

The earlier the physiotherapist can start the rehabilitation phase, the greater the opportunity to influence the overall outcome through careful assessment, individual treatment and establishment of a good rapport with the patient.

There are some general principles of physiotherapy when treating fractures, which must be remembered in every case. However, the treatments themselves must be made appropriate to the individual, particularly in the duration and type of exercises given. The number of repetitions should be calculated according to the patient's ability to carry out the exercise, although many therapists start with a combination of 'fives', e.g. five repetitions of the exercise held for 5 seconds, increasing either the number of repetitions or the duration as possible. If a patient with an acute fracture can only manage one successful repetition then this is much more acceptable then an incorrect movement or half-hearted attempt.

Physiotherapy assessment and treatment should never be regarded as a standard recipe (Chapter 3), as no two patients will ever be the same.

Acute unstable fractures

General points

Avoid any muscle contraction that will move the bone ends, thus inhibiting healing. It will increase pain and if vigorous may cause malalignment of the bone ends. This can occur when a strong muscle group is attached to the smaller fragment of the fracture, e.g. iliopsoas contraction on the proximal fragment of bone in a fracture of the upper shaft of the femur.

If a fracture is unstable it must be supported when exercises are done distal to it. For example, with a fracture of the humerus, the elbow, wrist and hand can be still exercised while the arm is held in the sling for support.

Joint motion

With any fracture, assisted active or passive movement is easier than active in the early stages, to increase the range of movement (ROM) and to give reassurance to the patient.

Following internal fixation, where possible, try to gain as much movement as possible of the joints to be immobilized in POP prior to its application. A good example of this is at the ankle, where often the internally fixed ankle is left in elevation without the POP until the swelling in the foot and ankle goes down and the range of dorsiflexion gets to neutral (plantigrade). Gentle movements and intermittent pressure can help to reduce the swelling and allow greater movement. Continuous passive motion (CPM) machines can also assist with this in between therapy sessions (Coutts et al 1989, Davis 1991).

Swelling

Active exercise distal and proximal to the fracture will help venous return and reduction of swelling, particularly if carried out in elevation.

Weight bearing

Full or partial weight bearing must not commence until some callus formation is seen on X-ray. Touch weight bearing may be allowed in some cases where non-weight-bearing is too difficult. It is important to get weight bearing as soon as possible to assist healing and to reduce the chance of osteoporosis, which has been shown to start from 2 weeks post-fracture (White et al 2003).

Walking with any walking aid at this stage must be safe, with good balance and co-ordination. If you are unsure whether or not the patient is safe then they must remain in hospital until they are. Non-weight-bearing can be very difficult for some patients and takes quite a time to get used to, particularly in elderly patients. It is in these instances that the surgeons may agree to allow touch weight bearing, to aid mobilization and release from hospital (if in doubt, check first).

Often pain and loss of function of the foot is one of the greatest problems when returning to lower limb weight bearing after removal of immobilization. While encased in a POP or immobilized with an external fixator, the joints of the foot become stiff, particularly the intermetatarsal joints, and the small muscles of the foot have not functioned properly. Thus when weight bearing is first attempted the foot is very painful and weight cannot be taken on it. Mobilization of all the foot joints and strengthening of the intrinsic foot muscles will assist ease of weight bearing.

Massage

Massage, with mobilization of the muscles and joints, especially in warm soapy water or with baby oil, will help to return the nutrition to the skin and give the patient reassurance and good sensory feedback. (The patient could do this at home.)

Function

Gentle functional movements will help the patient with any upper limb problems but lifting of heavy objects should be avoided until the callus at the fracture site is strong enough to do so.

Always use functional objectives and measurements that are particularly important to the patient.

Stable united fractures

General points

External fixators and internal fixation does not replace union of the bone: these are purely scaffolding devices until union takes place. Thus the bone should be treated with care, with limited weight bearing, until callus has strengthened the fracture site.

Excessive pain or fracture mobility after normal union times must be regarded as highly significant and if there is any doubt then the patient should be referred back to the orthopaedic surgeon as soon as possible.

Joint motion

Once a fracture has been stabilized (by cast brace, external fixator or internal fixation) then the range of motion at the joints proximal and distal to fracture can be regained. CPM machines can be used to help regain movement while the patient is hospitalized (Davis, 1991). Most CPM machines give support from the thigh to knee, ensuring no abnormal strain to the fractures of the shaft of femur or across the knee joint (O'Driscoll & Giori 2000).

Patients can undertake some simple accessory movements themselves and these assist the return of physiological motion and may help with pain relief. Union must be present before these are performed.

Strengthening

Do not apply excessive resistance across the fracture, either longitudinally from weight bearing or rotatory from muscle contraction, until the fracture and surrounding muscles are strong enough. For example, resistance to strengthen the rotators of the shoulder is usually given at the distal forearm; if the fracture is not united then this rotatory force can cause a re-fracture of the shaft of the humerus.

During strengthening exercises, do not suspend free weights distal to the fracture until after consolidation, particularly in the case of a fracture dislocation or transverse fracture near to a joint, as this causes an excessive traction force.

Suspension of weights over the unsupported joint to increase passive stretch may also be harmful with a fracture close to the joint, particularly for the knee and elbow, where longer levers are involved. An example of this is when the knee is in as full extension as possible, with the heel and the buttock supported but not the femur. A physiotherapist may add either manual pressure or weights over the knee joint to assist the stretch on the posterior capsule of the knee. It can be reasoned that, if there is a fracture near to a joint or an intra-articular fracture this may cause excessive stress in the anteroposterior direction, thus making it painful or prone to delayed union.

Muscle strength both at joints immediately proximal to and distal to the fracture and at joints further away may remain weaker for quite some time (up to 2 years). Bullock-Saxton (1994) indicated that fit young men with severe lateral ligament strain of the ankle still had proximal muscle function changes 2 years post-injury. Although this research was not undertaken on post-fracture patients, it can be assumed that the same principles apply to this category of patient. The more severe the injury the greater the risk of long-term problems, and the patient should be made aware of this.

All methods of strengthening can be introduced once the fracture has consolidated but from union until this time the fracture site should be supported while resisted exercises are done.

Once good isometric strength has been achieved, endurance training with small weights but large numbers of repetitions should commence first before power training (large weights, small numbers of repetitions). Isokinetic training can commence after union again provided the fracture is supported. Torque limits should be set into the test programme so that the patient cannot overwork.

Weight bearing

Weight bearing is increased as the fracture and muscle strength allow. Usually it is the patient who is reluctant to get rid of walking aids but you must ensure that the lower limb is strong enough to take and endure the increase in weight. Limb loading with a set of bathroom scales can be undertaken to ensure:

- correct load acceptance
- level of pain on loading
- the patient's confidence in the limb.

SUMMARY

All the above points must be borne in mind when administering the treatment programme. The physiotherapist has direct control over the treatment after fracture and may influence rehabilitation for good or bad. If there is any doubt about stability, position or overall performance then you should consult either senior physiotherapy staff or the doctors concerned.

REHABILITATION: THREE CASE HISTORIES

Rehabilitation will now be addressed using three case histories:

- A Colles fracture, after POP fixation (Case study 5.1)
- A fractured shaft of femur, after traction/internal fixation (Case study 5.2)
- A hip fracture, after internal fixation (Case study 5.3).

Before considering any of the case histories, or indeed the rehabilitation of any patient with a fracture, five general questions must be asked about the patient and the fracture.

1. What do I know about this fracture?
2. What should I find at this stage of the management if the fracture is healing normally?
3. What might go wrong with this fracture?
4. What do I know about this patient, particularly concerning his/her functional ability?
5. What are the expected overall outcomes for this patient, with this fracture?

Question 2 should be answered for both the current stage of fracture healing and for the future.

Question 4 will need to be addressed by a full subjective and objective assessment of the patient.

All questions should be answered for each of the patient's fractures. The questions can be taken in any order but all should be answered.

If all these questions can be answered then the physiotherapy treatment can be planned and any problems that might arise can be prepared for.

Rehabilitation following a Colles fracture

Now please return to Case study 5.1, Mrs Andrews, immediately post injury (p 98) and reread the scenario before proceeding.

Problem–solving exercise 5.2

Attempt to answer all the five major questions about Mrs Andrews and her Colles fracture.

(Answer at end of chapter.)

On reviewing the answer to the above exercise it is clear that we can only address questions 1–3 & 5 fully at this stage. Question 4 has been answered for the initial stage but a full functional assessment will depend on the results post removal of POP.

Case study 5.1: Mrs Andrews, removal of POP (2)

On review at 5 weeks the Colles fracture was deemed united, and the POP was removed. Mrs Andrews was then seen by the physiotherapy consultant in the clinic and given an initial assessment.

Observation

- (R) arm was held close to the body
- The skin around the hand, wrist and forearm was flaky, pale and dry
- (R) forearm was considerably thinner than the (L)
- Wrist was held in slight flexion and ulnar deviation
- Obvious thickening of the bone around the distal end of the radius and some soft tissue thickening around the dorsal aspect of the wrist.

Problem–solving exercise 5.3

Are these the normal signs of a fracture after removal of POP? Explain why.

(See end of chapter if you have problems.)

Following Mrs Andrews's initial quick assessment in clinic she has been given an appointment for the next day for outpatient physiotherapy. The next stage of the normal fracture healing pathway has been reached. A full subjective and objective assessment must be undertaken to answer question

4 in full; then we can set objectives for treatment. Now return to Chapter 3 on assessment and refresh your memory.

Problem–solving exercise 5.4

What would you need to ask this patient to complete question 4?

(Answer at end of chapter.)

Case study 5.1: Mrs Andrews, continued (3)

From what you have already been told about Mrs Andrews, some of these questions can be answered but we still need to know some details, as follows:

- Occupation – nil, retired post office manager
- Hobbies – bowls, knitting
- Home circumstances – widow, lives alone in a bungalow, friends have been helping with shopping
- Hand dominance – right
- Main problems:
  - Scared to move wrist through pain and apprehension
  - Arm feels weak and stiff
  - Worried about appearance of arm
  - Anxious to get back to bowls
- What has Mrs Andrews been doing with her arm – moving the shoulder up and down, stretching the elbow and moving the fingers. Has not been doing rotation of the shoulder and radio-ulnar joint and thumb, also has not been moved fully
- No other injury at the time
- Previous medical history – nil of note, no previous fractures, operations or serious illnesses.

Self-assessment question

- **SAQ 5.10** What would you assess in your objective examination?

(Answer at end of chapter, but try to come up with your own points first.)

Case study 5.1: Mrs Andrews, continued (4)

Major findings
Pain

Over the dorsal and radial aspects at end of range flexion, extension and radial deviation.

ROM – right	Active	Passive
Wrist		
Extension	0–5°	0–15°
Flexion	0–45°	0–50°
Ulnar deviation	0–20°	0–25°
Radial deviation	0–5°	0–5°
Radioulnar		
Pronation	0–60°	0–65°
Supination	0–5°	0–5°
Elbow		
Flexion	10–130°	10–130°
Extension	−10°	0°

Fingers
Flexion: tip of middle finger to 5 cm from 1st palm crease
Extension: with wrist in neutral to 20° at MCP joints.

Shoulder
Full movement.

(L) arm
No problems.

Muscle strength
All muscle on (R) wrist isometrically contract in the neutral position. Isotonically (R) biceps, triceps, deltoid, rotator cuff all Gd IV. Grip strength tested with a bulb grip dynamometer, records 2 kg pressure for the right hand using the large bulb.

Swelling
(R) hand 2 cm bigger than (L) at level of MCPs.

Sensation
Normal; (R) = (L) all tests

Dexterity
Able to grip a tennis ball, unable to pick up a 1 cm peg, hold a key or touch thumb to little finger.

Table 5.2 Treatment objectives

Patient's problems	Treatment objectives
Scared to move wrist due to pain and apprehension	Show the patient how to move without causing damage to the wrist and try to reduce pain
Arm feels weak and stiff	Encourage controlled movement of the wrist, radio-ulnar, elbow and shoulder joints
Worried about appearance of arm	Explain about general care of the skin
Anxious to get back to bowls, her main hobby	Explain the healing times and need to mobilize and then strengthen the arm before return to bowling

With this information we can now begin to plan Mrs Andrews's treatment, and the first step is to consider her main problems and put initial treatment objectives for them (Table 5.2).

Each time Mrs Andrews attends for physiotherapy these main problems should be reassessed and any further problems that may have arisen should be noted and addressed.

Problem-solving exercise 5.5

Describe how you would carry out each of the objectives in Table 5.2.

(Answer at end of chapter.)

The treatment to be carried out during outpatient sessions needs to be considered. This is based on the main problems, which are clearly related to joint stiffness after immobilization and thus are the main focus for treatment. Most of Mrs Andrews's concerns will be addressed during this consideration.

During the initial assessment it is also important for the physiotherapist to establish whether or not referral to the occupational therapist or social worker is necessary. If Mrs Andrews is having difficulties managing tasks around the house, then assessment by the occupational therapist might be useful. Some basic advice, especially in the kitchen, might help considerably. If greater difficulties were encountered further assistance could also be given, such as meals on wheels, district nursing (dressings, etc.) or care assistance, but Mrs Andrews does not need these.

Self-assessment question

- SAQ 5.11 How would you mobilize a stiff joint immediately after immobilization of a Colles fracture where union is complete?

Answer

If the patient is apprehensive ask him/her to hold just proximal to the wrist joint (i.e. across the fracture site) to gain reassurance while doing the exercises.

- Active/active assisted wrist exercises through as much range as possible, especially extension and radial deviation, making sure the exercises are clearly understood and could be repeated at home
- Gentle passive stretching to the long finger flexors and extensors, so stretching the soft tissues
- Maitland mobilization techniques: accessory GdI techniques to help with pain relief or GdII as the pain decreases, to increase range of motion. (Union must be achieved before mobilization techniques can be done.) (Coyle & Robertson 1998)
- Functional exercises that do not involve carrying objects, e.g. opening doors with that hand, washing up dishes, getting dressed using both hands
- Once range has been gained, strengthening exercises should be introduced to maintain the new range.

One of the greatest concerns for student physio-therapists is when to increase the number or type of exercises. For Mrs Andrews, there are five main points, which need to be reached to alter the exercise prescription:

1. All ranges of motion increase by more than 7°, but especially extension, radial deviation and finger flexion as indicated by measurement with a goniometer
2. Pain reduces at rest and does not increase with exercise, measured by a visual analogue scale
3. Strength increases in the grip and wrist extensors and a combination of these two in the functional position of the wrist, measured by a grip dynamometer
4. Swelling decreases in the hand using tape measure measurements
5. General hand function improves.

The patient should be aware that the wrist and hand may still become tired and ache for some time, particularly after use. As the exercises increase, the ache may return for a short time but will decrease with increased function, motion and strength.

Thus we can gradually increase first the number of exercises and then the type, i.e. introduce more active motion than active assisted or passive. We would gradually bring in longer lever arms and increase resistance, using small weights so endurance can be increased. Once the fracture has consolidated then greater resistance and full weight bearing can be introduced.

Finally, Mrs Andrews will be helped to return to her full function by introducing her to the techniques used for bowls. This can be started as a general exercise for the whole arm without a ball and then a small soft ball could be added. The size and weight of a ball would be increased to that of a bowls ball, as Mrs Andrews became more able.

Rehabilitation following a fractured shaft of femur

These injuries can only occur when considerable force is involved, given the strength of the femur and the surrounding muscle. Thus they predominantly occur in road traffic accidents, falls or after a violent twisting action. A fracture can also occur at the shaft of femur immediately below the tip of the femoral component of a total or partial hip replacement. This is because the metallic component is much more rigid than the underlying bone, so the bone takes added stress and a fracture can happen (Dandy & Edwards 2003, McRae & Esser 2002).

Because there is usually considerable violence involved, it is quite common to have associated injuries such as a fracture of the patella, posterior cruciate ligament rupture, posterior dislocation of the hip, or skin or vascular damage.

Case study 5.2: Mr Kingston, fracture shaft of femur, post-traction and internal fixation (1)

Mr David Kingston, a 30-year-old male, was admitted to hospital through A&E with a compound spiral fracture of the mid shaft of (R) femur after being involved in a road traffic accident (RTA), in which his motorbike was hit by a car, the previous evening. He was thrown from this motorbike and landed on his (R) side.

Subjective assessment

Social history: lives with wife and two children in a house with one flight of stairs (one banister (R) going up). Bathroom and bedroom upstairs. Unemployed bricklayer (1 year), wife works and he looks after the children (ages 5 and 7 years).

Smoking: 40 cigarettes a day.

Hobbies: riding motor bike and playing Sunday league football.

Drug history: nil.

History of present complaint: on admission a Denham pin was inserted in the (R) tibia and skeletal balanced traction was set up with 4 kg weight.

Case study 5.2: continued

Possibility of surgery in 3 days' time to insert an interlocking intramedullary nail. Patient cannot remember much about the accident but was not unconscious.

Painful (R) shoulder since RTA; no bony injury on X-ray.

Main patient problems:

- Pain in (R) thigh and shoulder
- Immobilization in hospital
- Family (he looks after the children while wife works)
- Inability to move (R) leg or arm.

Objective assessment

Observation

Patient's records: temperature 35°, blood pressure 110/70, pulse 65.

Patient: resting in the half lying position with skeletal traction and Thomas splint in situ suspended on an overhead beam. Leg held in full knee extension and ankle in plantarflexion and inversion. Clean dressing on each side of Denham pin, and over the lateral thigh where the femur pierced the skin. Swelling mid shaft of femur, down to and including the knee and around pin sites.

(R) arm is held in adduction and internal rotation with elbow flexion, no support in situ. No obvious deformity, swelling or bruising. Glucose intravenous drip in (L) arm.

Leg

Palpation: Lower leg feels cold, thigh warm, the dorsalis pedis pulse is present.

ROM – right	Active	Passive
Ankle		
Dorsiflexion	−30° to −20°	0–10°
Plantar flexion	30–40°	0–60°
Subtalar		
Inversion	10–20°	0–60°
Eversion	−10 to 0°	0–30°

Small foot joints	Cannot be tested	Full = to (L)
Toes	Full	Full = to (L)
Knee and hip	Cannot be tested	Cannot be tested
Patella	Cannot be tested	Full = to (L)

Muscle strength

Left
All groups Gd V

Right

Dorsiflexors	Gd II, pain at pin sites
Plantar flexors	Gd III pain stretch at pin sites
Inversion	Gd III
Eversion	Gd III
Quadriceps	Gd I – isometric only
Hamstrings	Gd II – isometric only
Glutei	Gd III – isometric only

Neurological signs
Sensation full (R) = (L)

Vascular signs
General fall in temperature, pulses all present, (R) = (L)

Chest
Auscultation: (R) expansion decreased as (R) arm is held by the body. Good air entry to all lobes, slight crackles in (R) and (L) bases.

Bed mobility
Not tested as very tired and uncomfortable.

Information about the shoulder is being withheld at the moment so as not to confuse the main facts about the leg.

From Mr Kingston's assessment, can you answer the five major questions?

(Answers at end of chapter.)

1. What do I know about this fracture?
2. What should I find at this stage of the management if the fracture is healing normally?
3. What might go wrong with this fracture?
4. What do I know about this patient, particularly his functional ability?
5. What are the expected overall outcomes for this patient, with this fracture?

The assessment of a patient with an acute fracture has to be limited to only the essential points. Any overactivity of the joints and muscles around the fracture site may cause movement of the bone ends and intense pain.

Reread Mr Kingston's assessment and compare it to that undertaken for Mrs Andrews and her more chronic state after being in POP for 5 weeks and the fracture having united. Bearing this in mind, we need to categorize the major points from the assessment into relevant and non-relevant.

Problem-solving exercise 5.7

Which do you think are the most relevant points from Mr Kingston's assessment and why?

Answer

- *Reduced bed mobility (chest and general)*: therefore risk of chest infection, particularly if going to theatre. Also susceptible to pressure sores because of lack of general mobility
- *Reduced ankle movement and strength*: therefore the soft tissue around the ankle may become contracted and he will not be able to walk correctly. Also, loss of the venous pump means potential vascular problems (deep vein thrombosis or pulmonary embolism)
- *Loss of quadriceps function and immobilization of the knee in extension*: inhibition of quadriceps due to pain, swelling and bruising. Lack of

control at the knee joint; along with immobilization of the knee in extension, this could lead to long-term loss of flexion. Knee kept in extension may also cause the patella to become adherent to the femur; this will have to be mobilized with isometric quadriceps exercises and passive movements
- *Potential shoulder problems* may limit the use of crutches.

These points become the main foci for the initial physiotherapy treatment and, if they are combined with the patient problems mentioned earlier (i.e. pain in (R) thigh and shoulder, immobilization in hospital, family problems and inability to move (R) leg or arm), then the physiotherapist and patient can work towards similar overall objectives. Of course, initially the physiotherapy treatment objectives were quite specific, and those of the patient more global.

In Mr Kingston's case he has indicated that he is concerned because he looks after the children while his wife works. This needs to be explored and if assistance is needed the physiotherapist should check with both the nursing and medical staff to ensure that the social work department has been informed. It may not be the role of the physiotherapist to initiate this contact but if the patient has revealed this concern then the therapist must pass it on to the appropriate people.

As mentioned earlier, the treatment must be made appropriate to the individual, particularly the duration and type of exercises given. Therefore the exercise regime will incorporate the following, and should be carried out after adequate painkillers have been administered:

- Isotonic exercise to the:
  - Ankle, dorsiflexion and plantarflexion
  - Subtalar and midfoot joints, inversion and eversion
  - Toe movements, flexion and extension, as often as possible
- Passive accessory movements:
  - Patella, inferior and superior, medial and lateral
  - Intermetatarsal joints, anteroposterior glide
  - Midtarsal joints, all movements

- Isometric exercises:
  - Quadriceps
  - Hamstrings
  - Glutei, extension and abduction of the hip
- Encourage bed mobility: bridging, moving up and down the bed using the other leg and getting up from supine to sitting
- Respiratory: deep breathing, coughing
- Upper limb strength: as able depending on the shoulder injury. Muscles needed for crutch walking are grip, wrist extensors, triceps, latissimus dorsi, deltoid, pectorals and trapezius and these should be concentrated on.

secretions can accumulate, thereby increasing the risk of infection, especially as Mr Kingston is a smoker.
- *Knee range*: now measurable as the patient is out of the Thomas splint.
- *Ankle and foot movements and power* should be checked against the preoperative assessment.

The greatest change in treatment objectives is that the knee and hip are now able to move and that Mr Kingston can get up without weight bearing. To allow Mr Kingston to go home he must have muscular control of both these joints and have adequate range of motion (70° of flexion and full extension at the knee).

Isometric exercises for quadriceps, hamstrings, glutei and iliopsoas can now be introduced through the range and, when these are stronger, isotonic exercises can be added. Friction-free surfaces can be used to gain active hip and knee flexion and extension and CPM can be used to gain passive motion when not in therapy sessions (Akeson et al 1984, Davis 1991).

Prior to crutch walking, Mr Kingston's (R) shoulder needs to be reassessed and, if strong enough, he may be able to transfer from bed to chair and then into standing. The intravenous drip will be in for 24 hours; this will dictate the time scale for walking but does not stop transfer to the chair.

Case study 5.2: Mr Kingston, continued (2)

After 48 hours on traction, a reassessment of the patient showed that Mr Kingston was in much less pain at the shoulder, thigh and pin sites. The range of dorsiflexion in the ankle had increased to the plantigrade position (0°) and muscle function at the ankle had increased to Gd IV, and quadriceps and hamstrings to an isometric Gd II. The shoulder joint could now be moved without severe pain.

It is quite common that, once pain has been controlled and the bone ends have been stabilized, movements and muscle strength start to return. This may take up to 2 weeks depending on the patient. The initial exercise programme can be continued, with the patient being encouraged to progress to doing all the exercises, as s/he is able.

As Mr Kingston's pain is reducing, a full examination of the shoulder can now take place. Six days after injury Mr Kingston went to theatre to have an interlocking intramedullary nail inserted.

Problem-solving exercise 5.8

What may happen and why, when a patient with a fracture of the lower limb gets up to either sit or stand for the first time?

(Answer at end of chapter.)

Self-assessment question

- **SAQ 5.12** What would you need to check after this type of surgery?

Answer

- *Chest function*: the general anaesthetic slows down the normal ciliary action and more

Problem-solving exercise 5.9

What would be the criteria for discharge for Mr. Kingston from a) the medical and b) the physiotherapy point of view?

Answer

a. All wounds have healed; fracture is stable, temperature not raised. No pain in calf or chest (indicators of deep vein thrombosis or pulmonary embolism). Adequate support at home.

b. • *Knee*: active knee range from 0–70°; quadriceps strength Gd III to straighten the knee from 70° flexion to 0° extension
   • Understands exercises fully
   • *Function*: safe non-weight-bearing on crutches in standing; independent walking; sit to stand, manages stairs either with crutches or safely on his bottom
   • Outpatient physiotherapy appointment made to local hospital
   • Patient aware of complications, especially: infection; deep vein thrombosis (calf pain with an increase in temperature); pulmonary embolism (chest pain, shortness of breath); persistent pain in thigh (possible loosening, re-fracture or infection); further or continuing loss of knee movement
   • Patient knows not to weight bear until return to the orthopaedic clinic, usually 6 weeks from fracture.

As Mr Kingston is returning home it may be appropriate for him to be seen by the occupational therapist to assess the home situation. This is not necessary or possible in all cases.

Mr Kingston was discharged, based on the above criteria, and is now on to the next stage of rehabilitation as an outpatient. From here on until the final stage of full functional ability, the treatment objectives will continue to progress until he can go back to his hobbies and potential work. Look back at the physiotherapy principles for a stable united fracture (page 108) and think how these would apply to Mr Kingston.

Problem-solving exercise 5.10

What would now be the treatment objective for Mr Kingston, with realistic time scales?

Answer

Minimum expected timescales are shown in parentheses.

• Maintain and increase the range of active and passive knee flexion 0–140° (4 weeks from start of outpatient treatment)
• Strengthen knee flexion and extension to Gd V; can only be full weight bearing after late union/consolidation (10–12 weeks post-fracture)
• Maintain and strengthen the muscles around the hips, particularly the glutei and iliopsoas on the injured side (10–12 weeks post-injury)
• Regain full soft tissue length particularly: quadriceps, hamstrings, iliopsoas, adductor mass, tensor fascia lata (4 weeks from start of outpatient treatment)
• Regain full proprioception at the knee
• Return to normal gait pattern: starts once partial weight bearing begins at 6 weeks, getting as near as possible to the normal pattern with crutches and then sticks (6–8 weeks post-injury), then with no support (10–12 weeks post injury)
• Return to squats, kneeling, and step-ups on injured limb; all can commence with partial weight bearing (6–8 weeks post-injury)
• Able to run, jump, independent standing on one leg: needs to be fully weight bearing (10–12 weeks post-injury)
• Return to playing football (12–24 weeks post-injury).

Rehabilitation following hip fracture

General information

There are two main areas containing four sites at which hip fractures occur:

• *Intracapsular (within the joint capsule) fractures* may be:
  – subcapital (i.e. at the base of the head of femur) or
  – transcervical (i.e. in the middle of the neck of femur)
• *Extracapsular (outside the joint capsule) fractures* may be:
  – intertrochanteric (i.e. at the base of the femoral neck between the trochanters) or
  – pertrochanteric (through both trochanters).

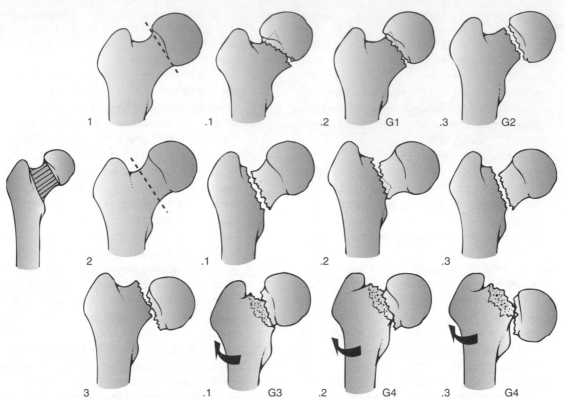

Figure 5.17   Hip fractures: neck region. 1: Minimally displaced subcapital fractures – 1.1, impacted with 15° or more of valgus; 1.2, impacted with less than 15° of valgus; 1.3, non-impacted fracture. 2: Transverse fractures – 2.1, basal; 2.2, adduction pattern; 2.3, shear pattern. 3: Displaced subcapital fractures – 3.1, moderate varus displacement with external rotation; 3.2, moderate displacement with shortening and external rotation; 3.3 marked displacement. (Adapted with permission from McRae & Esser 2002.)

Types of hip fracture are shown in Figs 5.17 and 5.18.

Displaced intracapsular fractures are the most difficult to treat and there are many surgical procedures for the surgeon to choose from. The commonest procedures include a dynamic hip screw, multiple pins, hemiarthroplasty and joint replacement.

Dandy & Edwards (2003) indicate that internal fixation should be considered for the younger, fitter patient with minimal bony displacement and that those who are older, unfit and with greater bone displacement require prosthetic replacement. Extracapsular fractures are usually managed with a dynamic hip screw or nail-plate with a long femoral plate.

Complications are common after hip fracture, many requiring revision surgery, including removal of internal fixation and secondary hemiarthroplasty or joint replacement. All the early and late complications mentioned previously (SAQ 5.9) may occur with these patients, particularly related to the post-surgical condition.

Fractures of the proximal third of the femur predominantly occur in people over the age of 50 years. A report on the 300 000 hip fractures in the USA during 1991 shows that 94% occurred in people over 50 years of age (US Congress Office of Technology 1994). The incidence of hip fracture, mortality and institutionalization varies with ethnicity and geography. Recently, Marottoli et al (1994) reported a hip fracture rate of 4.27% (120/2812 subjects) in Connecticut, USA. In the UK, in one English county, a discrepancy was found between the incidence of hip fracture in different ethnicities, with a 1.3:1 ratio of Asians to

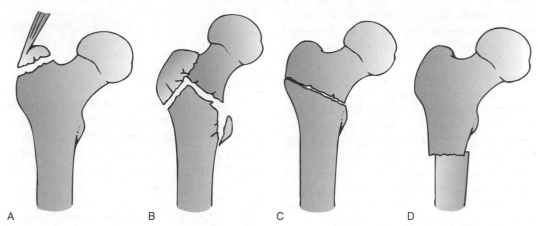

A   B   C   D

Figure 5.18   Hip fractures of the trochanteric region. A: Avulsion of the greater tuberosity. B: Pertrochanteric fracture. C: Intertrochanteric fracture between the trochanters. D: Subtrochanteric fracture. (Adapted with permission from Dandy & Edwards 2003.)

Caucasians in the hip fracture population (Calder et al 1994).

There is a general concern that the number of hip fractures is increasing, as the population lives longer, and that therefore the subsequent increase in financial costs of managing these patients will be immense. Cummings et al (1990) stated that, by the year 2040, 512 000 hip fractures will occur in the USA, with a management cost of $16 billion.

The prospective study of Marottoli et al (1994) from the USA established that, at 6 months post-fracture, 18% of their patients had died and 29% had been institutionalized. Seeman (1995) reports that a third of all hip fractures occur in men and that they have a greater mortality rate than their female counterparts. Dandy & Edwards (2003) states that, in the UK, 10% of older patients with hip fractures die within 6 weeks, 30% within 1 year and, of the remaining 70%, one-third do not return to their premorbid level of activity. The mortality rate also increases with revision surgery, to 28% in the first 6 months and 36% at 1 year (Keating et al 1993). Foubister & Hughes (1989) showed that 75% of patients with hip fractures treated in their unit in the UK returned home following surgery but of those with complications requiring revision surgery (3.7%) only 50% returned home (Keating et al 1993). These rates vary depending on the site of the fracture, with patients with displaced subcapital fractures having a poorer return to functional independence. There is

also a direct relationship between the rate of complications and functional outcome.

Thus it is not surprising to find that most acute orthopaedic, care of the elderly and rehabilitation wards have their fair share of patients with hip fractures. The demand for continuing care both at the patient's home and in care establishments has increased. Marottoli et al (1994) also indicated that the primary predictor for institutionalization was mental status; thus care must be provided because of decreased mental as well as physical ability.

Several schemes have been implemented to try to address these issues, all aiming to return patients to their own home or community as quickly as is feasible. In particular, many accelerated rehabilitation schemes are in operation that allow suitable patients to return home as quickly as possible after the fracture with the necessary level of care provided at home (Pryor & Williams 1989). Cameron et al (1994) studied the cost effectiveness of this type of scheme during 1989/90 and found it to be 38% more effective than conventional hospital care, releasing resources of up to 17%. Thus the accelerated schemes are financially better but the overall return of function may differ.

Williams et al (1994a,b) reported a prospective study on the outcomes of 120 women with hip fracture, mean age 79.9 years, who had all lived at home before the fracture and were discharged to home or nursing home care. Recovery of mobility continued during the 14 weeks post-fracture review, with the most rapid change between 2 and 8 weeks. The return of mobility in patients in short-stay nursing home care (less than 1 month) was equal to that of the home discharge patients, but the longer-term nursing home patients had a slower return or no change in mobility.

Those returning home showed a lower level of emotional distress such as anxiety, depression or manic behaviour than those going to nursing home care, either short- or long-term. However, in all groups the somatic mood distress was high, showing that the trauma of the fracture was highlighted more in physical terms, such as altered cardiovascular signs or functional issues.

Thus early discharge home schemes seem to assist return to function and are more cost effective but are dependent on good mental status and attitude, and of course adequate care at home. In this group of patients, return to independent mobility will be the main objective (Meeds & Pryor, 1990).

Thus the third case study is centred on this area.

Case study 5.3: Mrs Jones, fractured neck of femur (# NOF)

Present complaint

Mrs Jones, a 77-year-old lady, was admitted to hospital via casualty after a fall at home 2 days before. She was discovered by her neighbour lying on the floor, quite cold and unable to get up or walk.

Casualty report

Right leg externally rotated and shortened; on X-ray (R) subcapital # NOF. Early signs of hypothermia and dehydration.

Initial medical care

Skin traction with 3 kg of weight. For internal fixation with dynamic hip screw tomorrow, continue traction until then. Full team assessment and treatment as required.

Subjective assessment

Social history: Mrs Jones lives alone in a converted first floor flat with 24 steps to the front door. No steps inside the self-contained flat, which Mrs Jones owns. Independent prior to fall; no social service support at all.

Mrs Jones has one son and daughter-in-law who live 35 miles away with their two children. They visit occasionally and Mrs Jones spends a week with them twice a year.

Hobbies and interests: until 5 years ago Mrs Jones was a volunteer for the Red Cross and is still an active member of her local church. Enjoys reading, tapestry and listening to music.

Previous medical history: slight OA of the (L) and (R) hips and lumbar spine for previous 10 years. (L) Colles fracture 5 years ago, following a fall, with subsequent weakness and wrist stiffness since. Is able to use the hand functionally.

No other major illnesses or operations. Good eyesight with spectacles and good hearing.

Functional level prior to admission: functionally able about the flat but slower in the morning than in the afternoon. Cannot easily descend stairs, particularly in the morning, because of pain in her hips, but after a walk can climb the stairs more easily. Mrs Jones can walk slowly to the local shops and church, approximately 1 mile away, and occasionally used one stick.

Objective assessment

General posture

Patient lying slouched in bed, with skin traction on the (R) leg. No pillows under either leg; patient looks uncomfortable and in some pain.

Right leg is externally rotated and adducted in the traction and is a mottled colour and feels cold to the touch.

ROM (active)

Hips: Not tested due to patient's discomfort

	(R)	(L)
Knees	0–40°	0–95°
	Limited because of pain and traction	No pain
Ankle	10–80°	10–80°
	No pain	No pain

Passive movement of all joints or the spine Not tested.

Muscle power

	(R) Isometric only	(L) Isometric and isotonic
Gluteus maximus	1	4
Gluteus minimus/ medius	1	4
Quadriceps	1	4
Hamstrings	1	4
Ankle (isotonic)	5	5

Neurology
No numbness or altered sensation in either leg, although Mrs Jones reports that the right leg feels as though it has cramp.

Vascular
- Skin dry and cold on both legs. Right leg slightly mottled and bluish in colour
- Dorsalis pedis not palpable on either leg.

Respiration
- *Observation*: decreased expansion of both bases with the main movement occurring at the apexes
- *Auscultation*: decreased air entry to both bases with audible inspiratory wheeze.

Once again can you answer the five main questions about this patient? This time the answers will not be given separately but you can find them all in this chapter.

1. What do I know about this fracture?
2. What should I find at this stage of the management if the fracture is healing normally?
3. What might go wrong with this fracture?
4. What do I know about this patient, particularly their functional ability?
5. What are the expected overall outcomes for this patient, with this fracture?

Problem–solving exercise 5.11

Remembering that Mrs Jones is going to surgery the next day, what would be the physiotherapy treatment objectives at this time?

Answer
- Maintain respiratory function until after surgery
- Maintain venous return in the lower limbs
- Teach Mrs Jones how to assist with bed mobility if possible
- Try to maintain some muscle tone; it may not be practical to do this until after surgery
- Try to get to know and to reassure Mrs Jones prior to surgery.

Self–assessment question

- **SAQ 5.13** What are the major complications particularly associated with subcapital # NOF?

(Answer at end of chapter.)

When Mr Kingston's post-surgical recovery was discussed, the main emphasis was on the return of specific muscle strength and joint motion. With Mrs Jones the primary consideration is her return to functional independence and then secondarily the return of range of motion and strength around the hip.

This change in emphasis is justified by the description of function. In Mrs Jones's case, function is mainly geared towards getting in and out of bed, rising from sitting, standing independently, independent toileting, walking and stair climbing.

Mr Kingston, however, would not be classed as fully functional unless he was fit to work, to play sport, to play with the children and so on; therefore full range of motion and strength are needed. It could be argued that physiotherapy should help Mrs Jones to gain full range of motion and strength as well as the basic functional requirements. This of course is true, but the range of motion and strength required by Mrs Jones will be far less than that required by Mr Kingston and will be gained by concentrating on basic functional rehabilitation.

Now look back at the answer to SAQ 5.7 on the complications of bed rest (page 100). All these points are especially significant in any elderly patient with this type of fracture but the most important is getting Mrs Jones up and out of bed to increase her general mobility. When the fracture has been stabilized, sitting out of bed can commence on day 1 after the operation and once the drips and drains are out (day 2), walking is made easier. Assistance is obviously needed and it is advisable for two people with a walking frame to be used the first time walking is attempted. Alternatively the patient may be taken to use a set of parallel bars and, again with the assistance of two people, walking can commence. Mrs Jones may also need the assistance of a lifting device to help with toileting. The answers to Problem-solving exercise 5.8 should be taken into consideration: any patient with a fractured neck of femur will find getting out of bed difficult. Mrs Jones's condition has been made worse by the fact that she was lying on the floor for 2 days before being found.

Whatever type of rehabilitation programme Mrs Jones might be following, several other members of the multidisciplinary team need to be involved, including nursing staff, social workers, occupational therapists and the community liaison team. In a well organized rehabilitation set up all these members of staff would already be involved in Mrs Jones's care but if not, then this will need to be instigated. An accelerated rehabilitation programme would have its own team of care staff who liaise and continue care from the hospital to the home environment.

This team is made up of nursing staff, occupational therapists, physiotherapists and assistants as required.

On an accelerated rehabilitation programme Mrs Jones should be ready for discharge at approximately 1 week after the operation, providing the home circumstances are adequate.

Problem-solving exercise 5.12

What would be the criteria for Mrs Jones's discharge on the accelerated rehabilitation programme?

Answer

- Support arranged at home for general day-to-day living: family, meals on wheels, community liaison team, social services, etc.
- Assessment and support from the accelerated rehabilitation team, i.e. physiotherapist, occupational therapists, and nursing staff
- Home visit by occupational therapist and/or physiotherapist with the community liaison team
- Ability to walk short distances with the use of a walking aid (probably a walking frame at this time)
- Some limited functional goals such as washing, toileting, dressing herself
- No medical complications (see Problem-solving exercise 5.9a)
- Full co-operation from Mrs Jones and that she is happy with the arrangements.

As mentioned previously Williams et al (1994a, b) noted the greatest improvement in mobility to be between 2 and 8 weeks after operation; hence it is during this time that maximum rehabilitation support is needed whatever the environment of the patient. Patients kept in hospital at this stage may be moved to care of the elderly or rehabilitation wards to free up acute orthopaedic beds. The alternative is discharge to a nursing home for either short- or long-term care. This may be confusing for patients and recovery can be delayed until patients have time to settle again.

Progression from walking with two people and a frame varies dramatically. If there are no complications then Mrs Jones might be walking with sticks in 2–3 weeks. If any of the major complications develop then this objective would obviously be delayed. Thus the physiotherapist should base mobility gains on realistic objectives, which may be quite limited to start with, such as walk to the end of the bed with assistance of two people and the walking frame.

The goals for walking will then be to reduce the number of people assisting and then to try to gain total independence with the frame. Short frequent walks are more acceptable than a long walk once a day; hence co-operation among the nursing staff is essential to ensure continuity. The family can also be involved at the stage of independence with the frame, to allow them to see the progression but also to give additional encouragement when returning home. It may also be encouraging to introduce a timed walking assessment to give a true objective measurement outcome (Wade 1992, Worsfold & Simpson 2001).

Simpson & Salkin (1993) state that function rehabilitation should be geared towards getting in and out of bed, rising from sitting, standing independently, independent toileting, walking, stair climbing and eventually being able to get off the floor should another fall occur. Now that walking has been started for Mrs Jones, the other functions have to be initiated, such as independent toileting. This activity involves standing independently and moving from sitting to standing and vice versa, but usually in a confined space and to a lower seat. The need to turn the body through 180° is also required. Therefore this function does need to be considered separately from standing to sitting in a chair.

Each function needs to be broken down to specific components and each of these can be re-educated until the total function can be achieved. For example, rising from sitting requires four basic sequences:

1. Moving forward in the chair
2. Moving the body weight forward over the feet (flexion)
3. Lifting the bottom off the seat
4. Extension of the hips, knees and spine into standing (Ada & Westwood 1992, Butler et al 1991, Kerr et al 1991, Nuzik et al 1986).

If each of these sequences is practised until the patient is proficient at it, then the overall movement will be easier. Subsequently the repeated action will help improve muscle strength and endurance, range of motion and balance.

Time must be taken to ensure that Mrs Jones is aware of each of these stages and can recognize the correct movement.

Self-assessment question

- SAQ 5.14 Break down the functions of independent standing, getting in and out of bed and stair climbing, into the basic sequences.

Answer

Independent standing

1. Rising from sitting (as already mentioned)

2. Standing holding on to a walking frame while gaining balance
3. Hands off the frame, one at a time, maintain body weight equally on right and left legs
4. Reverse activities into sitting.

Getting in and out of bed

One of two ways: either with or without rolling on to one side.

Without rolling

Getting out of bed

1. Move towards the edge of the bed – may be easier to go to the non-affected side, but ideally it should be the side the patient is used to getting out of bed from
2. Sit up into half lying
3. Move feet over the side of the bed
4. Move bottom to the edge of the bed
5. Bend forward over the knees and stand up.

Getting into bed

1. Sit on the edge of the bed
2. Shuffle the bottom back as far as possible
3. Lean back on to the arms to the half sitting position
4. Move legs onto the bed, while in the half sitting position
5. Lie down.

With rolling

Getting out of bed

1. Move towards the edge of the bed on the non-affected side
2. With the legs together (a pillow can be placed between the legs to make this more comfortable) roll onto the side
3. Place the uppermost hand on the bed in front of the body and as the legs are being placed over the edge of the bed, push on the hand and the opposite elbow/hand to raise the body into the sitting position.

Getting into bed

Reverse the above procedure.

Stair climbing (no walking aids)

Ascending the stairs

1. Holding on with both hands, body weight on the affected leg, lift the non-affected leg, flexing at the hip and knee (static standing balance needed)
2. Place the non-affected leg on the step and lean forward over the foot
3. Extend the non-affected knee and hip, lifting the body weight up and place the affected leg on the step beside the non-affected leg (dynamic standing balance needed while raising the body weight).

Descending the stairs

1. In standing flex and hitch the affected hip (with knee straight) until it clears the step
2. Lower the affected leg and place on the step below, allowing the non-affected knee to bend in a controlled manner
3. Shift the body weight forward and laterally on to the affected leg while holding on to the banister
4. Lower the non-affected limb on to the step below.

Koval et al (1995) observed mobility recovery in patients with hip fractures at 12–18 months post-operation in a group of 336 community-dwelling patients who had all been ambulant prior to their fracture. Of these, 41% maintained their prefracture mobility, 40% remained ambulant but needed some kind of assisted device (stick or frame), 12% became independent walkers indoors but not outdoors and 8% were non-ambulant (numbers have been rounded so do not add up to 100%). These authors highlight a detailed scale of measurement of ambulation, which could be useful as a functional outcome measure for the physiotherapist.

The scale has seven categories:

1. Independent community walker
2. Community walker with a stick
3. Community walker with frame/crutches
4. Independent household walker
5. Household walker with a stick
6. Household walker with frame/crutches
7. Non-functional walker.

This study highlighted the fact that 59% of their subjects did not return to their prefracture mobility level, incorporating 34% who dropped one level, as defined above, 7% who dropped two levels, 4% who dropped three levels and 14% who dropped four or more levels (Koval et al 1995). The premorbid mobility level was predictive for the mobility outcome level at 12–18 months for all the patients and specifically for those in category 1. Thus the poorer the mobility scale prior to hip fracture the more likely the patient is to return to this level. The other major finding of this paper is that a rating of 3 or 4 on the general health status questionnaire (American Society of Anesthesiologists) was also a strong predictor of mobility outcome.

It is well known that following fracture of the neck of the femur in older people self-confidence is often lost and this hampers the rehabilitation outcome (Department of Health 2002, McQueen 2003). The fear of falling or being unsafe is prevalent and psychological support from both family and therapy staff is essential (Vellas et al 1997). Currently the role of hip protectors is being investigated to see if the number of falls and extent of injury is reduced by using these devices (Chan et al 2000, Kumar & Parker 2000). The hip protectors are made of padded foam to be worn under normal clothing or sewn into trousers or track suit bottoms and absorb the force of impact of the fall. The results show that the incidence of fractured neck of femur due to a fall is reduced when wearing the protectors (Kumar & Parker 2000) and that they are cost effective, particularly for the over 80 age group. There may be some doubt about their acceptance and compliance with their use but in most cases patients seemed to accept the hip protectors and wear them on a regular basis (Chan et al 2000). Although there is no research on the use of hip protectors following # NOF as a result of a fall, the pads should help to give the patient reassurance about sustaining further injury from a fall, particularly as they start to regain their confidence in walking.

Therefore Mrs Jones only has a 50:50 chance of returning to full function providing that there are no complications following surgery and she regains her self-confidence with no fear of falling.

The totally different emphasis and outcome for Mrs Jones compared with, say, Mr Kingston, means that the physiotherapist cannot work alone when the rehabilitation outcomes of a patient are more functionally based. Communication and negotiation with the patient, carers and other staff is particularly important.

Thus the physiotherapist has to change his/her role depending on the short- and longer-term rehabilitation outcome for the individual patient.

SUMMARY

This chapter has not tried to address the physiotherapy management of every fracture, as this would be impossible. However, the basic principles of physiotherapy management of patients with fractures have been addressed. As you apply these to other fractures, you will be able to undertake basic problem solving to help assess and plan the treatment of any patient with any fracture.

This chapter does not stand alone and there are links with those on soft tissue injury, rheumatic conditions and joint replacement. Many complications of soft tissue injury around the fracture site (e.g. tendon, ligament, muscle or nerve) have deliberately been omitted, as these are addressed in Chapter 6. Likewise the complications of fractures in patients with rheumatological conditions have not been covered here.

ANSWERS TO QUESTIONS AND EXERCISES

Self-assessment question 5.1 (page 91)

Answer follows question in text.

Self-assessment question 5.2 (page 94)

Answer follows question in text.

Self-assessment question 5.3 (page 97)

- **SAQ 5.3** A patient has been issued with a collar and cuff immediately after a fracture of the upper third of the humeral shaft. Which joints would you advise him/her to move?

Answer: Move all non-painful joints, i.e. interphalangeals, metacarpophalangeals, radioulnar joints, wrist, elbow (if possible but unlikely), gentle scapulothoracic movements and neck movements.

Self-assessment question 5.4 (page 98)

- **SAQ 5.4** How would the patient know if the POP was causing too much pressure and what advice would be given to them?

Answer:

- *Vascular signs*: distally the skin changes colour to a purple/blue; swelling may appear distal to the fracture or cast and will not reduce on elevation; distal segments of the limb may feel cold and clammy
- *Neurological signs*: altered sensation (paraesthesia) or numbness may occur in the distribution of the nerve root which is being compressed
- *Pain* may increase as a result of either vascular occlusion or nerve compression
- *Advice*: if any of these signs occur, elevate the part and return to the A&E department or GP as quickly as possible.

Self-assessment questions 5.5 and 5.6 (page 98)

Answers follow questions in text.

Problem-solving exercsise 5.1 (page 99)

- What type of support will be given for the arm, and what instructions should be given to the patient prior to review in 5 days time?

Answer: A high sling should be applied to support the hand and POP, in elevation. The patient should be instructed to:

- Observe for any signs of POP pressure (see answer to Self-assessment question 5.4)
- Keep the hand elevated to control oedema
- Observe for signs of infection, e.g. staining on the POP in the presence of an offensive smell; severe cases would have a discharge from the POP
- Keep the fingers mobile by putting the metacarpophalangeal and interphalangeal

joints of all fingers and the thumb through as full a range of movement as possible, increasing this as the pain and oedema decrease

- Remove the sling every hour, to exercise the shoulder into full elevation with full elbow extension and external and internal rotation
- Not get the POP wet
- Not scratch under the POP with long-stemmed items such as rulers or knitting needles (all these can scratch the skin and thus induce infection)
- Take regular painkillers, if and when necessary.

Self-assessment question 5.7 (page 100)

Answer follows question in text.

Self-assessment question 5.8 (page 105)

- **SAQ 5.8** What instructions should be given to a patient with a fracture of the lower third of tibia and fibula who is being sent home non-weight-bearing in a long leg POP cast from thigh to toes?

Answer:

- Keep the limb elevated either by lying down and placing the cast on a pillow or, on sitting, supporting the cast on a high footstool or chair
- Check that the toes do not turn a bluish colour or start to swell excessively
- Observe for infection, pressure areas at top and bottom of POP and excessive ongoing pain
- Keep toes moving through full range at all times
- Keep tightening the quadriceps, hamstrings and both anterior and posterior tibial muscles isometrically in the POP
- When standing up do not place weight down through the POP until medical or therapy staff indicate that this may be done
- Use the crutches for sit/stand, walking, and so on, as instructed prior to leaving hospital.

Self-assessment question 5.9 (page 107)

- **SAQ 5.9** Describe the immediate and longer term complications of fracture healing and rehabilitation.

Answer: *Immediate complications*:

- Infection
- Pressure sores
- Swelling/bruising distal to fracture
- Nerve, vascular, soft tissue damage
- Inability to reduce the fracture.

Postoperative complications:

- General immobility, thus pressure sores
- Reduced respiratory function
- Reduced vascular function
- Electrolyte imbalance.

Fat embolism: not common but if undetected can result in death. Microparticles of marrow fat appear in the circulation usually a few days after fractures of the shaft of femur or the pelvis. Severe hypoxia results from pulmonary insufficiency as the fat globules block the alveoli. Changes are also seen in the brain, kidney and skin. Noticeable by change in mood of the patient, drowsiness and then unconsciousness, tachypnoea (increased rate of respiration) and petechiae (small haemorrhages under the skin; Dandy & Edwards 2003).

Long-term complications: see text.

Problem-solving exercise 5.2 (page 110)

- Attempt to answer all the five major questions about Mrs Andrews and her Colles fracture.

1. *What do I know about this fracture?*

Answer: We have already outlined the type of fracture, its position and expected union and consolidation times and its initial management.

2. *What should I find at this stage of management if the fracture is healing normally?*

Answer: Given the case scenario at the start of treatment, then we expect to find a lady in a dorsal slab POP or a completed cast, supported in a sling. Instruction should have been given regarding exercise, skin care and 'do's and 'don't's. Mrs Andrews will be discharged from A&E and seen in the fracture clinic in 5 days' time for review and again in approximately 5 weeks' time. The POP should be removed at 5–6 weeks when initial physiotherapy assessment and treatment would be undertaken.

3. *What might go wrong with this fracture?*

Answer:

- Median nerve compression, carpal tunnel syndrome
- Rupture of extensor pollicis longus (at approximately 4–8 weeks)
- Potential for Sudeck's atrophy
- Malunion – it is often very difficult to reduce the distal fragment of the radius
- Joint stiffness, predominantly at the fingers, wrist and inferior radioulnar joints, but possibly also occurring at the shoulder and elbow (shoulder–hand syndrome)
- Alteration to the healing rate.

4. *What do I know about this patient, particularly concerning functional ability?*

Answer: Mrs Andrews is a 67-year-old lady who fell on to her outstretched (R) hand. Her functional ability is limited because of her POP and a full assessment is needed once the POP can be removed.

5. *What are the expected overall outcomes for this patient, with this fracture?*

Answer: If no complications arise, then in the next 4 months Mrs Andrews should have a functional wrist but may lack full movement, particularly extension and supination. Depending on her hobbies, she should gain full functional use.

Problem-solving exercise 5.3 (page 110)

- Are these the normal signs of a fracture after removal of POP? Explain why.

Answer: Yes, these are the normal signs of fracture after removal of POP. Following reduction, the wrist is immobilized in flexion and ulnar deviation to hold the bone ends in place, so it would appear in this position on removal from the POP. The thickening of the radius is due to callus formation and that at the wrist is due to the periarticular and intra-articular adhesion. The skin appearance is due to altered vascularization while in the POP, the skin losing its usual look and feel. The forearm is thinner because of muscle wasting on the palmar and dorsal aspects and this will emphasize the thickening at the radius and wrist. The patient will be scared to move the wrist and it will feel lighter and 'strange' immediately after POP removal; therefore it is not surprising that the patient holds the arm close to the body.

N.B. The patient may have held the arm close to the body for the last 5 weeks and therefore you need to check shoulder and elbow function.

Problem-solving exercise 5.4 (page 111)

- What would you need to ask this patient to complete question 4?

Answer:

- *Personal details*: age, occupation, hobbies, home circumstances (e.g. is there anyone to assist her?), hand dominance
- *Main problems now*, and what she has been doing with the arm since injury
- *History of present complaint*: how the fracture occurred and how it was managed, any other injuries at the time
- *Previous medical history*: especially history of osteoporosis, bone disease, diabetes, high blood pressure, respiratory disease, steroid use, major operations, previous fractures.

Self-assessment question 5.10 (page 111)

- **SAQ 5.10** What would you assess in your objective examination?

Answer:

- *Observation*: we already know the appearance of the wrist
- *ROM*: active, passive and accessory range of motion of shoulder, elbow, radioulnar joint, wrist joints and joints of the hand (active and passive movements to be measured with a goniometer/inclinometer)
- *Muscle power*: isometric muscle power across the fingers, wrist and radioulnar joints (this will not overstress the fracture at this stage and will not cause discomfort at the joints, where isotonic strength testing will). Need to test extensor pollicis longus especially. All measured either by use of the Oxford Scale of Manual Muscle Testing or a hand-held dynamometer. Isotonic strength of the muscles around the elbow and shoulder
- *Sensation*: light touch, hot/cold, proprioception, in the wrist and hand, especially median distribution

- *Dexterity of the hand*, i.e. differing types of grips, general hand function (if this is problematic then it may be necessary to refer Mrs Andrews for occupational therapist's assessment for help around the home)
- *Swelling*: measure general swelling at the lower border of the MCP joints.

Problem-solving exercise 5.5 (page 112)

- Describe how you would carry out each of the objectives in Table 5.2.

  Answer:

  Show the patient how to move without causing damage to the wrist and try to reduce pain

  Assisted active movements using the other hand, holding the fracture while doing shoulder and elbow movements, thus assisting with the 'good' arm. Gentle movement should help to reduce the pain but Mrs Andrews can help at home by soaking the hand in contrast baths (hot then cold) or by placing ice over the dorsal aspect of the hand.

  Encourage controlled movement of the wrist, radioulnar, elbow and shoulder joints

  As above but also the use of accessory movements, e.g. rotation of the wrist joint by compressing together the palmar aspect of the pisiform and the dorsal aspect of the head of the ulna, with the index and thumb of the opposite hand. Encourage combined movements, e.g. flexion/extension of the fingers and wrist, so stretching periarticular soft tissue as well as intra-articular adhesions.

  Explain about general care of the skin

  Massage in warm soapy water with some baby oil in it, and then continued use of moisturizer, oil or lanolin to help skin viability.

  Explain the healing times and the need to mobilize and then strengthen the arm before return to bowling

  At this stage the fracture has united and will be consolidated in another 6 weeks' time. Then lifting of a heavy bowls ball may be attempted, provided that the strength of Mrs Andrews's right hand has reached, and slightly exceeded, that of her non-dominant left hand, and also provided that adequate range of motion has been regained. If in doubt, ask Mrs Andrews to demonstrate the bowling action using her left hand, and to weigh the ball so that you know how much she has to lift.

Self-assessment question 5.11 (page 112)

Answer follows question in text.

Problem-solving exercise 5.6 (page 115)

- From Mr Kingston's assessment, can you answer the five major questions?

1. *What do I know about this fracture?*

   Answer: It is a spiral open fracture where the bone must have pierced the skin; this is unstable and needs to be reduced. A period of traction will be needed to allow the bone ends to be realigned and to ensure that the wound is not infected; it would normally be immobilized with internal fixation, using an intramedullary interlocking nail. Union time 6 weeks, consolidation 12 weeks.

2. *What should I find at this stage of management if the fracture is healing normally?*

   Answer: The objective assessment outlines a typical case. The patient is not able to move the limb a great deal; there is swelling and bruising of the thigh and knee. Sliding balance traction is in place, with no knee piece and 4 kg weight. The fracture is acute and still potentially unstable; there is a need to be cautious concerning over-vigorous exercise, particularly with regard to the hip flexors (iliacus and psoas major).

3. *What might go wrong with this fracture?*

   Answer:
   Initially:
   - Infection (osteitis) from open wound
   - Fat embolism
   - Overdistraction
   - Pressure sores from the Thomas splint
   - Nerve damage; may occur due to pressure on the common peroneal nerve at the head of the fibula (unlikely)
   - Vascular changes due to inactivity
   - Bone position might slip if strong hip flexion action is undertaken.

   Long term:
   - Joint stiffness at the knee (mainly flexion) and hip

- Reduced muscle power, quadriceps, hamstrings and anterior and posterior calf muscles
- Malunion (shortening of bone)
- Delayed union.

4. *What do I know about this patient, particularly concerning functional ability?*

Answer: Unable to function well at the moment. Reassess when initial trauma recedes, and some assistance will be needed at this moment. This limitation of movement and independence is a problem to this patient and he will need reassurance that function will return once the fracture has been internally fixed. Need to reassess for crutches later (after surgery).

5. *What are the expected overall outcomes for this patient, with this fracture?*

Answer: If no complications arise then Mr Kingston should regain full use of his leg, with full lower limb movement. This assumes that there are no wound or surgical problems. It will take at least 6 months and will depend on how severe the shoulder injury is. May play football once consolidation of the fracture site has occurred and full strength has been regained.

Problem-solving exercise 5.7 (page 115)

Answer follows question in text.

Self-assessment question 5.12 (page 116)

Answer follows question in text.

Problem-solving exercise 5.8 (page 116)

- What may happen and why, when a patient with a fracture of the lower limb gets up to either sit or stand for the first time?

  Answer:

  - The blood pressure drops dramatically – as a result of shock, not being in the upright position, and surgery. Therefore the patient may feel faint, dizzy or nauseous. This can be prevented by having a staged approach to the vertical position, sitting the patient for longer, first with the legs up and then down

  - The patient's leg may change colour to a purple/red engorged state and feel numb or

tingling. This is due to the sudden gravitational increase in blood in the lower leg; the venous pump is not used to coping with this as the limb has not been dependent. The limb needs to be placed vertically, over short periods of time of increasing duration, until the signs do not occur. Isotonic exercise to the foot and ankle will help with venous return, and should be encouraged with the limb dependent

- The leg may feel heavy. Again this is due to the increase in blood with the limb being dependent, but it is also because of lack of muscle control. Exercise will help this

- Balance, particularly in standing, may be unsafe. Again, as the patient has not been upright an adjustment of the normal balance mechanisms, i.e. spatial awareness and the vestibular system, is needed. Also, of course, the base of support is grossly reduced to one foot.

All these factors may be greater in patients with severe and/or multiple injuries, older people and those who have been on bed rest for longer periods of time.

Problem-solving exercise 5.9 (page 116)

Answer follows question in text.

Problem-solving exercise 5.10 (page 117)

Answer follows question in text.

Problem-solving exercise 5.11 (page 121)

Answer follows question in text.

Self-assessment question 5.13 (page 121)

- **SAQ 5.13** What are the major complications particularly associated with subcapital # NOF?

  Answer:

  - At surgery: avascular necrosis of the head of the femur, mainly due to the poor blood supply to that area; also intracapsular fractures can disrupt the blood supply at the cartilage margins or from the circumflex femoral arteries

- Non-union, because in some cases the femoral head cannot offer adequate fixation for the pins or the dynamic hip screw
- Postoperative confusion
- Infection (either of the wound, bone around fracture or urinary tract). Johnstone et al (1995) report that 12.5% of preoperative and 42% of postoperative hip fracture patients had a urinary tract infection (UTI), and this

occurred particularly in patients with subcapital fractures. Age and time delay to surgery also relate significantly to the presence of UTI.

Problem-solving exercise 5.12 (page 122)

Answer follows question in text.

Self-assessment question 5.14 (page 123)

Answer follows question in text.

References

Ada L, Westwood P 1992 A kinematic analysis of recovery of the ability to stand up following stroke. Australian Journal of Physiotherapy 38: 135–142

Akeson FC, Woo S, Amiel D, Coutts RD 1984 Physiology and therapeutic value of passive joint motion. Clinical Orthopaedics and Related Research 185: 113–125

Audit Commission 1995 United they stand: co-ordinating care for elderly patients with hip fracture. HMSO, London

Bromley I 1998 Tetraplegia and paraplegia. A guide for physiotherapists, 5th edn. Churchill Livingstone, Edinburgh

Bullock-Saxton J 1994 Local sensation changes and altered hip muscle function following severe ankle sprain. Physical Therapy 74: 17–31

Butler P, Nene A, Major R 1991 Biomechanics of transfer from sitting to the standing position in some neuromuscular diseases. Physiotherapy 77: 521–525

Calder SJ, Anderson GH, Harper WM, Gregg PJ 1994 Ethnic variation in epidemiology and rehabilitation of hip fracture. British Medical Journal 309: 1124–1125

Calliet R 1975 Scoliosis, diagnosis and management. FA Davis, Philadelphia, PA

Cameron ID, Lyle DM, Quine S 1994 Cost effectiveness of accelerated rehabilitation after proximal femoral fractures. Journal of Clinical Epidemiology 47: 1307–1313

Chan DK, Hillier G, Coore M et al 2000 Effectiveness and acceptability of a newly designed hip protector: a pilot study. Archives of Gerontology and Geriatrics 30: 25–34

Cheung K, Kwan E, Chan K, Luk K 2003 A new halo-pelvic apparatus. Spine 28: 305–308

Clark M, Watts S 1994 The incidence of pressure sores within a National Health Service Trust hospital during 1991. Journal of Advanced Nursing 20: 33–36

Coast J, Richards SH, Peters TJ et al 1998 Hospital at home or acute hospital care? A cost-minimisation analysis. British Medical Journal 316: 1802–1806

Coutts F, Hewetson D, Matthews J (1989) Continuous passive motion of the knee joint: use at the Royal National Orthopaedic Hospital, Stanmore. Physiotherapy 75: 427–431

Coyle JA, Robertson VJ 1998 Comparison of two passive mobilising techniques following Colles fracture: a multi element design. Manual Therapy 3: 34–41

Crawford Adams J, Hamblen D 1999 Outline of fractures. Churchill Livingstone, Edinburgh

Cummings SR, Rubin SM, Black D 1990 The future of hip fracture in the USA. Numbers, costs and potential effects of postmenopausal oestrogen. Clinical Orthopaedics and Related Research 252: 163–166

Dandy DJ, Edwards DJ 2003 Essential orthopaedics and trauma, 3rd edn. Churchill Livingstone, Edinburgh

Davis S 1991 Effects of continuous passive movement and plaster of Paris after internal fixation of ankle fractures. Physiotherapy 77: 516–520

De Laet C, Pols H 2000 Fractures in the elderly: epidemiology and demography. Baillières Best Practice and Research. Clinical Endocrinology and Metabolism 14: 171–179

Department of Health 2002 Older peoples' national service framework. Available on line at: http://www.doh.gov.uk/nsf/olderpeople/index.htm

Dinah AF 2002 Sequential fractures in elderly patients. Injury 33: 393–394

El-Shazly M, Dalby-Ball J, Burton M, Saleh M 2001 The use of trans-articular and extra-articular external fixation for management of distal tibial intra-articular fractures. Injury 32: S-D-99–S-D-106

Emami A, Mjoberg B, Karlstrom G, Larsson S 1995 Treatment of closed tibial shaft fractures with unilateral external fixation. Injury 26: 299–303

Fischer T, Koch P, Saager C, Kohut GN 1999 The radio-radial external fixators in the treatment of fractures of the distal radius. Journal of Hand Surgery 24B: 604–609

Foubister G, Hughes SPF 1989 Fractures of the femoral neck: a retrospective and prospective study. Journal of the Royal College of Surgeons of Edinburgh 34: 249–252

Gomberg BFC, Gruen GS, Smith WR, Spott MA 1999 Outcomes in acute orthopaedic trauma: a review of 130,506 patients by age. Injury 30: 431–437

Grundy D, Russell J, Swain A 1996 ABC of spinal cord injury, 3rd edn. British Medical Journal, London

Helber MU, Ulrich C 2000 External fixation in forearm shaft fractures. Injury 31: 45–47

Heslinga JW, Kronnie G, Huijing PA 1995 Growth and immobilisation effects on sarcomeres: a comparison between gastrocnemius and soleus muscles of the adult rat. European Journal of Applied Physiology and Occupational Physiology 70: 49–57

Johnstone DJ, Morgan NH, Wilkinson MC, Chissel HR 1995 Urinary tract infection and hip fracture. Injury 26: 89–91

Keating JF, Robinson CM, Court-Brown CM et al 1993 The effect of complications after hip fractures on rehabilitation. Journal of Bone and Joint Surgery 75B: 976

Kerr K, White J, Mollan R, Baird H 1991 Rising from a chair: a literature review. Physiotherapy 77: 15–19

Koval KJ, Skovron ML, Aharonoff GB et al 1995 Ambulatory ability after hip fracture: a prospective study in geriatric patients. Clinical Orthopaedics and Related Research 310: 150–159

Kumar BA, Parker MJ 2000 Are hip protectors cost effectiveness? Injury 31: 693–695

Lavini F, Renzi Brivio L, Pizzoli A et al 2001 Treatment of non-union of the humerus using Orthofix external fixators. Injury 32: S-D-35–S-D-40

Marks R, Allegrante JP, MacKenzie CR, Lane JM 2003 Hip fractures among the elderly: causes, consequences and control. Ageing Research Reviews 2: 57–93

Marottoli RA, Berkman LF, Leo-Summers L, Cooney LM Jr 1994 Predictors of mortality and institutionalisation after hip fractures: the New Haven EPESE cohort. Established Populations for Epidemiologic Studies of the Elderly. American Journal of Public Health 84: 1807–1812

McQueen JM 2003 Fall management and prevention: a day hospital perspective. British Journal of Therapy and Rehabilitation 10: 115–121

McRae R, Esser M 2002 Practical fracture treatment, 4th edn. Churchill Livingstone, Edinburgh

Meeds B, Pryor G 1990 Early home rehabilitation for the elderly patient with hip fracture. The Peterborough hip fracture scheme. Physiotherapy 76: 75–77

Nuzik S, Lamb R, VanSant A, Hirt S 1986 Sit to stand movement pattern. A kinematic study. Physical Therapy 66: 1708–1713

O'Connor D, Mullet H, Doyle A et al 2003 Minimally displaced Colles' fractures: a prospective randomised trial of treatment with a wrist splint or a plaster cast. Journal of Hand Surgery 28B: 50–53

O'Driscoll SW, Giori NJ 2000 Continuous passive motion (CPM): theory and principles of clinical application. Journal of Rehabilitation Research and Development 37: 179–188

Palmer S, Fairbank AC, Bircher M 1997 Surgical complications and implications of external fixation of pelvic fractures. Injury 28: 649–653

Pesco M, Altner P 1993 A protective Orthoplast splint in the treatment of a patient with Colles' fracture by external fixation. Journal of Hand Therapy 6: 39–41

Pryor GA, Williams DR 1989 Rehabilitation after hip fractures. Home and hospital management compared. Journal of Bone and Joint Surgery 71B: 471–474

Rieger H, Winckler S, Wetterkamp D, Overbeck J 1996 Clinical and biomechanical aspects of external fixation of the pelvis. Clinical Biomechanics 11: 322–723

Salihefendic R, Djozic S, Fazlagic S et al 1997 The use of the Sarafix external fixator for the treatment of war injuries. Injury 28: 242

Sato Y, Inose M, Higuchi I et al 2002 Changes in the supporting muscles of the fractured hip in elderly women. Bone 30: 325–330

Seeman E 1995 The dilemma of osteoporosis in men. American Journal of Medicine 98: 76S–88S

Simpson JM, Salkin SI 1993 Are elderly people at risk of falling taught how to get up again? Age and Ageing 44: 294–296

Swiontkowski MF, Chapman JR 1995 Cost and effectiveness in care of injured patients. Clinical Orthopaedics and Related Research 318: 17–24

Syed A, Agarwal M, Boome R 2003 Dynamic external fixators for Pilon fractures of the proximal interphalangeal joints: simple fixators for a complex fracture. Journal of Hand Surgery 28B: 137–141

Tetsworth K, Paley D 1994 Mal-alignment and degenerative arthropathy. Orthopedic Clinics of North America 25: 367–377

US Congress Office of Technology 1994 Hip fracture outcomes in people aged fifty and over. OTA-BP-H-120 US Government Printing Office, Washington, DC

Vellas BJ, Wayne SJ, Romero LJ et al 1997 Fear of falling and restriction of mobility in elderly fallers. Age and Ageing 26:189–193

Wade DT 1992 Measurement in neurological rehabilitation. Oxford University Press, Oxford

Weiner LS, Kelley M, Yang E et al 1995 The use of combination internal fixation in severe proximal tibial fractures. Journal of Orthopaedic Trauma 9: 244–250

White R, Schuren J, Konn DR 2003 Semi-rigid vs rigid glass fibre casting: a biomechanical assessment. Clinical Biomechanics 18: 19–27

Williams MA, Oberst MT, Bjorklund BC 1994a Post hospital convalescence in older women with hip fracture. Orthopaedic Nursing 13: 55–64

Williams MA, Oberst MT, Bjorklund BC 1994b Early outcomes after hip fracture among women discharged home and to nursing homes. Research in Nursing and Health 17: 175–183

Williams PE, Goldspink G 1978 Changes in sarcomere length and physiological properties in immobilized muscle. Journal of Anatomy 127: 459–468

Worsfold CC, Simpson JM 2001 Standardisation of a three-metre walking test for elderly people. Physiotherapy 87: 125–132

Chapter 6

Soft tissue injuries

Anne-Marie Hassenkamp

CHAPTER CONTENTS

OBJECTIVES

By the end of this chapter you should:

- Have an insight into and overview of the classification of soft tissue injuries, the average healing times, the different managements and common complications
- Understand and be able to implement the assessment of a patient with a soft tissue injury
- Be able to identify how to problem solve for and with a patient in relation to assessment and treatment for a patient with a soft tissue injury irrespective of the exact nature and site of the injury or the medical management
- Have an understanding of the latest physiotherapy guidelines.

KEYWORDS

Soft tissues, classification, management, complications, physiotherapy management, long-term outcome, soft tissue injury guidelines.

Prerequisites

Make sure that you have familiarized yourself again with the physiology of soft tissue healing and the medical management of soft tissue injuries.

For that you might find the following texts helpful:

- Dandy DJ 1998 Essential orthopaedics and trauma, 3rd edn. Churchill Livingstone, Edinburgh
- Crawford Adams J, Hamblen DL 1995 Outline of orthopaedics, 12th edn. Churchill Livingstone, Edinburgh
- Another useful text for background reading is Anderson MK, Hall SJ 1995 Sports injury management. Williams & Wilkins, Baltimore, MD
- Shirley Sahrmann's work (Sahrmann S 2000 Diagnosis and treatment of movement impairment syndromes. Mosby, St Louis, MO) is absolutely essential for any physiotherapist working in the musculoskeletal field.

INTRODUCTION

About the connective tissues

Connective tissues are one of the four principal tissues in the body and their general functions include (Clancy & McVicar 1995):

- Protection for delicate organs, which they surround
- Provision of a structural framework for the body
- Supporting and binding of other interconnecting tissue types within organs
- Transportation of substances from one region to another
- Internal defence mechanism against potential pathogenic invaders
- Storage of energy reserves.

True connective tissues have a viscous matrix and two types of cell:

- *Fixed cells*, which have either a homeostatic, repair function (e.g. fibroblasts and fibrocytes), a homeostatic defence function (e.g. macrophages) or a storage function (e.g. adipocytes)
- *Wandering cells*, which mostly have a defence function (e.g. macrophages).

They also contain three different kinds of fibre:

- *Collagen fibres*: long, straight, stiff and strong and give the tissue tensile strength
- *Reticular fibres*: made of reticulin and interwoven between the collagen fibres, adding flexibility to the properties provided by the collagen
- *Elastic fibres*: made of elastin, stretchable and give the tissue some elasticity (Clancy & McVicar 1995).

Having looked at the different fibres that make up connective tissue it is important to recognize that some of them are true connective tissues while others are specialized for different functions: (Clancy & McVicar 1995).

True connective tissues (as discussed above) consist of:

- a viscous matrix
- fixed or wandering cells
- collagen, reticulin or elastin fibres.

Vascular connective tissues consist of:

- Blood
  - matrix – plasma
  - cells – leukocytes, erythrocytes, thrombocytes
  - fibres.
- Lymph
  - matrix – lymph
  - cells – leukocytes
  - fibres.

Skeletal connective tissues consist of:

- Blood
  - matrix – inorganic salts of calcium
  - cells – osteocytes
  - fibres – ossein.
- Cartilage
  - matrix – chondrin
  - cells – chondrocytes
  - fibres – elastin and collagen.

Adipose connective tissues consist of:

- Blood
  - matrix – interstitial fluid with high lipid content
  - cells – adipocytes
  - fibres – collagen (rare).

As mentioned before, connective tissues are only one of the four principal tissues. The others are:

Epithelial tissues, which deal mainly with:

- protection
- transport (across membranes)
- lining of internal cavities
- secretion (e.g. sweat, tears).

Muscle tissue, which includes:

- skeletal (striped, voluntary)
- smooth (non-striped, involuntary)
- cardiac.

Nervous tissue, which consists of:

- neurons (conducting and receiving stimuli)
- neuroglia (protecting neurons).

In summary, therefore, one can say that there are four principal tissues, which differ according to their special function and hence their location.

> **Self-assessment questions**
>
> - **SAQ 6.1** How are connective tissues classified?
> - **SAQ 6.2** The physiological functions of collagen fibres lead clearly to the biomechanical properties the body expects soft tissues to have. What are they?
>
> (Answers at end of chapter.)

The soft tissues that we as physiotherapists will be dealing with are mainly ligaments, fasciae, muscles and their tendons, bursae, capsules, nerves and their sheaths. Clearly, such a group of different anatomical entities has a wide variety of functions. These can be briefly summarized as:

- Ligaments secure and allow movements of joints
- Muscles are responsible for movement, stability, strength
- Bursae and capsules generally support, nourish and protect vulnerable or heavily used joint regions
- Nerves allow for rapid communication of the body with all its parts.

As with almost all other tissues and systems in the body, injury of soft tissues can occur through trauma, overuse (particularly of a repetitive kind), disease and chemical agents such as inflammatory processes. This variety of different functions and causes for injury often makes soft tissue injury an everyday occurrence as well as being a feature of, for example, big road traffic accidents. It also means that this kind of injury or damage happens very frequently and hence to most people in a variety of ways.

Stages of healing

Before the management issues can be discussed in more detail, it is necessary to look at the different stages of healing. For this the reader is referred to Evans (1980) and Clancy & McVicar (1995).

The process is understood to involve three major stages: injury, inflammation and repair, or the inflammatory phase, the proliferative phase and finally the remodelling or maturation phase. Evans (1980) explains that, although these phases are definitely separate, they do overlap to a certain extent. The most important signs of inflammation therefore are *calor* (heat), *rubor* (redness), *dolor* (pain) and *tumor* (swelling).

Dandy (1998) and the physiotherapy soft tissue injury guidelines (ACPSM 1999) summarize it like this:

1. After the injury the torn fibres bleed, the space fills with clot and the surrounding vessels dilate. This is the time of calor and rubor. Inside the dilated capillaries, the rate of blood flow slows.

   White blood cells invade the clot after about 4 hours. The heat and redness take a few hours to develop. They are caused by a rise in local tissue temperature, which increases the metabolic demands of the area leading to vasodilatation. The pain (dolor) is caused by chemicals released at the site of injury by the dead and dying cells acting on the bare nerve endings of pain fibres.

   As the swelling increases the pressure in the tissues rises and hence pain can also be caused by increased tissue pressure. The swelling is a consequence of the increased permeability of the blood vessel walls, caused by the release of chemicals by the damaged cells. This swelling is mostly quite fluid (inflammatory exudates) and contains a large number of inflammatory cells and a high concentration of protein. This has two major effects:

a. It contains fibrinogen, which takes part in the fight against infection. The rest of the inflammatory exudates will result in scar tissue

b. The presence of protein increases the osmotic pressure of the tissue fluid in the injured area, hence starting to suck out more fluid from the local capillaries and into the tissues.

The swelling therefore starts to appear about 2 hours after injury and can continue until 4 days. If swelling occurs immediately, it is often a sign of bleeding into the joint.

2. During the first 2–3 days, the wound margins fill with macrophages, which remove dead tissue. Fibroblasts and capillary buds appear and the clot is replaced with granulation tissue.

3. Between 3 and 14 days, the fibroblasts form fibrous tissue, vascularity diminishes and the scar contracts to 80% of its original size. After 14 days the wound is healed soundly enough to withstand normal stresses but does not regain its full strength until 3 months.

4. Between 2 weeks and 2 years, the fibrous tissue contracts further. The wound, which is a dull purplish colour at first, gradually becomes pale. Scars on the flexor aspect of joints produce tight contractures but those on the extensor aspect of joints stretch and leave ugly white scars.

From this it becomes clear, therefore, that a few hours, 2–3 days, 3–14 days and 2 weeks post-injury are important landmarks in the management of soft tissue injuries that will be directly related to treatment goals.

Desrosiers et al (1995) demonstrated in a study looking at injured canine anterior cruciate ligaments that mechanical stimulation as provided by physiotherapy was essentially the only factor able to improve ligament healing. They found that the scar tissue was aligned with the ligament fibres rather than being perpendicular to it. This clearly results in a more elastic and tensile ligament.

Connective tissues are unique among the tissues of the body in that, because of their fibre make-up

and distribution they are much more deformable than other tissues. Each of the connective tissues mentioned earlier has unique mechanical properties depending on its function, e.g. those structures made up of more elastin than collagen are able to deform more than those with more collagen than elastin. These latter fibres, being stiffer and less able to deform on demand, are more prone to tearing earlier.

What happens to a ligament once it becomes stretched? The stress–strain curve will give some help with this. Stress may be either tensile if a material is stretched or compressive if its ends are pushed together. Strain on the other hand implies a change in length. Smith (1995) identifies strain as the amount of force needed before collagen becomes strained and elongated. Initially, she suggests, the slack is taken up before stress and strain become proportional to each other. This means that the more force is applied to the ligament the more it deforms in response to this demand. Elongation happens here and no damage has been caused, meaning that the tissues can go back to neutral once the force is released. This is referred to as elasticity.

The ability to slowly deform under a constant load for a limited amount of time and then return to the starting point – provided the original forces decrease – is known as creep.

However, if the force continues to increase, microfailure starts to occur, leading to a flattening of the curve. This indicates that the fibres cannot deform any more and the plastic range of the tissues has been reached. Actual break-up of the tissues will occur after plasticity has been reached if the load continues. Recovery to the status quo is now no longer possible but a healing cycle involving fibrosis will take place. Smith (1995) points to the importance of connective tissue being a dynamic structure, which is able to respond to applied forces with a series of plastic changes.

Fibrosis or scarring will happen in a very disorganized way, with fibres pointing into any direction. In order to influence the alignment of these fibres, stresses simulating functional activities have to occur. Reynolds et al (1996) established that this remodelling process of collagen is much quicker and more effective soon after the injury, reducing massively after 2 months and being virtually nil after 1 year. This is a very important time scale for rehabilitation.

CLASSIFICATION OF SOFT TISSUE INJURIES

1. **Ligaments/tendons**. The differentiation here refers to the loss of stability incurred (Fig. 6.1):
   - *Sprain*: stability is not affected
   - *Partial rupture*: some fibres are torn and hence there is some loss of stability but some fibres are still intact, e.g. subluxation
   - *Complete rupture*: loss of stability and continuity of ligament has occurred, e.g. dislocation.

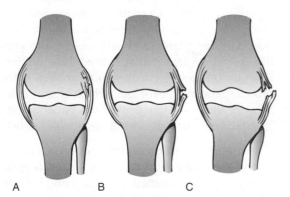

Figure 6.1 Grades of ligament injury: (A) sprain; (B) partial rupture; (C) complete rupture. (Adapted with permission from Dandy 1990.)

2. **Muscles** can be injured through:
   - crushing
   - laceration
   - ischaemia
   - ectopic ossification (Fig. 6.3).
3. **Nerves** can be affected by:
   - division
   - stretching
   - crushing.
4. **Blood vessels** can be injured by (Fig. 6.2):
   - division
   - stretching
   - spasm
   - crushing.

Self-assessment question

- **SAQ 6.3** What is the difference in classification of injuries between ligamentous injuries on the one hand and injuries to blood vessels, muscles and nerves on the other?

(Answer at end of chapter.)

As mentioned earlier in the text, soft tissue injuries can have a multitude of different causes,

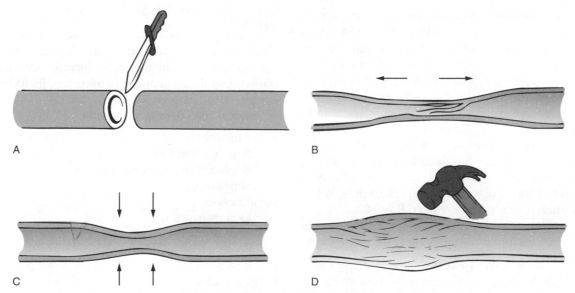

Figure 6.2 Types of injury to blood vessels: (A) complete division; (B) stretching; (C) spasm; (D) soft tissue damage to the wall. (Adapted with permission from Dandy 1998.)

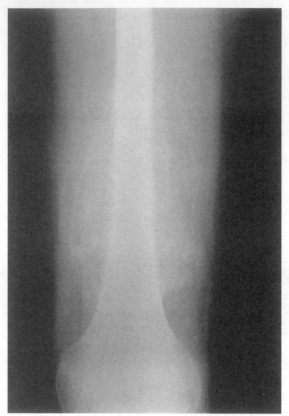

Figure 6.3 Ectopic ossification within muscle following fracture. (Reproduced with permission from Dandy 1998.)

e.g. a road traffic accident, sports injury, simple everyday activity like walking along the street. They can occur alone but of course often occur in conjunction with other, more serious injuries. Soft tissue injuries that occur in the presence of fractures are often classified in a different way from the above-mentioned list. This classification depends on the surgical principles and on the individual prognosis for each trauma. In the Anglo-American literature these combined bony and soft tissue injuries are classified according to Gustillo (Dandy 1998) as open fractures 1–3 and the subclassification of grade 3 lesions as A, B and C.

Injuries may occur not only for a multitude of different reasons but also in many different ways:

- *Through a direct or indirect cause.* A direct cause might be, for instance, a blow to the arm resulting in a painful deltoid muscle, while an indirect cause would hint towards a secondary fact,

e.g. a subluxation of a joint resulting in severe stretching of the ligamentous and capsular fibres surrounding it.

- *Through an underlying pathology.* Several disease processes are known to involve collagen fibres, e.g. rheumatoid arthritis, which can result in tears of the upper cervical ligaments. It is known that age affects tendons and ligaments and makes them more prone to failure under mechanical loading (Astrom & Rausing 1995).

- *Through stress or fatigue.* This overuse factor is often seen in sports injuries or people who repetitively perform a particular movement, e.g. using a keyboard. Repetitive stress injury (RSI) is a classic long-term overuse problem, although it is as yet unclear if that is the whole picture. Another frequently encountered problem is the muscle-patterning problem, which is seen in all areas of the body (particularly in patients with low back pain or long-standing shoulder pain).

The importance of these different causes lies of course in the assessment on the one hand (e.g. do you only assess the immediate region and investigate the mechanical nature of the injury or do you explore lifestyle issues and a precise medical history?) and treatment management on the other.

MANAGEMENT OF SOFT TISSUE INJURIES

This is basically either conservative or surgical.

Conservative considerations include immobilization, mobilization and rehabilitation, including advice.

Surgical considerations include:

- For ligaments
  - Repair when torn
  - Replacement or reconstruction
  - Shortening
- For nerves
  - Decompression
  - Repair when torn
  - Freeing (neurolysis)
  - Grafts
- For muscles
  - Reattachment
  - Transposition

- For tendons
  - Reattachment
  - Transfer
- For capsules
  - Resection
  - Splitting.

Immobilization or protection

Once the injury has occurred and bleeding is still in progress, any movement is going to be severely painful.

Depending on the location and extent of the injury, immobilization can either be partial or complete. It is designed to protect the injured tissues from undue stress, which may disrupt the healing process and delay rather than promote healing (ACPSM 1999). This can be achieved by several different means:

- Elastic bandage (partial)
- Tubigrip (partial)
- Strapping (partial)
- Plaster of Paris (complete)
- Slings
- Splints
- Crutches
- Bed rest.

Partial immobilization

This is:

- very specific to a particular anatomical region, e.g. the ankle joint, and will not involve the related neighbouring joint (in the case of the ankle, the knee joint) – when using Tubigrip only the forefoot and the ankle up to midcalf will be covered

- very specific to the plane of movement involved; it will therefore assist the function of the injured structures. In the case of a twisted ankle due to an inversion injury the strapping will therefore involve the lateral and inferior aspect of the joint rather than the joint as a whole.

Tubigrip/elastic bandage

The advantage of Tubigrip or an elastic bandage is that on the whole it is affordable and easily managed by the patient because its application is very general and does not require any anatomical precision. It can also be used immediately while the injured area is still swelling or while the injury is too painful to allow the detailed examination necessary for more precise techniques.

Strapping

This is usually even cheaper and often more comfortable than Tubigrip as it is less bulky. It needs to be applied very precisely to be of any use and to be comfortable. It can be applied once the swelling is subsiding. This management needs much more specialized help (and enough time to teach the patient) to be effective. It is essential that strapping (in contrast to, for example, Tubigrip) is checked regularly for signs of skin damage caused by the adhesive tape. Attention to possible continuing swelling has to continue as a matter of urgency and safety.

Complete immobilization

Plaster of Paris (POP) affords complete immobilization but at times its disadvantages outweigh the obvious advantages: clearly, if a complete tear of a ligament (tendons tear very rarely!) has caused severe instability of a region a POP cylinder supporting that region might be the only option – especially if there has been surgical repair. It is important to remember, though, that immobilization severely weakens soft tissues and hence makes them more prone to re-injury. In a famous study, Noyes et al (1974) immobilized the knees of monkeys in POP casts for 8 weeks. The resultant weakening of the anterior cruciate ligament took 9 months to recover. Instead of complete POP immobilization continuous passive motion (CPM) is currently accepted as the treatment of choice when the promotion of the healing is a primary outcome. Refer to Amiel et al (1995), Beaupre et al (2001) and Chen et al (2000) for a more detailed discussion of the effects of CPM.

The subsequent management will obviously depend on the kind of immobilization chosen initially and therefore has to be included in the goal setting as it will affect the overall outcome.

Self-assessment question

- SAQ 6.4 A patient with a slight sprain of the wrist is managed with a Tubigrip over the radiocarpal joint. What areas/joints would you need to include in your assessment and treatment?

(Answer at end of chapter.)

LIGAMENTOUS INJURIES

Case study 6.1: John Brown (1)

John Brown is a 25-year-old man and a keen hobby footballer. Yesterday, while playing football, he was tackled and fell. Although he immediately felt pain he was able to play on, but his pain got much worse once he stopped playing. He now complains of a sharp pain on the medial aspect of his right knee, which increases on extension.

Self-assessment question

- SAQ 6.5 What would you expect in terms of objective findings when examining John Brown's knee? (You might need to refer back to Chapter 3.)

Answer

- *Look*: This is a very new or acute injury and hence you expect to see strong reddening of the affected area (due to the dilatation of blood vessels and increased permeability of vessels). This reddening is going to be quite localized over the medial aspect of John's knee.
- *Feel*: there is going to be a localized swelling over the injury site that feels warm to the touch.
- *Test*: all movements will be uncomfortable actively and passively alike because of the inflammatory process in that region.
- Flexion is full (though painful) but extension is the really aggravating movement, resulting in a

very localized sharp pain on the medial aspect of the knee. This pain radiates along a narrow band of about 5 cm from the femur to the tibia (i.e. along the site of the medial collateral ligament).
- Medial distraction of the knee is very painful but lateral distraction is only moderately uncomfortable.
- No signs of instability have been elicited.

The meaning of the problem to John

John is young and a keen footballer – although clearly not as fit as he could be. It might be that his entire social life is linked to his sporting activities or that he lives up on the third floor without a lift.

Remember that the meaning of the injury to the patient is often the most important aspect to find out in an assessment.

Self-assessment question

- SAQ 6.6 What kind of question would you feel most comfortable with and what do you think is important to elicit in order to get a feel for the remits of rehabilitation?

(Answer at end of chapter.)

Case study 6.1: John Brown, continued (2)

John can only walk with a pronounced limp, leaning on an umbrella.

The most likely diagnosis is going to be a medial collateral ligament sprain of the knee.

Classic signs for that injury are:

- Immediate pain at injury but able to continue to play (impossible with a muscle injury), with worse pain at rest
- Pain in the closed packed position of the knee, which stretches the medial collateral ligament
- Stable knee (hence a sprain and not a rupture)
- Localized pain (ligaments of the knee do not refer pain)

- It is clear that any joint examination is never done in isolation but needs to involve related structures, e.g. for the knee the other components of the closed kinetic chain have to be included (hip and foot). For a more detailed background on examination procedures the reader is referred to Hertling & Kessler (1996).

Management

The conservative treatment of soft tissue injuries consists of either protection and rest, or mobilization, ice, compression and elevation. These are therefore abbreviated as PRICE or MICE.

The guidelines on soft tissue injury management (ACPSM 1999) are clear about the importance of these during the first 72 hours after the injury. It makes sense to be guided by the particular stage of injury/inflammation. As long as wound edges are gaping and bleeding any increase in movement and hence tension will delay the inflammatory process and hence protection and rest seem to be the logical advice to give. If on the other hand you are only able to see the patient after 3 days when granulation has occurred, then it seems to make sense to start immediately with some mobilization to encourage the forming scar to be laid down in the line of stress, i.e. in the way that body needs to be used in future. Buckwalter (1995) discusses the arguments for treating soft injuries with rest or activity.

Problem–solving exercise 6.1

Using the examination and assessment findings and relating them to the different stages of the inflammatory cycle, what would be the first line of John's management? After you have worked through this exercise for yourself, compare your answers with those in the following section.

Initial management for John Brown

1. He should first be given some protective bandage/Tubigrip. Rest for the first 24–36 hours post-injury will help to protect the sprained ligament

from further damage. Advice should be given on minimizing stair climbing, sitting in deep chairs, etc., as all of these require very strong muscle contractions, which might interfere with the healing process.

2. An icepack will help minimize further haemorrhage and swelling. This John should be using several times a day for short periods (20–30 min) on top of a wet towel to prevent a burn.

3. Compression can be applied via an elastic bandage or even a splint. This should extend to about 10 cm superiorly and inferiorly beyond the knee. Always apply compression from distal to proximal.

4. Elevation should be encouraged to prevent fluid stasis, which would obviously prolong swelling and hence the inflammatory process. Ideally, elevate the injured part above the level of the heart.

In addition John should be given a pair of crutches for a few days (remember that he seemed to indicate problems with weight bearing by leaning on an umbrella). This will help to distribute the forces generated by walking and therefore protect his knee during the early stages of healing.

With John's injury the compression element was achieved by using an elastic bandage. This aim could also be achieved by the use of Tubigrip, which is an elastic stocking-like tube. It is more expensive than the bandage and requires good hand and arm movement and strength to apply it. Its advantage, though, is in the even pressure throughout that is applied.

A very important aspect of John's early management is emotional support. The suddenness and painfulness of a soft tissue lesion can knock all the confidence out of a sportsperson. He will need reassurance about the nature of the injury, the possible timescale and the hoped-for realistic outcome.

Self-assessment question

- **SAQ 6.7** What do you base your assumptions on timescale and outcome on?

(Answer at end of chapter.)

Subsequent treatment

Clearly, John is a keen sportsman who will want and need to achieve a high level of flexibility and strength as quickly as possible. This is one reason for starting his rehabilitation soon, the other being the quality of the scar. Fibrous tissues need to be laid down in the line of stress and use, which will only happen if the ligament is encouraged to simulate exactly that. John therefore needs to start moving his knee as fully as possible as soon as the pain and swelling allow (after about 2–3 days).

He can begin with gentle autoassisted and then active exercises maintaining range of movement (ROM; don't forget the non-affected parts of his body) and isometric contractions first of quadriceps, later of hamstrings and hip muscles (holding the contraction to the count of 10) for the maintenance of strength. These are carried out several times a day (?every hour if John agrees).

You might want to try some ice and frictions after the first 3 days to ensure a good-quality scarring process. These are done by rubbing the fingers transversely (i.e. in a right angle towards the orientation of the ligamentous fibres) and can only be tried once the internal bleeding has completely stopped.

Frictions involve enough pressure to include the patient's subcutaneous tissues in the movement. The main action seems to be a counter-irritation and hence an increase in local blood supply. Therefore the manoeuvre must never be attempted until the acute inflammatory stages have subsided.

After a few days (3–5) John should be weight bearing, walking normally and only using his Tubigrip if the swelling has not totally subsided.

After about 1 week he should be able to start with gentle jogging, walking on uneven surfaces (to help proprioception), then beginning exercising on stairs and finally to start with short 'stop–start' sprints to really load his knee and to give him the confidence that he will be all right at speed (playing football) and at awkward angles.

The management of the acute lesion therefore has the aim of (Hertling & Kessler 1996):

- Decreasing pain and swelling
- Preventing deformity and protection of the joint
- Preventing stiffness
- Preventing muscle atrophy and tight adhesions
- Regaining strength and confidence.

Electrotherapy

You might wish to consider several different electrotherapy modalities in John's management. Carley et al (1985) discuss the use of electrotherapy for the acceleration of wound healing in a randomized controlled clinical trial. The reader is also referred to Low & Reed (1994) for an extensive discussion on this area and how it relates to healing times and quality of scar tissues. Tim Watson's work (1996, 2000) is another area of important reading.

Review point

John has a clearly defined simple sprain of a knee ligament, surely one of the most frequent soft tissue injuries.

Before you move on, be sure you are certain about the important aspects of this case:

- How did it happen?
- Did it necessitate an abrupt stop of the activity? What was the reason for this?
- Was there any swelling? Why?
- How did the pain behave on movement and weight bearing?
- What were the pertinent findings that helped you to identify the structure in question?
- What pathological processes influenced the timescale of the healing?
- What key aims did the management have and how did these relate to the healing timescale.

Problem–solving exercise 6.2

How would these principles [see text] help you with the assessment and treatment of a patient with a simple sprain in a non-weight-bearing region of the body, e.g. a sprain of the interphalangeal joint (collateral ligament) of the second digit on the dominant hand?

Include in your deliberations the likely cause (?which movement) of this injury.

The following problem is equally often seen in practice:

Case study 6.2: Gemma Jackson (1)

Gemma Jackson is a 35-year-old woman who tripped on the pavement on her way to work, resulting in a severe inversion sprain of her ankle. Her pain is so severe that an ambulance is called and she is seen in the Accident and Emergency (A&E) Department. A stress X-ray (plantarflexion and inversion) demonstrates that although no fractures have been sustained a partial ligamentous rupture has occurred. This might result in some instability.

Self-assessment question

- **SAQ 6.8** How would an X-ray be able to demonstrate that diagnosis?

(Answer at end of chapter.)

Case study 6.2: Gemma Jackson, continued (2)

When you see Gemma (coming straight from A&E), she complains of severe pain on the lateral aspect of her ankle. On examination it becomes apparent that she is unable to move the ankle in any way or weight bear on it.

Self-assessment question

- **SAQ 6.9** Remembering John's sprain and treatment, how would you approach Gemma's treatment?

Answer

Gemma clearly also has a severe ligament injury and hence the initial aims are the same as John's. The PRICE regime is applied to reduce pain and swelling. Instead of just severely overstretching the ligament, as John had done, Gemma has acquired a partial rupture, resulting in some instability of the ankle joint. In order to protect the joint from further damage therefore it is necessary to augment the stability of the joint by supplementing the injured lateral ligaments of the ankle (calcaneofibular ligament, bifurcate ligament and/or dorsal calcaneocuboid ligament). This can be achieved by strapping the ankle in slight eversion. The lower leg needs to be shaved and Friar's balsam, etc. applied to the skin to protect it from the sticky tape. Then use some adhesive spray on the area, again to protect the skin as well as to increase the stickiness of the tape. Sometimes some adhesive weaving underlay is useful to reduce the problems with the adhesiveness.

A horseshoe-shaped piece of felt or foam rubber should be used to fill in the submalleolar depressions prior to the strapping so that the tape will be able to obtain equal pressure and to reduce the risk of a haematoma forming. The basket-weave adhesive tape strapping should always be applied from the medial aspect of the leg, passed under the heel with the foot held in eversion and extended up the lateral aspect of the leg under slight tension in order to pull the ankle into slight eversion.

If this strapping has been applied well, inversion, eversion and rotation of the ankle will be limited.

Caution with strapping:

- Never strap before an assessment has been completed
- Strapping is not a first aid measure
- Never strap if you are unsure of the injury
- Check skin sensation
- Never strap if there is an open wound
- There is little research into the effect of bracing and taping (Barkoukis et al 2002).

In contrast to John, who only needed a locally applied bandage or Tubigrip, Gemma needs to have support covering her foot and her lower leg up to the knee in order to effectively combat swelling.

Therefore, ligamentous injuries, which interfere with the stability of the joint because that joint is anatomically even more reliant on its ligaments for stability, benefit from being strapped as part of the PRICE regime.

Self-assessment question

- **SAQ 6.10** What is the rationale for the PRICE regime in this case? How long would you advise the patient to persist with this approach? Are there any contraindications to this treatment? (See below.)

Problem-solving exercise 6.3

Once the PRICE regime can be progressed, what will be your treatment aims? Refer back to John's story if you need help in order to understand where John and Gemma are similar and where they differ.

Progression of treatment

This will involve the following:

- Ice and frictions (be sure the internal bleeding has completely stopped)

- Passive movements (accessory as well as physiological) in order to maintain full ROM – think of the scar quality at all times!

- Active exercises to improve ROM and strength; don't forget the non-affected regions

- Gentle weight bearing aiming to progress to full weight bearing within a few days

- Wobble board. Because of the force of the inversion injury, articular nerve fibres and their mechanoreceptors, which play a part in the reflex stabilization of the ankle joint, have been separated. Gemma needs much more help than John with building up her neuromuscular

co-ordination. This can be achieved by frequent use of the wobble-board, first in one movement plane then progressing to all possible planes. Readers are referred to Freeman & Wyke (1967) for more early background reading on this. The effect of strength and speed of torque development in the ankle is a huge research area and Robinovitch et al (2002) describe the specific combinations of baseline ankle torque, rate of torque generation and peak torque that are required to attain rebalancing after a trip/near miss. Proprioception is a very difficult concept, which seems to have functions that are sensory and those that are not. Stillman (2002) discusses the terms proprioception, kinaesthesia, motor control and balance in his readable papers

- Gentle trampolining

- Gentle jogging

- Any functional activity that fits in with Gemma's lifestyle (refer back to the subjective part of the assessment)

- Active strengthening exercises involving the calf, ankle and foot muscles; this is necessary for security in the region

- Core stability work (O'Sullivan et al 1997).

Signs for more caution would be:

- Persistent pain
- Swelling that recurs regularly.

Remember that it will take quite some time for the ligament to achieve its maximum elastic and tensile strength after an injury like this (refer back to the healing timescale if you are unsure of this). You need to caution Gemma about loading the ankle too soon in a position where it needs to rely a lot on its lateral ligaments (e.g. walking on rough ground in unsupportive shoes, walking barefoot on the beach, etc.).

It is of great importance to advise Gemma (as well as John) of the need to continue with her stretches and strengthening exercises for many weeks if not months in order to influence the scar as long as it still changes. This will ensure the strongest possible ligamentous repair and hence decrease the likelihood of a secondary injury due to a poor primary repair.

For more detail on the assessment techniques and the biomechanical considerations and rationale refer to Hertling & Kessler (1996).

Review of the literature on treatment of ankle soft tissue injuries

Ogilvieharris & Gilbart (1995), in a superb review, examined the English-language medical literature on soft tissue injuries of the ankle published between 1966 and 1993. A total of 84 articles were analysed reporting the treatment results of 32 025 patients. The authors concluded that non-steroidal anti-inflammatory drugs (NSAIDs) shortened the time to recovery and were associated with less pain. Active mobilization appeared to be the treatment of choice. Ice and Diapulse were also reported as being helpful while ultrasound, diathermy, aspiration and injections were not identified as particularly helpful. Again, the earlier quoted work by Tim Watson will be helpful to you at this point (Watson 1996, 2000). Robertson & Baker (2001) present an excellent review on the effectiveness of ultrasound and concluded that there was little evidence that active ultrasound was more effective than placebo ultrasound for treating people with pain or a range of musculoskeletal injuries or for promoting soft tissue healing.

Problem-solving exercise 6.4

David is a 35-year-old graphic artist who tripped over uneven paving stones in the street and fell on to his dorsiflexed right hand. He felt a tearing sensation in his wrist and was immediately aware of severe pain. His hand and the carpus were displaced backwards momentarily before it snapped back into place. He took himself off to the local A&E Department, still in severe pain. On examination and X-ray it became clear that he had not fractured any bones in the fall but that he had sustained a carpal subluxation. Reduction was not necessary.

David is referred immediately to you. You find that the wrist and carpus are hugely swollen.

Self-assessment question

- SAQ 6.11 What do you expect to find on examination? (remember the internal swelling and hence the increased pressure in the carpal tunnel)? (See text.)

Problem-solving exercise 6.5

Reminding yourself of the principles of John's sprained and Gemma's partially torn ligament how would you deal with David?

What are your treatment aims?

How would you progress treatment? (Remind yourself of the healing timetable). Refer back to both John and Gemma for details of the physical treatment.

David is completely dependent on his hand professionally. How will you incorporate this aspect into your management?

Case study 6.3: James Low

James Low is a 46-year-old accountant who injured his ankle during a charity parachute jump. The force of his injury was so severe that it resulted in a complete rupture of the lateral ligaments of his ankle, leading to gross instability. A doctor he sees in the A&E Department of the local hospital makes this diagnosis.

The doctor will have arrived at this diagnosis by

- grasping the calcaneus and then fully inverting the foot passively; this, in contrast to an ankle with an intact lateral ligament, will result in a fairly large range of movement as the talus is now able to wobble in the mortise. As with all other ligamentous tests it is necessary to test the uninjured side in order to get a feel for the 'normal' state of the ligamentous apparatus. This is vital, as it is well recognized that wide individual variations exist with regards to ligament laxity. You therefore always need to establish what is normal before you are able to discern what is abnormal.

- a stress X-ray with the ankle in plantar flexion and inversion, which will demonstrate tilting of the talus.

The best management for these injuries still seems to be under discussion. Surgical repair is regarded as second choice and usually consists of either the repair of the ligament or the reinforcement of the lateral aspect of the ankle by transferring the tendon of peroneus brevis or by a free graft of plantaris (Dandy 1998).

On examination, weight bearing will be impossible because of:

- severe pain and swelling
- instability of the ankle.

Remembering Gemma's management, you know that strapping will be able to reinforce a ligament but is not strong enough to take on the role of main stabilizer by itself. Hence a plaster cast is the preferred option in order to give protection to the injured site. This will most probably be a Litecast below-knee plaster (refer to Chapter 5 for more details on the different plaster materials and rules of application) with the ankle in slight eversion. Remembering the healing timetable, you will see that this plaster will have to be on for a minimum of 3–4 weeks in order for fibrous tissue repair to take place.

James will be independent in a walking plaster and might wish to use a stick for security.

After about 4 weeks the plaster is removed and James is referred to physiotherapy.

Problem–solving exercise 6.6

What do you need to find out before planning your management of James's ankle? Refer back to the healing timetable and to Gemma's and John's treatment for similarities and differences. You might also wish to re-read the post-POP management concerns raised in Chapter 5.

An answer is given in the following section, but try to work this out for yourself first.

Further assessment of James Low

1. Pain

After 4 weeks in plaster pain should not be a great feature as long as the ankle is not being moved; it might become a problem that needs addressing once weight bearing and exercises start.

2. Swelling

This will be a major problem as lack of movement in the plaster and hence very reduced absorption will have resulted in a fibrosing of the original haematoma; it will be hard and cold to the touch.

3. Range of movement

This might very well turn out to be the major issue. After 4 weeks in the plaster the soft tissues (ligaments, joint capsules, membranes, etc.) will have shortened virtually into all directions but the worst will be plantarflexion and inversion. There will be very little difference between active and passive ROM.

4. Mobility

James has lost a lot of his neuromuscular control around the ankle, plus strength, and therefore cannot weight bear through his ankle with ease. Hence he is in danger of re-injuring the ankle. He will find himself to be more vulnerable and much less mobile than before the removal of his plaster.

5. Social set-up

As an accountant, James sits at a desk most of the day but his office is on the first floor of a house without a lift. He is unmarried and lives alone. His home is a bungalow with a small paved garden. He usually takes the bus to work. James's hobbies are mostly intellectual pursuits rather than sports.

Self-assessment question

- SAQ 6.12 How would you now address the above five points in your treatment plan? (After you have tried this question for yourself, check your answer against the approach described in the next section.)

Physiotherapy treatment of James Low

1. Mobility

Clearly, James needs some help with this as long as his ankle is as stiff as it is at the moment. He should therefore be given a pair of crutches for a few days and taught partial weight bearing (PWB), including going up and down stairs, in order for him to be able to be independent.

2. ROM

James needs to start with gentle active physiological movements. This is important in order to take account of the lack of elasticity in the soft tissues at this time. Passive movements could quickly overstretch the joint and hence result in re-injury. He should do these for a few days to get some proprioception and movement back into the joint.

The next step will be for James to continue with his active exercises while you introduce accessory movements, particularly stressing inversion and plantarflexion (e.g. Maitland grades III and IV) as far as joint irritability allows (refer back to Chapter 3 for details). It is likely that this concentrated stretching of the fibrosed scar (i.e. into joint resistance) will result in some treatment soreness. This can be countered by finishing each treatment with some accessory movements of a lower grade (i.e. I or II) to stimulate the mechanoreceptor and hence engender some pain relief.

The concentrated stretches will result in a low-grade inflammatory reaction as some scar fibres tear. Electrotherapy might therefore be a useful pain-reducing modality at this point but make sure you go back to the earlier quoted evidence on this aspect.

Bearing in mind the tissue healing timetable, you will remember that inflammation always goes along with some pain and definitely swelling. Hence, ice, compression (elastic bandage) and elevation after treatment will be good advice for James.

Can you see that he could now be treated like Gemma as regards his physical injury? What psychosocial clues have you picked up, though, that would lead you to a different treatment plan?

3. Social set up

James clearly needs some advice on how to use his body. He likes doing things that require a low level of activity and hence he is quite unfit. This is compounded by his stressful and sedentary job. James must therefore be introduced to an exercise regime and be given a sound rationale for it (the biomechanics of soft tissue and their need for stretching and movement in order to remain elastic and tensile). This will allow him to be at less risk during sudden physical stresses.

Summarizing ligamentous injuries

- You need to be aware of the anatomy and biomechanics of the injured region in order to assess the region and predict a possible outcome.

- You need to be aware of the healing timetable of tissues in order to know if you are dealing with an inflammatory (acute) or a repair (chronic) situation. This will direct you to the relevant approach.

- It is of maximum importance to employ a long view and advise the patient on long-term care as the scar is going to continue to change long after the patient has been discharged from physiotherapy. Concerns about the quality of the scar tissue (i.e. linking the exercises and stretches to the way the region is going to be used later on) are of greatest importance.

- Always refer to the guidelines on soft tissue injury management (ACPSM 1999).

Complications

Compartment syndrome

This can be a very serious secondary occurrence after any tissue injury. As the tissue swells up it needs space to expand. If this is not possible the tissue will become ischaemic very quickly and hence will be destroyed.

The different compartments to remember are (Dandy 1998):

Forearm
- The ventral compartment includes:
  - the median and ulnar nerve
  - the radial and ulnar artery
- The dorsal compartment includes:
  - the posterior interosseous nerve
  - no major vessels.

Lower limb

- The anterior tibial compartment contains:
  - the anterior tibial artery
  - the deep peroneal nerve
- The superficial posterior compartment contains:
  - no important nerves or vessels
- The deep posterior compartment contains:
  - the posterior tibial vessels and nerves
  - the peroneal artery
- The peroneal compartment contains:
  - deep and superficial peroneal nerves.

It is absolutely essential to check for signs of ischaemia (white colour, cold to touch, no distal pulses (if relevant) and severe pain) in patients with a history of trauma and suspected deep swelling.

Recurrent instability

If the self-treatment after discharge is not adequately executed, an often seen complication of ligamentous sprains or ruptures is recurrent instability. This is particularly frequently seen in the ankle joint but is also common in the knee and the elbow.

The major causes for this are cited as:

- Functional instability, due to a massive previous injury resulting in an interruption of the reflex arc and hence resulting in a loss of reflex stabilization of the joint
- Inadequately treated sprains, due to weakness of the surrounding muscles and shortening of the ligaments
- Problems of the distal anatomical regions
- Undiagnosed causes (Corrigan & Maitland 1983).

MUSCLES AND TENDONS

So far we have looked at ligamentous injuries only and now we need to look at how muscle injuries might differ. The worked examples of the previous section are needed as a background for these.

The focus here will be particularly on:

- lateral epicondylitis of the elbow as an example of an overuse injury
- supraspinatus tendinitis as an example of an injury precipitated by degeneration
- hamstring strain as an example of direct trauma.

Problem-solving exercise 6.7

Focusing on overuse or degeneration of soft tissue, what do you imagine the main differences to be from cases of trauma (e.g. the previous case studies)?

What are the hallmarks of injury and do they apply to degenerative processes and overuse?

In order to help you with these points you might wish to re-read the details on the inflammatory processes in healing and then remind yourself of the stress–strain curve and the ability to deform. You need also to remind yourself of the factors that influence (negatively or positively) these processes.

Lateral epicondylitis

Case study 6.4: Alison Hunt

Alison Hunt is a 54-year-old secretary who has developed a severe pain on the lateral aspect of her elbow over the past 2 months. It is uncomfortable most of the time but it particularly interferes with her hobby of playing tennis. Although not 100% sure she feels that the onset was connected with her club league tournament. On closer investigation she remembers a forceful mis-hit that resulted in some local pain.

She now complains of pain over the lateral aspect of the elbow radiating distally into the forearm and into the wrist and dorsum of her hand. A diagnosis of lateral epicondylitis has been made.

Self-assessment question

- SAQ 6.13 Thinking about John and Gemma, what do you expect to find on observation? What will be similar and what will be different with regard to:
  a. observation
  b. testing?

Answer

a. Clearly you are looking for signs of inflammation because, although the injury is chronic (history of 2 months), Alison is likely to re-injure her elbow by continually using it. Hence you would expect to find redness, swelling, tenderness and heat. In contrast to Gemma and John there will be no internal bruising due to a sudden disruption of fibres but there might very well have been internal bleeding due to avulsion of single tendon fibres off their insertion.

b. The cause of the problem is meant to be in the tendon region of a muscle. Pain therefore will not be provoked by testing the joint (i.e. either stability or stretch of ligaments) but by contracting the affected muscle, hence increasing the tension on its point of insertion to bone.

Self-assessment question

• SAQ 6.14 Having established that you are dealing with a muscle tendon problem, what muscles do you know to insert into the lateral epicondyle and what tests therefore could you think of to test your hypothesis?

Answer

The common extensor group.

• Resisted extension of the wrist in order to provoke the common extensor muscle group will result in pain and might even demonstrate some weakness
• Resisted radial deviation with the fingers extended (hence the extensors stretched and therefore pulling on their insertion) will be painful
• Resisted elbow movements (i.e. testing more proximal muscles) will therefore be unaffected
• Functional activities involving the wrist, e.g. shaking hands, twisting open jam jars, will all reproduce the pain
• Passive extension of the elbow will be slightly limited as well as painful because of the shortening and hardening of tendon fibres at their insertion
• The upper limb tension test (ULTT) might prove positive.

We have said that Alison's problem is not due to sudden trauma but due to the painful and shortened scar resulting from overexerting or overstretching the common extensor muscle group.

Self-assessment question

• SAQ 6.15 This is clearly not an acute picture as in the previous case studies but an acute incident on top of a chronic condition. Remembering the previous case studies, how would you approach Alison's treatment? You need to remember the tissue-healing timetable for this. After you have worked out your answers to this question, read the next section.

An approach to the treatment of Alison Hunt

1. Rest   This clearly is a problem that re-starts every time the old injury pattern recurs. Hence Alison must be advised to stop all activities that exacerbate her problem. This can be very difficult and she might need a lot of support and information in order to be motivated. Often, rest is the most important ingredient for the problem to limit itself. If Alison finds it impossible to rest the elbow enough to break through the aggravating mechanical pattern, a plaster back-slab can be used to enforce rest.

2. Hydrocortisone injections   This powerful anti-inflammatory treatment can work very quickly provided the hydrocortisone is injected into the exact anatomical spot. The injections are associated with a much more pronounced and long-lasting anti-inflammatory effect than NSAIDs. They can in fact halt the healing process by virtually eliminating the inflammatory response. Most doctors therefore believe that steroids have no role in the treatment of acute soft tissue injuries. However, in chronic soft tissue injuries a steroid injection can result in quick pain relief, although there is a risk of weakening the tendon, which can lead to rupture in weight-bearing tendons. Some relief can be expected but it is often only temporary (Almekinders 1999).

3. Ice and deep friction   This may be followed by ultrasound.

4. Accessory mobilizations   These are used to gain full end-range of extension.

5. Mills manipulation   This is rarely successful in the long run (Corrigan & Maitland 1983).

6. Advice and education
This should cover:

- the cause of Alison's problems and the effect the biomechanics have on the region
- the use of her arm, including looking at her tennis technique
- the need to avoid overuse of a particular region and hence the need to 'cut up' long activities and interweave them with others
- the fact that long arm stretches and neck movements could be sensitizing manoeuvres
- general strengthening of the neighbouring region
- sensitive support while Alison is exploring other ways of doing her job.

Are you clear about the similarities and differences between the ligamentous injuries on the one hand and muscle/tendon overuse on the other? If not, go back over the case studies.

Supraspinatus tendinitis

This is a very frequent complaint. The mechanism of injury seems to be overuse or trauma on top of a degenerate tendon. Because of the degeneration aspect of this condition patients often describe a history of flare-ups and remissions over a long time span, often over many years.

Pain is felt over the lateral aspect of the arm, sometimes radiating into the deltoid region. Rarely will the pain extend down to the elbow. Night pain is common. Look up the anatomy of the rotator cuff and remind yourself of its important function (e.g. Hertling & Kessler 1996) before continuing.

Self-assessment question

- SAQ 6.16 On examining a patient with supraspinatus tendinitis, which movements will be particularly painful? Why are they painful and how will they need to be tested?

Answer

- Active abduction is painful, particularly on resistance or even during an isometric contraction. Usually pain occurs as an arc roughly between 60 and 120° of abduction; bringing the arm back to neutral from full abduction elicits pain in the same region and therefore classically the patient drops the arm to a pain-free zone when starting to experience the pain (i.e. the arm is being dropped from about 120° to about 50°). This coincides with the tendon being compressed between the acromion superiorly and the greater tuberosity inferiorly
- External rotation will be painful
- There is usually some wasting to be noticed over the supraspinatus area
- The rotator cuff is very involved in the scapulohumeral rhythm and therefore a supraspinatus tendinitis is going to alter this.

Self-assessment question

- SAQ 6.17 Now that you know the signs and symptoms of this condition, come up with a reasoned plan for its management. Then compare your approach with the one presented in the following section.

Management of supraspinatus tendinitis

Treatment includes the following:

1. Rest: movements that are known to aggravate the problem (i.e. abduction and external

rotation) must be avoided to allow the healing process to start

2. Injection of corticosteroid around the tendon to help with the chronically exacerbated inflammatory process (Almekinders 1999)

3. Ice and deep frictions followed by ultrasound. Brosseau et al (2002), in their review of the efficacy of frictions for treating tendinitis, were unable to identify a significant effect in favour of this treatment avenue. They came to the conclusion that more high-powered trials will have to be conducted before the effectiveness of this treatment modality can be ascertained

4. Accessory movements that move the humeral head away from the acromion (always starting from a pain-free position):
   a. posteroanterior movements of the humeral head
   b. longitudinal movements of the head caudally
   c. quadrant position with very gentle movements

5. Strengthening of the other parts of the rotator cuff

6. Working on the other parts and planes of the kinetic chain.

This condition is going to take a long time and a lot of patient education before it is dealt with. Because of the degenerative nature of the underlying cause it often recurs and therefore occasionally requires surgical decompression of the tendon by either removing the outer end of the acromion or splitting the coracoacromial ligament. These procedures increase the subacromial space and therefore give the tendon more space to move around in, which should result in less 'rubbing' of the tendon against the roof of this tight space and hence less scarring.

Hamstring strain

Here neither overuse nor degeneration seems to be the underlying problem but usually a direct blow to the muscles or a very forceful contraction. The patients therefore are invariably active and athletic people.

A typical history might include a strenuous activity during which the patient suddenly feels something give way, resulting in an ache. After a few hours, the pain and hence loss of mobility are marked.

The diagnosis will be a partial rupture of some muscle fibres either in the muscle belly or closer to the musculotendinous junction.

Self-assessment question

- **SAQ 6.18** You now know the history and the signs and symptoms of this problem. You might need to look up the exact anatomy and biomechanics of the hamstrings before testing the injury site and then devising a management plan. After you have done that read the following section on testing and management.

Tests for hamstring injury

- Both sites are going to be aggravated by *resisted knee flexion*. This will only confirm the hamstring muscle as the culprit, it will not differentiate between the musculotendinous junction and the muscle belly.

- *Straight leg raise*. If this is full, you know that the insertion of the muscle into the ischial tuberosity is at fault. If this is limited you can be pretty certain that the problem lies within the muscle belly rather than near the tendon.

- *Hip flexion with the knee bent* takes all the tension off the hamstrings and therefore is pain-free – as long as it is done passively.

- *Neural tension tests.*

Management of hamstring injury

- *Rest.* Take weight off the injured region in order to avoid re-injury but encourage gentle active movement without weight bearing to speed up the resorption process of the haematoma for about 2–5 days

- *Ice, frictions and ultrasound over injury site* (remember John regarding contraindications to this treatment in the early stages of healing)

- *Strength.* After about 3–5 days start with gentle exercises through the 0–90° range, perhaps using a wall pulley. This will allow for a controlled increase in resistance. Include quadriceps in the strengthening regime as the ratio of flexor and extensor strength is vital for good and safe function. Slowly add increased weight bearing to the resistance regime.

- *Control.* Devise short start–stop regimes to increase the flexibility of the muscles

- *Endurance.* Use of a bicycle (vary the height of the seat to get different parts of the muscle to work more), stairs, swimming, etc.

- *Education.* This is undoubtedly the most important aspect of the rehabilitation. The following aspects should be covered:
  - Information about the anatomy, biomechanics and mode of injury
  - Information about the healing process, particularly the late stages, and the importance, therefore, of long-term aftercare
  - Exploration of training style/life style (i.e. how does this person want to use their body?)
  - Warm-up and warm-down procedures.

Remember that the relationship you develop with the patient is going to be gate-way to a successful or failing rehabilitation phase.

By now you should be clear about the similarities and differences between ligamentous and musculotendinous injuries. If not, please go back to the case studies and try to identify these points.

Adhesive capsulitis

In contrast to the mechanical stressors underlying the previously mentioned conditions, adhesive capsulitis of the shoulder (or 'frozen shoulder') involves an underlying inflammatory process of the glenohumeral capsule that results in thickening and contraction of the capsule. Apart from severe pain this leads to marked restriction of ROM in the shoulder.

It seems that middle-aged women are mainly affected; there is no trauma that has caused it and the onset is more often gradual over several weeks than suddenly overnight.

The exact underlying cause has not yet been identified but it has been noted that this condition virtually never recurs at the same site. It is as if an 'immunization' had happened.

Self-assessment question

- **SAQ 6.19** Remembering the capsular attachments of the glenohumeral joint which movements would you expect to be particularly limited?

(Answer at end of chapter.)

Treatment of adhesive capsulitis

As a rule of thumb, treatment (apart from pure pain-killing methods not involving movement) should not be started unless the night pain has disappeared. This can easily take 4–6 months after onset, with the whole course lasting for about 18 months.

After that, treatment needs to focus on (Hertling & Kessler 1996):

- *Pain control* (ice, mobilization techniques in low grades and electrotherapy or acupuncture)
- *Range of movement*:
  - accessory movements grades III and IV to increase range – caudad longitudinals in as much flexion as can be tolerated
  - posteroanterior/anteroposterior accessory movements
  - stretching
  - auto-assisted active exercises (using a walking stick that is grasped by both hands but guided by the non-affected side)
- *Strength*: isometric exercises into flexion, abduction and adduction, internal and external rotation proprioceptive neuromuscular facilitation (PNF) patterns within the kinetic chain directions.

Electrotherapy is usually not helpful in the rehabilitation of this condition unless it is tried for pain relief in the early stages (e.g. transcutaneous electrical nerve stimulation, TENS).

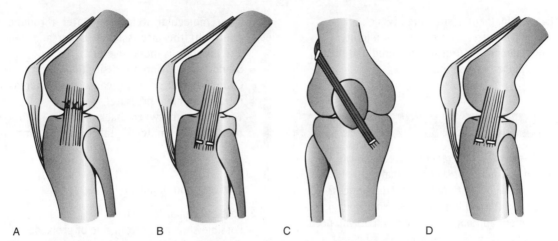

Figure 6.4 Surgery to ligaments: (A) repair; (B) reattachment; (C) replacement with tendon or prosthesis; (D) advancement of ligament attachment. (Adapted with permission from Dandy 1998.)

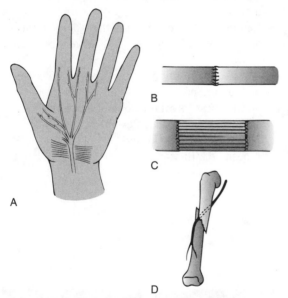

Figure 6.5 Surgery to nerves: (A) decompression; (B) repair; (C) grafting; (D) neurolysis, where tethering of the nerve to bone or other tissues is released by operation. (Adapted with permission from Dandy 1998.)

SURGICALLY REPAIRED SOFT TISSUES

The chapter so far has dealt with the conservative treatment of soft tissue injuries; the second part will introduce some thoughts on the surgical repair of these tissues (Dandy 1998).

Surgical procedures carried out on ligaments include (Fig. 6.4):

- Repair when worn
- Replacement or reconstruction
- Shortening.

Surgical procedures carried out on nerves include (Fig. 6.5):

- Decompression
- Repair
- Freeing (neurolysis)
- Grafting.

Ligament repair

Case study 6.5: Emily Jones

Emily Jones is a 21-year-old student who dislocated her right thumb in falling on a dry ski slope. She immediately felt something 'go' and now complains of severe pain, swelling and bruising.

On examination active movements cannot be tolerated because of pain, and on testing the joints passively, her thumb appears to be unstable. Hence a complete rupture of the medial collateral ligament is suspected (which one would expect after a dislocation of a joint).

The ligament is surgically repaired and the hand is placed in a splint.

Problem-solving exercise 6.8

Identify the main difference between Emily's problem and John's or David's. What do they have in common and what are the vital differences? How should these differences influence your management approaches? How much do you need to know about the surgery itself? (See below.)

Nerve decompression

Case study 6.6: Steve Morris (1)

Steve Morris has a long history of backache, which troubles him periodically. Bed rest for a few days followed by wearing a corset until the muscle spasm had gone has always dealt with his problem. He is 40 years old and works as a computer analyst.

He and his family moved house 3 weeks ago and 2 weeks ago he developed his back pain again. Instead of being helped by his usual routine his pain got worse and started to travel down into his buttock and leg, now involving the posterior aspect of his thigh and leg and radiating into the lateral aspect of his ankle and foot.

An acute lumbar nerve root compression by an intervertebral disc is suspected.

Self-assessment question

- SAQ 6.20 What would you be looking for in Steve to help clarify this diagnosis?

Answer

Subjectively, you might expect:

- Pain worse in the morning (as the proteoglycans in the nucleus have taken in 8.8 times

their molecular weight in water throughout the night the disc is much larger and hence the prolapse is more severe)
- Standing and lying are easier than sitting
- Coughing and sneezing cause pain (increased intra-abdominal pressure)
- Time lapse between back and leg pain (as the nuclear material takes some time to extrude).

Objectively, you might find:

- Loss of lumbar lordosis
- Possible shift away from side of prolapse
- Flexion and side flexion to side of pain are the most painful test movements
- Passive straight leg raise increases pain (as the already stretched dura is stretched even more
- Neurological deficit in the dermatomes and myotomes of the S1 nerve root, as shown by:
  - loss of sensation (lateral aspect of ankle, foot and posterior calf)
  - weakness (plantar flexion of ankle and toes, hip extension, knee flexion)
  - loss of reflex (ankle jerk)
- A positive MRI scan.

Case study 6.6: Steve Morris (2)

Steve is being operated on to decompress his S1 nerve root.

This is often done via microsurgery, which only resects the bit of intervertebral disc that is causing the compression. On the whole this means that the stability of the spine is not interfered with as the superficial (erector spinae) and deep (multifidus) stabilizing muscles of the spine have not been cut.

Self-assessment question

- **SAQ 6.21** Postoperative regimes obviously vary according to the practice of different surgeons but, taking into account what you now know about wound healing and tissue healing, devise a reasoned plan for Steve's management. After you have set out your own plan, compare it with the following section.

Treatment of Steve Morris

1. Rest In order to give the wound a good chance to lay down scar tissue, Steve will need to stay in bed for about 2–4 days. To help resorption of the postoperative haematoma and circulation in general, he should move his toes, ankles and knees (below about 60° of flexion so as not to move his lumbar spine too much).

2. Mobility Once he is allowed out of bed, Steve should walk and stand rather than sit, to put the least amount of pressure through the operation site.

3. Range of movement Once the inflammatory process has passed and the scar tissue has begun to be laid down, it is important that Steve starts, very gently, to use his back as he wants to use it later on, i.e. he must start to bend it. This will encourage the fibroblasts to be laid down in the alignment of stress rather than in a perpendicular fashion contracting the whole region. Straight leg raises have to be performed regularly to prevent the nerve root from becoming stuck down in adhesions.

4. Strength Isometric and isotonic back extensor exercises should be done from about the fourth day. Abdominal exercises must be started later (after 5–6 days) as the contraction of the muscles involved increases the intra-abdominal and intradiscal pressures enormously. They need to be in good shape, however, in order to contribute to the muscular corset of the trunk which will lead to greater safety later on.

5. Education Again this is the most important aspect of Steve's rehabilitation.

- You need to be able to motivate Steve (refer back to the subjective assessment section in Chapter 3) to become involved in a back care regime for his spine.
- For this, he needs to know about his spine; the relevant anatomy and biomechanics; the effect of loading it in different positions; the contribution muscle strength can make and the way in which strenuous, long-lasting tasks need to be split up.
- You need to impress on Steve that the healing process can take up to 2 years and that the quality of the healing process is in his hands once you have empowered him.

SUMMARY

This chapter has aimed to give you an insight into some areas of soft tissue injuries. As you will have appreciated this is a very large and complex sector of medicine where surgeons and therapists often overlap and cooperate in order to achieve the best outcome for the patient.

Use the worked example case studies to help you with problem solving in other settings you will be confronted with. Be clear what is characteristic for each setting and what are general features. It is not necessary to know every particular syndrome that can occur in this area but it is important for you to be able to recognize the vital aspects of a person's set of problems and identify in which way they are special.

ANSWERS TO QUESTIONS AND EXERCISES

Self-assessment question 6.1 (page 135)

- **SAQ 6.1** How are connective tissues classified?

  Answer: According to their loose or dense fibre distribution and by the type of fibre they possess (elastin, reticulin, collagen).

Self-assessment question 6.2 (page 135)

- **SAQ 6.2** The physiological functions of collagen fibres lead clearly to the biomechanical properties the body expects soft tissues to have. What are they?

  Answer: Strength, flexibility, elasticity.

Self-assessment question 6.3 (page 137)

- **SAQ 6.3** What is the difference between the classification of ligamentous injuries on the one hand and injuries to blood vessels, muscles and nerves on the other?

Answer: Ligamentous injuries are classified by the resultant interference with stability while injuries to the other tissues are classified according to the mechanical or chemical cause of injury.

Self-assessment question 6.4 (page 140)

- **SAQ 6.4** A patient with a slight sprain of the wrist is managed with a Tubigrip over the radiocarpal joint. What areas/joints would you need to include in your assessment and treatment?

Answer: Inferior and superior radioulnar joints, carpal bones and intercarpal joints.

Self-assessment question 6.5 (page 140)

Answer follows question in text.

Self-assessment question 6.6 (page 140)

- **SAQ 6.6** What kind of question would you feel most comfortable with and what do you think is important to elicit in order to get a feel for the remits of rehabilitation?

Answer: If you have problems answering this question go back to Chapter 3 to refresh your mind.

Problem-solving exercise 6.1 (page 141)

See following section in text.

Self-assessment question 6.7 (page 141)

See information in text.

Problem-solving exercise 6.2 (page 142)

How would these principles [see text] help you with the assessment and treatment of a patient with a simple sprain in a non-weight-bearing region of the body, e.g. a sprain of the interphalangeal joint (collateral ligament) of the second digit on the dominant hand?

Include in your deliberations the likely cause (?which movement) of this injury.

Answer: The mechanism could be, for instance, twisting something against very strong resistance, or a fall on to the distal part of the dominant hand. Non-weight-bearing reduces the time of healing on the one hand , but the dominance in functional tasks lengthens the timescale and complicates the outcome. (See information in this and previous chapters, especially Chapter 3.)

Self-assessment question 6.8 (page 143)

- **SAQ 6.8** How would an X-ray be able to demonstrate that diagnosis (of partial ligament rupture)?

Answer: The joint surfaces of the ankle joint are gapped further than normal (hence the stress X-ray: a conventional anteroposterior X-ray would not demonstrate this).

Self-assessment question 6.9 (page 143)

Answer follows question in text.

Self-assessment question 6.10 (page 144)

See text.

Problem-solving exercise 6.3 (page 144)

See information in text.

Problem-solving exercise 6.4 (page 145)

See information in text.

Self-assessment question 6.11 (page 145)

See text.

Problem-solving exercise 6.5 (page 145)

See information in text.

Problem-solving exercise 6.6 (page 146)

See the following section in the text.

Self-assessment question 6.12 (page 146)

See the following section in the text.

Problem-solving exercise 6.7 (page 148)

See the advice following the questions in the text.

Self-assessment question 6.13 (page 148)

Answer follows question in text.

Self-assessment question 6.14 (page 149)

Answer follows question in text.

Self-assessment question 6.15 (page 149)

See the following section in the text.

Self-assessment question 6.16 (page 150)

Answer follows question in text.

Self-assessment question 6.17 (page 150)

See the following section in the text.

Self-assessment question 6.18 (page 151)

See the following sections in the text.

Self-assessment question 6.19 (page 152)

- **SAQ 6.19** Remembering the capsular attachments of the glenohumeral joint, which movements would you expect to be particularly limited [in adhesive capsulitis]?

 Answer:
 - External rotation – most limited
 - Abduction – second most limited
 - Internal rotation and flexion – virtually free.

Problem-solving exercise 6.8 (page 154)

See information in text.

Self-assessment question 6.20 (page 154)

Answer follows question in text.

Self-assessment question 6.21 (page 155)

See the following section in the text.

References

ACPSM 1999 Guidelines for the management of soft tissue (musculoskeletal) injury with Protection, Rest, Ice, Compression and Elevation (PRICE) during the first 72 hours. Chartered Society of Physiotherapy: London

Almekinders LC 1999 Anti-inflammatory treatment of muscular injuries in sports. An update on recent studies. Sports Medicine 28: 383–388

Amiel D, Chiu CR, Lee J 1995 Effects of loading on metabolism and repair of tendons and ligaments. In: Gordon SL, Blair SJ, Fine LJ (eds) Repetitive motion disorders of the upper extremity. American Academy of Orthopaedic Surgeons, Rosemont, IL: p 217–230

Anderson MK, Hall SJ 1995 Sports injury management. Williams & Wilkins, Baltimore, MD

Astrom M, Rausing A 1995 Chronic Achilles tendinopathy. Clinical Orthopaedics and Related Research 316: 151–164

Barkoukis V, Sykaras E, Costa F, Tsorbatzoudis H 2002 Effectiveness of taping and bracing in balance. Perceptual and Motor Skills 94: 566–574

Beaupre LA, Davies DM, Jones CA, Cinats JG 2001 Exercise combined with continuous passive motion or slider board therapy compared with exercise only: a randomised controlled trial of patients following total knee arthroplasty. Physical Therapy 81: 1029–1037

Brosseau L, Casimiro L, Milne S et al 2002 Deep transverse friction massage for treating tendinitis. In: Cochrane Library, Issue 4. Oxford: Update Software

Buckwalter JA 1995 Should bone, soft tissue and joint injuries be treated with rest or activity? Journal of Orthopaedic Research 13: 155–156

Chen B, Zimmerman JR, Soulen L, DeLisa JA 2000 Continuous passive motion after total knee arthroplasty: a prospective study. American Journal of Physical Medicine and Rehabilitation 79: 421–426

Clancy J, McVicar AJ 1995 Physiology and anatomy. A homeostatic approach. Edward Arnold, London

Corrigan B, Maitland G 1983 Practical orthopaedic medicine. Butterworth, London

Crawford Adams J, Hamblen DL 1995 Outline of orthopaedics, 12th edn. Churchill Livingstone, Edinburgh

Dandy D 1998 Essential orthopaedics and trauma, 3rd edn. Churchill Livingstone, Edinburgh

Desrosiers EA, Methot S, Yahia LH, Rivard CH 1995 Response of ligamentous fibroblasts to mechanical stimulation. Annales de Chirurgie 49: 768–774

Evans P 1980 Healing at cellular level. Physiotherapy 66: 256–259

Freeman MAR, Wyke BD 1967 Articular reflexes at the ankle joint. British Journal of Surgery 54: 990

Hertling D, Kessler R 1996 Management of common musculo-skeletal disorders: Physical therapy principles and methods, 3rd edn. JB Lippincott, Philadelphia, PA

Low J, Reed A 1994 Electrotherapy explained, 2nd edn. Butterworth-Heinemann, Oxford

Noyes FR, Torvic PJ, Hyde WB, DeLucas JL 1974 Biomechanics of ligament failure. 2. An analysis of immobilisation, exercise and reconditioning effects in primates. Journal of Bone and Joint Surgery 56A: 1406–1418

Ogilvieharris DJ, Gilbart M 1995 Treatment modalities for soft tissue injuries of the ankle – a critical review. Clinical Journal of Sports Medicine 5: 175–186

O'Sullivan PB, Twomey LT, Allison GT 1997 Evaluation of specific stabilising exercise in the treatment of chronic low back pain with radiologic diagnosis of spondylolysis or spondylolisthesis. Spine 22: 2959–2967

Reynolds CA, Cummings GS, Andrew PD, Tillman LJ 1996 The effect of non-traumatic immobilization on ankle dorsiflexion stiffness in rats. Journal of Orthopaedic and Sport Physical Therapy 23: 27–33

Robertson VJ, Baker KG 2001 A review of therapeutic ultrasound: effectiveness studies. Physical Therapy 81: 1339–1350

Robinovitch SN, Heller B, Lui A, Cortez J 2002 Effect of strength and speed of torque development on balance recovery with the ankle strategy. Journal of Neurophysiology 88: 613–620

Sahrmann S 2000 Diagnosis and treatment of movement impairment syndromes. Mosby, St Louis, MO

Smith N 1995 Physiotherapy practice: its relevance to healing and sports injuries. British Journal of Therapy and Rehabilitation 2: 301–305

Stillman B 2002 Making sense of proprioception. Physiotherapy 88: 646–667

Watson T 1996 Electrical stimulation for wound healing. Physical Therapy Reviews 1: 89–103

Watson T 2000 The role of electrotherapy in contemporary physiotherapy practice. Manual Therapy 5: 132–141

Chapter **7**

Rheumatic conditions

Karen Atkinson

OBJECTIVES

By the end of this chapter you should:

- Have an overview of rheumatic disorders
- Be aware of the problems and issues experienced by patients with rheumatic conditions
- Have an overview of the assessment of patients with rheumatic disorders
- Recognize how to problem solve during the assessment and treatment of patients with rheumatic conditions irrespective of the disease process or extent of medical intervention
- Understand how physiotherapy management is related to pharmacological intervention
- Be aware of the types of physiotherapy intervention possible with a range of patients with rheumatic conditions, utilizing a functional approach and including patient education
- Start to appreciate the different perspective which needs to be adopted when working with children as opposed to other groups of clients
- Begin to understand the implications of chronic disease for the patient including biomedical, psychological and social factors
- Have an overview of the roles of the members of the healthcare team in the management of patients with rheumatic conditions.

KEY WORDS

Rheumatology, connective tissue disorders, pharmacological management, physiotherapy management, osteoarthrosis (OA), rheumatoid arthritis (RA), ankylosing spondylitis (AS), juvenile idiopathic arthritis (JIA), healthcare team, patient education, function, implications of chronic disease.

Prerequisites

In order to obtain most benefit from this chapter you should have read the introductory chapters of the book. These provide background information about the problem-solving approach, change in the musculoskeletal system, recognition of these changes and clinical reasoning. It is particularly important to have read the section in Chapter 2 on the structure and function of articular cartilage.

Reacquaint yourself with the features of normal synovial joints and connective tissue (bone and cartilage are particularly important). Use any anatomy book for this, but for detailed information see, for example, Gray's Anatomy Package Book/CD-ROM, 38th edn (1998), Churchill Livingstone, Edinburgh. For a brief overview see Dandy DJ, Edwards DJ 2003 Essential orthopaedics and trauma, 4th edn. Churchill Livingstone, Edinburgh, chapter 3.

Familiarize yourself with the changes that occur during inflammation and revise the cardinal signs. Make sure you understand the mechanisms involved in the development of oedema and how this can affect function.

INTRODUCTION

The approach taken in this chapter is somewhat different from that taken in others. Here we are concerned with enabling patients to manage problems they are experiencing as a result of a disease process, whereas in the majority of other chapters we are considering the consequences of various types of trauma. As you have seen, the consequences of trauma can be extensive and may involve a number of complications, but for most patients this is isolated to one area of the body. For patients with rheumatic conditions, however, you will find that the situation is usually different in that they may have to manage more widespread problems due to the general systemic changes that can occur as a result of the disease process. These problems may have an impact on how patients react to treatment and can affect levels of motivation and compliance. Patients with RA, for example, often experience fatigue for much of the time and this has obvious implications for their ability to manage activities of daily living and may also reduce the amount and intensity of exercise that they can undertake. Your role as a physiotherapist often involves enabling the patient to function as effectively as possible within the limits of the disease.

The range of interventions used in the management of patients with rheumatic diseases can help to alleviate, but cannot abolish, the effects of these conditions. Many patients have to manage pain, limited function and reduced quality of life despite undergoing extensive treatment. Other measures are necessary, therefore, to enable patients to develop personal strategies. These strategies have to address both the effects of the disease and patients' roles in what are often complex management regimens tackling the issues they experience as a result of their condition. The enabling measures vary widely depending on the patient's requirements and the resources available but could include patient education, various complementary therapies and/or counselling. There is considerable evidence that informed patients who actively participate in their treatment and assume some responsibility for management have better outcomes, have greater self-efficacy and use fewer medical resources than those patients who are more passive (Bernhard 2001). Physiotherapists are often important links for patients in this process. They should be able to provide relevant and up-to-date information or at least be able to direct patients to the available sources, for example, relevant websites, literature and self-help groups.

It is possible to view our role here within the context of rehabilitation. This can be defined as: 'a process of active change by which a person who has become disabled acquires and uses the knowledge and skills necessary for optimal physical, psychological and social function' (McLellan 1991). This is a useful definition as it reminds us of three key concepts:

- It is the individual patient who remains at the centre of the process and actively determines the management agenda.
- The collaboration between the patient and the skilled professional healthcare team members whose knowledge and experience enable goals to be achieved.
- The central role of education in rehabilitation.

Physiotherapists encounter patients with rheumatic disorders in all areas of practice and across all age groups. In many cases the primary problem experienced by the patient will be due to the arthritis. At other times, however, the arthritic changes may be a secondary, but nonetheless significant problem, affecting how much the patient is able to do. Consequently, it is important that all physiotherapists have a working knowledge of problem solving and a background of clinical reasoning in the assessment and treatment of patients with rheumatic conditions.

A tremendous amount of research is carried out in the field of rheumatology and as a result the literature is extensive. If, for example, you were to perform a search just relating to RA and drug therapy, limited to the last 2 years, your efforts would yield well over a thousand references. It is easy to get lost in an avalanche of information and we are therefore seeking to provide you with a basis from which to approach this field. In recent years a great deal has been discovered about the aetiopathology of the rheumatic diseases as well as the mechanisms that occur during pharmacological treatment. In the field of physiotherapy, treatment approaches have also developed, especially in relation to the use of exercise and the application of physical agents such as ice and electrotherapy modalities.

Overall management of rheumatic conditions is a complex topic in which fashion and opinion still compete with evidence-based practice (Wollheim 1999). Many of the interventions that physiotherapists use in the management of patients with arthritis are in themselves fairly routine. It is, however, the clinical reasoning in relation to when particular interventions would be most effective, combined with patient education and its application to functional activities that are the essential focus for you. This approach also needs to be fully integrated with the individual patient's requirements and perceptions, any pharmacological management and the intervention of other members of the healthcare team.

THE RHEUMATIC DISORDERS

Over 100 distinct rheumatic diseases have been identified. The list is not static, with some problems becoming less common (e.g. acute rheumatic fever), new diseases emerging (e.g. Lyme disease and the rheumatic consequences of HIV infection), new concepts being described and some diseases being redefined in the light of further research (Christian 1992).

It is not the purpose of this chapter to try and cover all of these diseases, but to provide a framework for you to access when assessing and treating patients with rheumatic disorders. Many of these patients present with very similar signs and symptoms irrespective of their particular condition. It is essential, however, to remember that there may be considerable individual variation in the patients' ability to perform necessary and pleasurable activities as a result of these disease processes owing to different physical, psychological and social factors (Harvey 2003).

Rheumatic disorders can also be referred to as 'connective tissue syndromes', a term indicating the more wide-ranging aspects of these conditions. It is commonly expected that someone with 'arthritis' will have joint problems, and indeed many patients do have severe joint signs and symptoms. A large number of these disease processes do, however, affect connective tissue throughout the body, not just bone and cartilage. As a result of this, patients often experience marked systemic effects. There are also some connective tissue syndromes in which the joints are not affected at all.

It is often the case that those patients with rheumatic conditions that you will interact with most commonly will be experiencing their most overt problems as a result of the articular symptoms. It is essential to remember, however, that patients may also have to manage additional difficulties caused by background symptoms such as fatigue, gastrointestinal problems, anaemia and neuropathies.

Medical research continues to search for the causes of the rheumatic disorders and is gradually formulating a better understanding of the various disease mechanisms (Bernhard 2001). Some are much better understood than others. For example the mechanisms causing gout were described in the 1950s and 1960s, and because of this drugs have been developed that are able to prevent its occurrence. With a disease such as RA, however, it is proving much more difficult to discover all the details of aetiology and pathogenesis that might lead to its prevention. It has been understood for many years that the cause of RA is multifactorial, including genetic make up, the immune response of the particular person and some inciting agent. More recent work suggests, however, that the idea of an inciting agent or trigger factor may be

misconceived and that the cause of RA may partly be chance, i.e. random gene combination or mutation (Edwards 2002). But there are so many variables that at present it is not possible to be sure of the exact cause. If the cause of a disease is not clear it will inevitably be more difficult to prevent its occurrence. Further research leading to better understanding of the disease mechanisms should in turn lead to more effective interventions. For the moment, however, many of these diseases remain chronic and incurable.

Examples in the form of case studies are used in this chapter to represent common disorders that you, as a physiotherapist, will be likely to encounter in clinical practice. By using the principles that you learn here, you should be able to formulate basic, coherent problem lists and plans of treatment in collaboration with patients you meet who have rheumatic conditions.

Self–assessment question

- **SAQ 7.1** What are the three key concepts underlying the rehabilitation process as defined earlier? (See above.)

Review point

Before going on to read about the drugs used in the management of rheumatic conditions, review the information so far. Try to think how your approach to patients experiencing problems as a result of these diseases may have to be different from that used with patients who have sustained a fracture or soft tissue injury.

PHARMACOLOGICAL MANAGEMENT

It is likely that any patient referred to you with problems due to a rheumatic condition will be taking medication. In some cases, such as patients with RA, 'polypharmacy' is the norm. In other words, the patient with active disease will probably be taking a number of different drugs to combat various elements/effects of the disease. It is not the aim of this chapter to provide detailed pharmacological information but to give you an overview of the types of drugs available for the management of rheumatic conditions. There are many drugs on the market already and new ones are being produced all the time. It is not necessary for you to know about every one but it is important that you know where to find out about the drugs if you come across unfamiliar names when reading patient notes or carrying out an assessment. There is a great deal of information on this to be found on rheumatology websites as well as in reference books such as MIMMS or the British National Formulary. What you do need to be aware of is the different categories of drugs that may be used, their effects and possible side effects. This is important, as a patient's pharmacological management often has a bearing on his/her ability to co-operate with your treatment and this in turn will affect the efficacy of that treatment.

It is almost inevitable that patients who seek help because of musculoskeletal disorders will be experiencing pain. Relieving pain adequately can prove to be a very great therapeutic challenge, not least because the experience of pain varies greatly from one individual to another (University of Southampton 2002). Patients expect that pharmacological therapy will alleviate their pain and improve other symptoms that they experience. It is generally accepted that drugs will help to reduce pain, swelling and inflammation and in so doing will preserve joint integrity and function (Sterling 1990, Swezey 1990a). Symptoms arising from established deformity and secondary degenerative change, however, will not respond (Butler 1990). Many of the drugs do cause adverse reactions due to either their pharmacological effects or to the patient's hypersensitivity. These reactions can be mild and the patient can often continue to take the drug with dose reduction but on some occasions the effects are severe and the treatment has to be stopped altogether. Disease modifying antirheumatic drugs (DMARDs), for example, have a long list of potentially dangerous side effects and can only be used safely if monitored carefully (White & Cooper 2002).

Analgesics

Pain is 'an unpleasant sensory and emotional experience associated with actual or potential tissue damage' (Magliano & Morris 2002). In general terms it functions to prevent further injury and to allow healing. It is the commonest symptom in rheumatology and can arise by a number of different mechanisms that can be included under the headings of inflammation and mechanical derangement (Turner-Stokes 1993). It is important that the origin of the pain is pinpointed as far as possible in order that management is correctly targeted and effective (Magliano & Morris 2002).

Pain is usually the symptom uppermost in the patient's mind and sometimes analgesics will be prescribed in order to combat this, or they may be given as an adjunct to other drugs (such as non-steroidal anti-inflammatory drugs (NSAIDs) and DMARDs for symptomatic relief. Only a very small proportion of patients will find analgesics alone sufficient to control their symptoms (SIGN 2000). As a result of experiencing chronic pain, some patients with rheumatic conditions may also have to manage complex psychosocial issues. These patients can sometimes be helped by cautious use of antidepressants as the drugs have an analgesic effect independent of their antidepressant properties (Magliano & Morris 2002).

Centrally acting analgesics exert their effect on the central nervous system. Opioid analgesics are substances with opiate-like pharmacological effects. They target the brain and stimulate inhibitory spinal pathways. They also inhibit the discharge of peripheral nociceptors. These drugs can, therefore, reduce the perception of pain but have the tendency to cause nausea, constipation and drowsiness. Weak opioids can be used in combination with paracetamol. These drugs are often prescribed but have on occasions been reported by the patients to be unhelpful (Magliano & Morris 2002, Turner-Stokes 1993).

A number of patients with chronic pain use cannabis for its analgesic and euphoria-inducing effects. This is occurring while the political debate around the legalization of cannabis continues. Cannabinoids are currently being produced by pharmaceutical companies following drug trials and the first cannabis spray is expected to be available by the end of 2003. In the first instance, however, this will only be prescribed to patients with multiple sclerosis. There are concerns that, because the active ingredients are being isolated, the side effects will be more common and the drugs might be too strong. They contain over 95% of tetrahydrocannabinol whereas, in its more natural form, the drug has approximately 20% of this active substance (Glynn 2003). As a physiotherapist, you may come across patients with rheumatic conditions who use cannabis to manage their pain levels.

Quite often, the anti-inflammatory properties of the other varieties of drugs used in the management of rheumatic conditions have an analgesic effect in themselves.

Non-steroidal anti-inflammatory drugs

There is much evidence available to show that NSAIDs are effective and provide symptomatic relief of pain and stiffness, but they have no effect on disease progression. They can be tailored to fit the individual patient's needs and lifestyle (SIGN 2000, Pipitone & Choy 2003). These are often the first agents to be employed in many rheumatic conditions combining pain-relieving effects with an additional benefit of reducing inflammation.

The mode of action is probably multifactorial but a key mechanism is the interference with the formation of inflammatory prostaglandins by inhibiting the two cyclo-oxygenase enzyme (Cox-1 and Cox-2) pathways (McKenna 2000, Pipitone & Choy 2003, SIGN 2000). Cox-1 synthesizes prostaglandins that regulate normal physiological processes such as protection of the gastrointestinal mucosa, maintenance of renal function and so on. Cox-2 has been identified in a number of areas such as the central nervous system and the renal cortex but its role is not currently established. In relation to rheumatic conditions, however, its major role appears to be in the development of an inflammatory response.

Understanding of these physiological processes explains why NSAIDs are effective in reducing inflammation but also why their use is limited by their toxicity to the upper gastrointestinal tract (Kill 2002, McKenna 2000). The problem here can be illustrated by the following findings: 'Thirteen

of every 1000 RA patients who take NSAIDs for 1 year have a serious gastrointestinal complication' (SIGN 2000). This means that the annual mortality attributed to adverse gastrointestinal effects is four times that of individuals not taking NSAIDs.

The newer Cox-2-selective NSAIDs have been shown to have better gastrointestinal safety profiles and should be used in patients with risk factors for gastrointestinal complications. Risk factors include advanced age, history of ulcers, higher doses of NSAIDs, use of corticosteroids, cigarette smoking and alcohol consumption (Pipitone & Choy 2003, SIGN 2000). These new NSAIDs (e.g. meloxicam and celecoxib) appear to be as effective as conventional agents (e.g. ibuprofen and diclofenac) and the gastrointestinal complications are comparable to those of placebo (Magliano & Morris 2002).

Self-assessment question

- **SAQ 7.2** An NSAID will suppress the classical features of inflammation – what are these features?

These drugs are indicated where joint or soft tissue inflammation causes pain, stiffness and swelling. In the acute situation a few days of treatment will usually quickly control symptoms, after which the dose can be reduced or the drug stopped altogether. In chronic conditions the initial dose should be low and several drugs should be tried to find the one best tolerated by the patient (Thompson & Dunne 1995). Many patients may try up to three different agents before finding one that suits them, as there is individual variability in response, the reasons for which are still uncertain (Furst 1990, Thompson & Dunne 1995). Toxicity is a major limiting factor and the side effects are related to dose and duration of therapy. The common side effects are gastrointestinal toxicity, as mentioned earlier, fluid retention and hypertension. Other less common but potentially serious side effects are renal disease and hypersensitivity, including asthma. Less serious side effects include headache, dizziness, tinnitus and rash (SIGN 2000).

Because of these problems, the long-term use of this type of drug may be contraindicated.

Disease–modifying antirheumatic drugs

These are drugs that have a beneficial effect on the course of many rheumatic diseases as well as providing symptomatic relief (SIGN 2000). They are described as remission-inducing agents but, even though there has been a great deal of research, some of the mechanisms by which these drugs work are still not well understood. It is known that they slow the rate of progression of joint damage that occurs as a result of inflammation. The levels of inflammatory markers and elevated platelet count are reduced by DMARDs (but not by NSAIDs) and these factors are linked to better long-term outcome. DMARDs can reduce symptoms and disease activity and can enhance functional status and quality of life (Pipitone & Choy 2003, SIGN 2000, White & Cooper 2002).

Approach to treatment and monitoring

Disease-modifying antirheumatic drugs have been used in the treatment of inflammatory arthritis for decades. The traditional 'pyramidal' approach to treatment, based on the use of symptomatic drugs first, with subsequent addition of DMARDs if their effects are inadequate, has now been rejected. The current thinking is that that they should be introduced as soon as possible in order to preserve maximum functional outcome and reduce eventual disability. Treatment with DMARDs needs to be sustained in order to maintain disease suppression (SIGN 2000). Once the maintenance dose for a DMARD has been established, that dose will continue indefinitely or until side effects or lack of efficacy require the drug to be discontinued or the dose to be increased.

It must be noted, however, that these drugs have relatively high levels of toxicity and, as with NSAIDs there is variability in response and so the most appropriate one needs to be chosen in order to maximally reduce symptoms with minimum side effects. Recently, newer, more potent drugs with a better safety profile have become available (Pipitone & Choy 2003). It is essential, however, to closely monitor the effects of treatment with DMARDs at all times but especially in the early stages, when drug reactions are more likely to occur. Most general practitioners only have a small number of patients on DMARDs and so are unlikely to be familiar with all of the side effects.

To help in standardization of monitoring and to enhance local practice, the British Society for Rheumatology has produced the National Guidelines for the Monitoring of Second-Line Drugs. It is important that the choice of DMARD is discussed with the patient and that information is available covering the therapeutic effects, side effects and monitoring procedures. In some cases the patient is provided with a shared-care booklet where both the hospital and community-based nurses and doctors can record monitoring results. This is usually kept by the patient so that all staff members involved in his or her care have access to an easily interpreted record of sequential results (White & Cooper 2002).

Disease-modifying antirheumatic drugs are slow to take effect and the patient may not notice any change for 6 weeks to 3 months or longer after starting to take them. As a physiotherapist, you should be aware of this when assessing a patient, ensuring that you discover when a particular drug was started. This will give you a truer picture of any changes in the patient's symptoms. There is an increasing trend to use DMARDs in combination, that is, to start another without stopping the currently used one. At present, however, the balance of evidence of the benefit of this therapy does not support the use of DMARDs in combination (SIGN 2000).

Efficacy and toxicity

Research suggests that sulfasalazine, leflunomide, penicillamine, intramuscular gold and methotrexate are similar in efficacy in the treatment of rheumatic disorders. Less-effective drugs include hydroxychloroquine (an antimalarial drug) and auranofin. A beneficial effect on radiological progression has been shown with all DMARDs except hydroxychloroquine. Antimalarials and auranofin have relatively low toxicity but their efficacy is only moderate. Gold has higher toxicity rates and a greater percentage of patients have to stop this therapy. Sulfasalazine and methotrexate are the current drugs of choice because of their more favourable efficacy/toxicity profiles (Pipitone & Choy 2003, SIGN 2000). A list of common side effects due to DMARDs can be seen in Table 7.1.

Corticosteroids

The anti-inflammatory effects of these drugs in producing symptomatic relief is well established, although recent studies show that benefits are not long-term. Corticosteroids can be used as 'bridge therapy' to provide relief from symptoms during the period when DMARDs are building up to their full effectiveness, which can be as long as 6 months with some drugs. Low-dose corticosteroids have also been shown to slow the progression of radiographic changes in early RA. When the drug is discontinued, however, articular damage continued at the pretreatment rate (Pipitone & Choy 2003, SIGN 2000, Wollheim 1999).

As with many of the drugs used in rheumatic conditions there are side effects, which in this case include fluid retention, hyperglycaemia, premature atherosclerosis and osteoporosis. Because of the time-limited clinical and functional effects and the marked adverse reactions with long-term use, it is not recommended that oral corticosteroids are routinely prescribed. If they are felt to be necessary, the lowest possible dose should be used for the shortest possible time and patients must be monitored for adverse effects (SIGN 2000).

Local corticosteroid injections

Steroid injections can alleviate pain and swelling. In conjunction with appropriate NSAID therapy and splinting, they can help in the effective management of rheumatic conditions. The steroids are rapidly taken up by the synovium and improvement may be seen within hours and can be maintained for weeks or months. Occasionally, the synovitis does not recur.

The sorts of rheumatic condition that respond well are RA, reactive arthritis, connective tissue disorders such as systemic lupus erythematosus, psoriatic arthritis, other types of seronegative spondyloarthropathies and the inflammatory stages of OA (Golding 1991). Intra-articular injections can allow local treatment of inflamed joints while minimizing unwanted systemic effects. They can also be used, as with oral or intramuscular corticosteroid therapy, to provide relief from symptoms pending the onset of DMARD effects. Even patients whose overall disease control is good can experience localized pain and swelling in one or more joints; injections can, therefore, be useful in these situations (Pipitone & Choy 2003, SIGN 2000).

Table 7.1 Established disease-modifying antirheumatic drugs and some side effects

Drug	Common/minor side effects	Rare/severe side effects
Hydroxychloroquine	Nausea, diarrhoea, headaches, skin reactions	Retinal toxicity, haematuria, proteinuria
Sulfasalazine	Nausea, diarrhoea, headache, mouth ulcers, rash	Leukopenia (decreased white blood cell count), thrombocytopenia (decreased platelets), allergic hepatitis
Methotrexate	Nausea, vomiting, diarrhoea, mouth ulcers, rash, hair loss, headaches, depression	Leukopenia, thrombocytopenia, allergic pneumonitis (rare), liver disease
Intramuscular gold	Mouth ulcers, rash, jaundice	Leukopenia, thrombocytopenia, proteinuria (protein in the urine), colitis, peripheral neuropathy
Penicillamine	Nausea, loss of taste, rash, reversible fall in platelet count	Bone marrow suppression, proteinuria, haematuria, autoimmune diseases
Auranofin	Nausea, diarrhoea, mouth ulcers, rash	Leukopenia, thrombocytopenia, hepatitis (rare)
Leflunomide	Nausea, vomiting, diarrhoea, anorexia, mouth ulcers, hair loss, headaches, dizziness, skin reactions, hypertension	Leukopenia, anaemia, thrombocytopenia, severe liver dysfunction (rare)

Modified from SIGN 2000, White & Cooper 2002 and Pipitone & Choy 2003.

Pharmacological management is central in the treatment of rheumatic disorders and has a marked effect on both the patient's condition and how s/he responds to the other types of treatment that may be available. It is extremely important for you to remind your patients that they should not stop taking their drugs or change the dosage when they start to attend for physiotherapy. If they do this it will be impossible for you to ascertain whether it is your intervention or other factors which are responsible for causing any improvement or deterioration.

Self-assessment question

- **SAQ 7.3** Briefly review the types of drug used in the management of rheumatic conditions. What are the benefits and disadvantages of each type? (See above.)

OSTEOARTHROSIS

Osteoarthrosis, which has already been mentioned a number of times, is the commonest joint disorder. It is strongly associated with ageing and is a major cause of pain and disability in the elderly population (Doherty et al 2001). It was previously considered to be an exclusively degenerative disorder that was a result of wear and tear in elderly joints. More recent work, however, suggests that this is not the case and that the pathological processes in OA are more dynamic in nature. It is not a single disease process but rather the outcome of a range of processes and disorders that can eventually lead to structural and functional failure of one or more synovial joints (Nuki 2002). Presently there are no interventions that are known to alter the long-term outcome of this condition, but appropriate simple management can help to alleviate the problems that it causes and will in turn benefit the patient with OA (Doherty et al 2001, Hutton 1995).

Osteoarthrosis occurs with great frequency throughout the world. X-ray evidence has shown OA changes in the joints of 40–60% of the population over the age of 35. As mentioned earlier, this percentage increases with age, reaching as much as 85% in those individuals aged over 75. More women show changes, particularly in the hand and/or knee, than men, particularly after the age of 50, but men are more frequently affected under the age of 45 (Nuki 2002). By the age of 50, however, X-ray changes of OA are seen in the lumbosacral area in 90% of the population (Kaufman & Sokoloff 1992).

Even though X-rays show these changes, it is interesting to note that the correlation between symptoms and radiographic evidence is poor. Some people with clear OA changes on X-ray will experience no symptoms while other individuals may have pain suggestive of OA in the absence of any radiographic findings (Nuki 2002).

Osteoarthrosis can affect both the axial and peripheral joints but some joints are often involved while others are rarely affected (Hutton 1995). Up to 25% of people over 65 years of age have OA in the knee or hip, which are the principal large joints to be affected. Generally the prevalence is greater in the knee joint (Doherty et al 2001). OA is progressive and the underlying pathological processes are both destructive and productive. It is the balance of these processes that dictates the rate of progression of the joint damage. The whole joint is involved, including subchondral bone, ligaments, capsule, synovial membrane, articular cartilage and the muscles surrounding the joint (Nuki 2002). There are also secondary inflammatory changes, which contribute to the destructive mechanisms. A classification of OA can be seen in Box 7.1.

Although OA is conventionally classified as primary, secondary or endemic it is becoming clear that all types involve multiple aetiological factors. These can be described as systemic or constitutional risk factors and local biomechanical risk factors. The systemic/constitutional factors that may increase susceptibility to OA include age, gender, genetic factors, racial predisposition and bone density. These, along with others such as injury, obesity, deformity and muscle weakness, can operate as local biomechanical risk factors that may determine the site and severity of the condition (Doherty et al 2001, Nuki 2002). The genes responsible for OA have not yet been identified, although work is being carried out on this. Some

Box 7.1   Classification of osteoarthrosis

1. Primary (idiopathic) osteoarthrosis
   Localized – hands and feet, knee, hip, spine or other joint
   Generalized – three or more joint areas
2. Secondary osteoarthrosis
   a. Post traumatic
   b. Congenital/developmental
   c. Localized – hip disease (e.g. Perthes disease), mechanical and local factors (e.g. obesity, hypermobility, valgus/varus deformity)
   d. Pre-existing bone and joint disorders, e.g. rheumatoid arthritis, Paget's disease, avascular necrosis
   e. Metabolic disease, e.g. haemophilia, gout
   f. Miscellaneous other diseases, e.g. neuropathic arthropathy, endocrine disorders
   g. Occupation/recreation-related
   h. Immobilization
3. Endemic, i.e. only found in a certain population or in a certain region

Adapted from Kaufman & Solokoff 1992, Doherty et al 2001 and Nuki 2002.

of the risk factors mentioned above, e.g. obesity, trauma and repetitive adverse loading (in the lower limb), are, however, potentially avoidable.

Pathological changes in osteoarthrosis

Before moving on to this section, it would be advisable to read the section on articular cartilage in Chapter 2 if you have not done so already. This provides the 'normal' background on which to superimpose the changes that occur in this pathological process.

In ageing joints, the metabolism, enzymatic modelling, collagen synthesis and the nature of the surrounding tissues remain normal (Bland 1993). As you are already aware, however, changes occur in articular cartilage with increase in age. These include a decrease in water content, some reduction in the tensile strength and stiffness of collagen (but the collagen fibre network is largely intact), decrease in proteoglycan synthesis and decreased

cartilage thickness. These changes are, however, distinct from those that occur in OA. Here the water content is increased, tensile strength is greatly decreased, the collagen fibre network is grossly disrupted, proteoglycan synthesis increases and the cartilage thickness initially increases and later decreases. Many of the tissues in and around the joint become thicker, hyperplastic and hypertrophic. This can result in increasing clinical deformity (Kaufman & Sokoloff 1993, Nuki 2002).

In OA there is damage to the chondrocytes and, as mentioned earlier, there are multiple mechanical and biological factors that can contribute to this. Three possible mechanisms are postulated by which the alterations in cartilage may develop:

- Abnormal mechanical forces that induce the failure and loss of cartilage
- Increased bone stiffness preceding and causing cartilage damage
- Chondrocyte dysfunction.

Chondrocytes make up about 5% of the total cartilage mass. They are responsible for synthesizing and secreting the bulk of the rest of the cartilage (proteoglycans, link proteins, collagen type II and hyaluronic acid; they also regulate breakdown of the cartilage with proteolytic enzymes). Exercise, movement and force upon the joint are essential for maintenance of the cartilage. It has been found that changes similar to OA can occur during immobilization, although the cartilage returns to normal when normal weight bearing resumes. If the joint is subjected to vigorous exercise at this stage, however, the cartilage does not return to its normal state and the OA type changes can be accelerated (Bland 1993).

Hyaline cartilage has a shock-absorbing function within the joint. Joint failure results from an imbalance between, on one side, the forces acting through the joint and the chemical processes occurring in the cartilage and, on the other side, the capacity of the cartilage to resist and repair any damage. This joint failure can happen in two ways either through excess loading damaging initially normal tissue or abnormal cartilage being further damaged by normal levels of mechanical stress (Fig. 7.1; Nuki 2002).

Once the chondrocytes are damaged, matrix breakdown results from release of chondrocytic

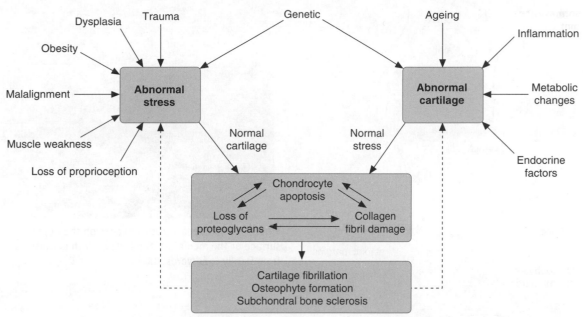

Figure 7.1 Possible mechanisms for the development of osteoarthrosis. (Redrawn with permission from Nuki 2002.)

enzymes and, overall, the development of OA seems to be an imbalance between synthesis and breakdown of cartilage; attempts to repair the damage are followed by a failure in the system. There is loss of cartilage and the underlying bone, leading to a reduction in normal joint function. The primary cause of this loss of tissue is the degradation of proteoglycans and collagens by active proteases. In OA the most likely source of these proteases is the chondrocytes themselves (Cawston & Rowan 1998). The effect of this is that the chondrocytes synthesize type I and III collagen at the expense of the normal type II.

At the beginning of the pathological process there is great metabolic activity but as the process advances the chondrocytes fail and this activity decreases. This is what causes the decrease in proteoglycans, which in turn increases stiffness in the cartilage so causing it to become more susceptible to mechanical disruption (Cawston & Rowan 1998, Kaufman & Sokoloff 1993, Nuki 2002). The smooth surface of the cartilage is breached and collagen fibres break. Roughening (fibrillation) occurs and friction on this surface during joint movement causes particles to be released that are then absorbed by the synovium. This triggers an inflammatory response that is probably due to the release of intracellular enzymes. This is experienced by the patient as stiffness or aching in the joint some time after exercise rather than at the time movement is occurring (Dandy & Edwards 2003).

All the joint tissues depend on each other for health and function. Insult to one impacts on the rest. The OA process involves the production of new tissue, bone as well as cartilage, and remodelling of joint shape (Doherty et al 2001). The subchondral bone is abnormally active with an increase in bone density and in the number of cells present. New spurs of bone (osteophytes) form at the joint margins (Fig. 7.2) and these can restrict movement (Dandy & Edwards 2003).

Bone beneath the hyaline cartilage becomes hard and dense, and there is often some change in the shape and congruity of the articular surfaces. This in turn alters the line through which weight passes across the joint so that different areas of cartilage begin to experience greater stresses. As the cartilage fails, the bone beneath is exposed and becomes hard and 'eburnated'. Without the articular cartilage to enhance movement, friction increases and weight transmission is uneven. Because of overloading in some parts of the joint, microfractures

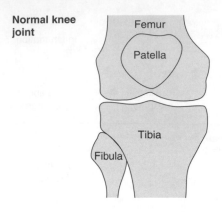

Normal knee joint

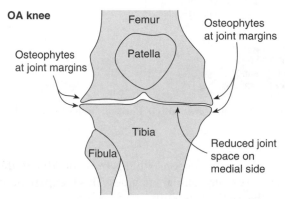

OA knee

Figure 7.2 Formation of osteophytes at joint margins.

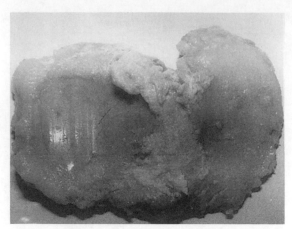

Figure 7.3 Osteoarthrotic changes on the upper surface of the medial tibial plateau. (With permission from Dandy & Edwards 2003.)

can occur. These heal with callus, making the bone even harder, denser and less resilient, so increasing the potential for further microfractures to occur. Synovial fluid can enter cracks in the bone and form subchondral cysts (Dandy & Edwards 2003).

The photograph in Figure 7.3 shows exposed bone and osteophytes on the upper surface of the medial plateau of the tibia (this has been removed during an operation for total knee replacement).

If the disease continues to advance, the joint becomes more and more disorganized with decreased joint space and formation of osteophytes at the joint margin. As the joint surfaces are worn away the ligaments become lax, leading to instability and deformity (Fig. 7.4).

Primary osteoarthrosis

In primary OA, the first joints to be affected are often small joints in the hand such as the interphalangeal

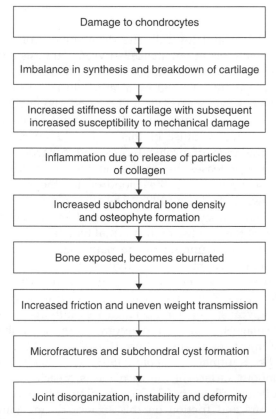

Figure 7.4 Summary of possible joint changes in osteoarthritis.

joints, the first carpometacarpal joint and occasionally the intercarpal joints; and the first metatarsophalangeal joint in the foot. There are also nodes that appear over the interphalangeal joints called Heberden's nodes (distal) and Bouchard's nodes (proximal); these are usually painless (Kaufman & Sokoloff 1992). The development of Heberden's nodes in middle age is a marker for a strong genetic predisposition to develop OA in the knee joint as part of the generalized condition (Doherty et al 2001).

Generalized 'nodal' OA tends to most commonly affect white women during the fifth and sixth decades, presenting in a polyarticular manner. This is the perimenopausal period and suggests a link to oestrogen deficiency as an important risk factor for the development of the condition (Nuki 2002).

There is a difference in the progression of OA in weight-bearing and non-weight-bearing joints. The upper limb joints can be painful and range of movement may be lost. Problems do, however, tend to be less disabling as the joints are seldom under load. More disabling problems tend to occur in the larger weight-bearing hip and knee joints and the spine (Dandy & Edwards 2003).

Inheritance is a major factor in predisposition to large joint OA and up to 25% of people over 65 years of age have OA in the knee or hip (Doherty et al 2001). In the elderly population OA of the knee is the most common cause of disability. The pathological changes generally occur in the medial compartment. X-ray changes and clinical findings parallel each other, which is unusual in OA, where the radiographic evidence generally predates clinical manifestations (Kaufman & Sokoloff 1992). Pain is well localized to the anterior or medial aspects of the knee and upper tibia. Patellofemoral pain is more noticeable when going up and down stairs or hills. If the patient experiences pain in the posterior aspect of the joint this would suggest a popliteal cyst (Doherty et al 2001).

In OA of the hip the pain begins insidiously, is usually bilateral and maximal in the anterior groin area with variable radiation to the buttock and anterolateral thigh, knee or shin regions. Referred pain is usually diffuse. Occasionally, a patient will complain of low back pain initially if a flexion contracture of the hip has increased the lumbar lordosis. OA of the hip is more common in men (Dandy & Edwards 2003). In both hip and knee OA the patient may exhibit antalgic gait, which is jerky and asymmetrical as a result of unequal weightbearing, i.e. less time spent on the painful side (Doherty et al 2001).

Within the spine degenerative changes can occur in the intervertebral discs and in the synovial joints. Symptoms most frequently begin at around 55 years of age. Initially pain is often mild, intermittent and localized. As the degenerative changes progress, however, pain may increase in intensity and be associated with muscle spasm (Ray and Cowie 2002). There is little correlation between changes in the intervertebral disc and clinical signs in either the cervical or lumbar areas. Most individuals have some X-ray changes from the age of 35. When the synovial joints are affected, however, symptoms do tend to occur more commonly (Kaufman & Sokoloff 1992, Ray and Cowie 2002).

Secondary osteoarthrosis

Box 7.1 provides a summary of the numerous possible causes of secondary OA. This offers some explanation as to why a wider range of joints are affected by secondary OA than by primary OA.

Joint abnormality due to previous trauma may predispose a patient to premature, localized OA changes. Examples of this could be malalignment following a fracture through the joint surface or soft tissue damage such as meniscus injury or damage to a cruciate ligament. The risk of developing OA is increased threefold following major knee injury (Nuki 2002). Irregularities within joints can also be due to genetic or developmental problems such as Perthes disease, epiphyseal dysplasia or slipped epiphysis (Dandy & Edwards 2003). Inflammatory arthritis also causes damage to the articular surfaces, which can predispose to premature changes of OA.

There does seem to be some correlation between OA in certain joints and specific occupations and/or leisure pursuits. Not all of the work has been conclusive but, for example, miners seem to develop OA in the hips, knees and spine; foundry workers in the elbows; fingers, elbows and knees are affected in dockyard workers; farmers, firefighters and construction workers develop OA in the hips and knees; and people in occupations that involve a lot of knee bending, squatting, kneeling and heavy lifting develop problems in their knee joints. Jobs involving repetitive pinch grip predispose to the development of OA changes in the distal interphalangeal joints (Kaufman & Sokoloff 1992, Nuki 2002). Conversely, as mentioned earlier, immobilization can also adversely affect the cartilage, initiating OA-type changes.

There seems to be a correlation between certain types of metabolic or endocrine disorders and OA changes. Age, sex, race, heredity and obesity are also implicated in the development of OA but this may be as true for primary disease as for secondary. Obesity is now a well established risk factor, particularly in OA of the knee joint. It precedes the development of knee OA with a 40% increase in risk for every 5 kg increase in weight. Conversely, commensurate decreases in incident knee OA have been shown for every 5 kg weight loss, demonstrating that obesity is a modifiable risk factor (Nuki 2002). This is an important point for physiotherapists to be aware of when providing advice for patients with OA in lower limb joints who are overweight.

Self-assessment questions

- **SAQ 7.4** Which joints are the most commonly affected in primary OA?
- **SAQ 7.5** Review the possible causes of secondary OA. (See above sections for answers.)

Problem-solving exercise 7.1

Using the information that has been provided so far, try to work out the clinical features you might expect to find when assessing a patient with OA. If you are not sure, or wish to see if you are on the right lines, remember you can check your ideas later in the chapter under the relevant section; an answer is also given at the end of the chapter.

ASSESSMENT OF THE PATIENT WITH OSTEOARTHROSIS

Case study 7.1: Mrs Stamford (1)

Mrs Stamford is a 70-year-old lady who is attending for outpatient physiotherapy for the first time with a diagnosis of OA knee. She has noticed increasing pain with decreased mobility in her left knee joint for the last 5 years. This has only caused her problems in the preceding 6 months and seems to be getting worse. She walks with one stick in her left hand.

Problem-solving exercise 7.2

Decide what you need to find out during your assessment of this patient:

a. During your subjective assessment
b. During your objective examination.

Write down a checklist of what you feel would be appropriate questions and examination techniques.

Case study 7.1: Mrs Stamford, continued (2)

On assessment the following information was obtained:

Subjective assessment

This retired teacher has had increasing problems with pain and loss of movement in her left knee for the last 5 years but has only experienced significant functional problems in the last 6 months. These seem to be increasing in severity.

The pain is continuous but is worse on movement and locomotion. It often disturbs her sleep. The pain is well localized to the anteromedial aspect of the knee and upper tibia.

Her knee feels particularly stiff in the morning but loosens up after about 15 minutes when she starts to move around. Generally, however, she describes the left knee as 'stiff' in comparison to the right.

She identifies her main problem as being unable to walk far enough, because of pain and stiffness, to perform her everyday living and leisure activities such as shopping, walking the dog, visiting friends and housework (particularly walking up and down hills or stairs, when she experiences more pain in the patellofemoral area). She bought the walking stick herself and finds it helps a little, but has been given no instruction in its use.

Social history: widow, living alone in a terraced house half a mile from the nearest shops, unable to drive. Bathroom and bedroom upstairs. Four steep steps to front door. Two grown-up children living away, neighbour helps with shopping once a week.

Hobbies: walking and bowls. Unable to take part in these activities for last 6 months.

Drug history: takes aspirin as necessary for the pain. Has never taken steroids.

Past medical history: nil of note. General health good.

Objective assessment

Observation
Mrs Stamford walks with a stick, favouring her left leg. She found getting up from the chair difficult after sitting in the waiting room. She had some problems removing her shoe and tights from her left leg. The left knee joint looks enlarged and there appears to be some swelling. The bulk of the quadriceps looks reduced. She holds her knee in slight flexion when on the plinth. Slight genu varus deformity (Fig. 7.5).

Skin colour/condition: normal

Thickening around the joint line.

Right knee: nothing abnormal discovered.

Examination
Range of movement
- Right knee active and passive full range
- Left knee active: extension minus 5°, flexion 80° with pain throughout range increasing towards maximum flexion
- Left knee passive: extension minus 5°, flexion 90° with discomfort at end of range
- There is coarse crepitus on movement
- Full range of movement in hips and ankles, equal right and left with no discomfort.

Swelling (measured at base of patella)
Left 40 cm; right 34 cm.

Muscle bulk:
- 5 cm above base of patella – left 35 cm; right 39 cm
- 15 cm above base of patella – left 40 cm; right 48 cm.

Muscle strength
Quadriceps and hamstrings on left Gd IV; all other groups Gd V both sides.

Stability
Laxity of the joint is obvious on testing the collateral ligaments, with an increase in pain on the medial side on varus stress.

Palpation
- Left knee tender on palpation anteromedially and posteriorly
- Soft effusion but no increased temperature.

Functional assessment
Mrs Stamford has some difficulties with washing and dressing the lower half of her body. Walking distance is limited by pain and she goes up and down steps one leg at a time. The therapist observed that both the patient's ability to move from sitting to standing and back, and her bed mobility are affected by the pain and stiffness.

You now have a great deal of information about this lady and her particular issues. The next step is to sift out the main problems that you would wish to address when discussing your ideas for management with the patient. Before going on to this, let's review the main areas involved in assessment that are used to establish the initial database. This acts as a precursor for identifying specific problems and the goals of treatment in relation to the patient's needs. It also aids in the design of an appropriate treatment plan in partnership with the patient.

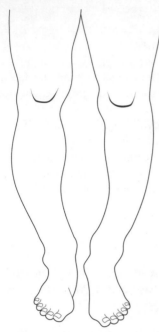

Figure 7.5   Genu varus deformity at the knee joint.

Assessment guidelines

It is important that you are alert and that you listen and respond to the questions and needs of the patient during the assessment. It should be an interactive session relating to the patient's goals. These will be dependent on various factors such as age, lifestyle and the stage of the disease process. The time of day that the assessment occurs and the level of patient activity just prior to it should also be taken into account.

Subjective information

Demographic details and history of the present condition

- Diagnosis
- Onset, including symptoms, rate of progression and whether it is better or worse at present
- Joints affected
- Main problems as described by the patient, e.g. pain levels/behaviour, stiffness, loss of function. (Some of these could be assessed using visual analogue scales or numerical rating scales.)

- Functional ability (various functional scales may be used for this part of the assessment)
- Systemic problems (this will not be an issue for the patient with primary OA)
- Any previous treatment and its effect (not for the patient in this case study).

General health and past medical history

Medication/drug history

- Present drugs, including dosage and effects
- Past drugs taken with any side effects, reasons for stopping. Has the patient taken steroids in the past?

Splints

Not relevant for this patient.

Social history

- Occupation
- Hobbies
- Accommodation
- Family/carers
- Any external support agencies involved, e.g. social services or voluntary organizations.

Objective information

General observation

- Appearance
- Gait.

A lot can be learned from observing how a patient gets up from the chair in the waiting room, walks through to the treatment area, turns to look at the physiotherapist, prepares for the physical examination, gets on to the plinth and so on. These observations can then be used as cues to personalize the questioning during the subjective part of the assessment.

Joints involved

- Observation of any apparent swelling/effusion, colour changes, skin condition, deformity and so on
- Physical examination to discover amount of swelling and muscle wasting, range of movement/stiffness, end feel, crepitus, stability, muscle power and extent/nature of any deformity

- Palpation to ascertain temperature, skin condition, type of effusion, thickening, tenderness, muscle spasm and any sensory disturbances.

It is important to try and differentiate where the pain is coming from. In general, pain of joint origin is characterized by discomfort throughout range whereas that from tendons or bursae can be isolated by palpation and are more likely to occur during part of the range of movement. Muscular pain can be indicated by local tenderness or by discomfort on a particular movement. It is likely to be aggravated by active contraction (Caldron 1995).

Extra-articular manifestations
Not relevant for this patient.

Functional assessment

- Activities of daily living assessment, e.g. stairs, transfers, washing, dressing, walking, occupation, housework, hobbies, driving, etc. as appropriate

- Health assessment questionnaires such as the Arthritis Impact Measurement Scale (AIMS) could be used. These take psychosocial and general wellbeing issues into account as well as functional problems (Hutton 1995, Rheumatic Care Association of chartered Physiotherapists 1994).

This would be an excellent opportunity for you to check back to the list you made in response to Problem-solving exercise 7.2. See how many of the areas of the assessment you managed to come up with independently and fill any gaps by using the information above. By this point in the process you should have a good picture of the patient and her specific issues. Only thorough enquiry and physical examination can determine causation and severity of pain, degree of disability and the impact of the OA on the patient's life (Doherty et al 2001).

The general format given above will provide you with an overall structure to use in the assessment of most patients with rheumatic conditions in the clinical setting. Assessment practices will vary from centre to centre, but on the whole these are the areas that should be covered by the physiotherapist. Some departments will have their own ready-printed sheets or booklets to fill in as the patient is questioned and examined, which can be very useful as a prompt particularly for students and newly qualified staff.

> ### Problem-solving exercise 7.3
>
> Use the information given in the case study to try and identify this patient's main issues. Then go on to think about the goals of physiotherapy management that you could use in order to design your treatment plan.

CLINICAL FEATURES OF OSTEOARTHROSIS

By now you should have a good idea of the different clinical manifestations of OA that are of relevance to the physiotherapist. This section gives a brief overview.

Clinically patients experience gradually developing joint pain with stiffness, enlargement of joint size and limitation of movement. The usual symptoms that cause the patient to seek treatment are the pain and loss of function as these are the ones that have a marked effect on lifestyle. In the later stages there may well be instability and deformity.

Pain

The pain of OA is typically of insidious onset and is variable so the patient may describe good days and bad days. Later on it becomes continuous and may disturb sleep. Patients with chronic pain may describe non-restorative sleep, night pain, fatigue and low mood, which can compound the pain and disability (Doherty et al 2001). The pain is mainly related to movement and weight bearing: it may continue for a while after activity but is generally relieved by rest (Dandy & Edwards 2003, Doherty et al 2001). There is no nerve supply to the hyaline cartilage but other periarticular structures, bone and capsule are richly innervated and these give rise to the pain. If there is a secondary inflammatory response in a particular patient then this may also release substances that act as pain mediators, e.g. prostaglandins and cytokines (Hutton 1995, Kaufman & Sokoloff 1992).

The patient may describe the pain as localized or very diffuse and it can be referred to an unaffected joint, for example to the hip from the back, to the groin and knee from the hip or from the knee up the thigh and into the hip area.

Stiffness and limitation of movement

The terms stiffness and limitation of movement are used separately here as if describing different concepts. Stiffness is a difficult phenomenon to define and is described in varying ways by patients. What they describe as 'stiffness' is often a collection of factors, which may include some link with pain, muscle weakness and/or limitation of movement at a joint. It is a multifaceted feature of many rheumatic conditions and, although patients appear able to assess its severity, they have difficulties with definition and are often ambiguous in the terms they use. The reason that we emphasize this is that it is important for you to spend some time investigating the patients' perceptions of the state of their joints, i.e. the subjective aspects; as well as carrying out the objective tests.

Some physiotherapy departments may use questionnaires to find out about these points, an example of which can be seen in Figure 7.6. This is particularly related to the hand but could be adapted for any stiff joint/area of the body. It uses a series of visual analogue scales to look at the ease and quality of movement, a list of descriptors to ascertain what factors the patient associates with stiffness and then some functional questions to ask about specific activities. It also provides an opportunity for the patient to describe his/her main problems.

Limitation of movement usually occurs slowly as the joint surfaces change shape and osteophytes form. Patients may not notice the change in the amount of movement until it affects function. Pain often prevents the patient moving through full range and this could result in shortening of soft tissue structures so leading to further loss of movement and deformity. Limitation of movement, although an element of stiffness, can be measured more objectively and the results recorded. The results of both objective and subjective tests do, however, make up part of the initial data base that you will later use to ascertain whether any changes have occurred as a consequence of your intervention.

If there is joint laxity, the patient may have a sense of instability and be unwilling to move fully which, again, combined with the pain will decrease mobility.

Loss or alteration of function

All the factors mentioned so far will tend to change the patient's ability to carry out functional activities. As with the loss of movement this process can be insidious, with patients subconsciously restricting their actions to those permitted by the affected joint(s). They may walk shorter distances, only go upstairs when absolutely necessary or not work for as long or as hard without a pause.

This process tends to be self-perpetuating. With decreased activity the muscle power will decrease accordingly so causing the joint to be less stable. This puts more stress on the joint structures so increasing pain, limitation of movement and possibly deformity. Deformity in one joint will inevitably have an effect on adjacent areas of the body. Signs and symptoms may, therefore, extend over time. For example, if a patient has OA in the hip joint, which consequently becomes fixed in a degree of flexion, the level of the pelvis may drop on that side in order for the heel to reach the floor or the lumbar lordosis may increase, so leading to low back pain and other related problems.

Many patients experience disability as a result of secondary weakness. If there is timely and appropriate intervention from the healthcare team it may be possible to enable the patient to maintain satisfactory functional levels and to avoid or at least postpone potential problems.

X-ray appearance

It is important for you to be able to recognize the common changes of OA on radiographs. The main features are:

- Narrowing of joint space
- Sclerosis (increased density) of the bone on the weight-bearing surfaces
- Formation of osteophytes at joint margins
- Possible appearance of subchondral cysts
- Changes in the shape of the bone and possibly deformity.

Hand Questionnaire

This questionnaire makes up part of the assessment of your hand. The information your physiotherapist obtains from it will be used to help formulate a treatment plan tailored specifically for you. It is easy to fill in, it consists of placing a mark on several scales, choosing from a list of words and answering some simple questions. Please complete it and hand it in before you leave the department. Thank you.

1. Please place a mark on the following scales at the point you feel appropriate for the state of your hand at the moment. When you try to make a fist with your affected hand:

(a) How fully can you move it?

No movement   Full movement

(b) How easily can you move it?

Extremely easily   With great difficulty

(c) How painful is it?

Not painful at all   The worst pain I can imagine

(d) How stiff does it feel?

Extremely stiff   No stiffness

2. Please place a ring around any of the words below that describe the way your hand feels:

Limited movement   Painful   Tight   Rigid

Weak   Tense   Stuck   Hurts   Inflexible

Sore   Immobile   Aches   Solid

3. The following questions apply to everyday activities, please circle Yes or No as appropriate:

(a) Can you EASILY write with a pen/pencil?   Yes   No
(b) Can you EASILY turn a key in a lock?   Yes   No
(c) Can you EASILY tie the laces on a pair of shoes? Yes   No
(d) Can you EASILY button an article of clothing?   Yes   No
(e) Can you EASILY open jars of food?   Yes   No

4. What activity would YOU describe as most difficult due to your hand problem?

_____

_____

_____

_____

_____

Thank you for filling in this questionnaire. Remember to hand it in BEFORE you go home today.

Figure 7.6   An example of a questionnaire that could be used to investigate hand stiffness in patients with rheumatic conditions.

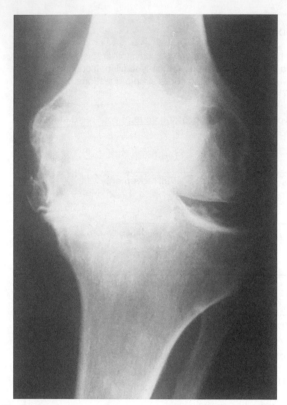

Figure 7.7   X-ray of an osteoarthrotic knee joint. (With permission from Dandy & Edwards 2003).

Many of the above features can be seen in the X-ray of an OA knee joint in Figure 7.7.

IDENTIFICATION OF PATIENT PROBLEMS AND GOALS OF MANAGEMENT

Review point

At this stage you have sufficient information to identify the range of difficulties that this patient may have. Review your response to Problem-solving exercise 7.3 and keep these points in mind as you read the following section.

As part of the overall process of assessment, you must use your skill and judgement in problem solving. Initially this will help you to decide whether the patient might be helped by treatment and/or a self-care programme. In Mrs Stamford's case you would probably decide that she would benefit from this type of intervention. With some patients, however, the joint changes and associated problems have progressed to such an extent that physiotherapy intervention would be of no benefit. In this situation surgery may be the only way of relieving the patient's pain and improving function. If this is the case, then you may have to refer him/her back to the consultant or general practitioner.

In Mrs Stamford's case the problems that you should have identified from the information given were as follows:

- Pain
- Stiffness/limitation of movement
- Muscle weakness
- Functional difficulties – particularly gait problems such as walking any distance and going up and down stairs, steps and hills.

In the light of these identified problems, therefore, what goals might you decide on in partnership with Mrs Stamford? (Please note that the goals below are framed using professional terminology; remember that this needs to be phrased differently when you discuss the goals with your patient)

1. Reduction of pain
2. To maintain or increase (if possible) range and ease of movement
3. To maintain or increase (if possible) muscle strength
4. To correct deformity (if possible) or prevent any further deformity occurring
5. To maximize functional potential and maintain or increase exercise tolerance
6. To educate, advise and support the patient with regard to her condition
7. To encourage the patient to take on responsibility for self-care and self-management.

As necessary, these goals of treatment should be formulated in liaison with other members of the healthcare team. It is important to remember, however, that the patient is the key here and the goals must take her requirements into consideration. Participative goal setting avoids professional dominance (Harvey 2003) and moves us away from the 'medical model' of health where the patient has a passive role and the professional assumes the position of power in the therapeutic relationship.

Goals should be explicit, achievable and challenging and they also need to be recorded. It may be useful to use SMART goals (S, specific; M, measurable; A, achievable; R, realistic; and T, time-limited). Once you have formulated the written management plan you can share this with the patient (Harvey 2003).

> ### Review point
>
> Does the list of problems and goals of treatment that you came up with earlier match the ones that we have suggested? If you did not manage to come up with all of them, don't worry. Check the ones you missed and make sure you understand them. If you came up with all of the ones mentioned above and more – well done! Make sure that any extras you thought of are realistic and relevant to this patient and that you had not started to consider issues concerning management. That's the next step.

> ### Self-assessment question
>
> - **SAQ 7.6** What changes might you expect to see on an X-ray of a patient with OA? (See above.)

GENERAL MANAGEMENT PRINCIPLES FOR PATIENTS WITH RHEUMATIC CONDITIONS

A very important point to remember when treating patients with any rheumatic condition is that no intervention can influence the disease progression. The principles of management you use here should be the same as for any chronic disease, with education being a key element. It is important for healthcare professionals to work together and with patients to identify realistic expectations of intervention. This can enable patients to develop a sense of control over the disease and ensures that identical, and not conflicting, advice and information is provided. This takes a team approach (Doherty et al 2001, Hutton 1995).

When considering management in all types of rheumatic condition you should remember several points:

- The time course of the disease, i.e. it is a chronic condition for which (in most cases) there is no 'cure'

- The variability of the disease from time to time in the same patient and the variability from patient to patient. Many of the conditions are phasic, with exacerbations and remissions. Thus it is sometimes difficult to know whether the intervention is beneficial or whether the patient is entering a slightly 'better' phase. The effect that drugs have on the condition must also be considered when evaluating intervention.

> ### Review point
>
> This may be a good time to briefly review the timescales involved for drugs (especially DMARDs) to take effect.

- Optimal management involves the combined healthcare team – usually no one person can meet all the requirements that may be involved in the patient's management. Effective and comprehensive care can only be provided when the specific problems of the patient, the resources available and the patient's environment are taken into account. The elements that you were introduced to in the movement continuum theory of physical therapy (Cott et al 1995; see Introduction) are relevant here and will help you to consider patients in a more holistic way. A team approach has been shown to be effective in optimizing the management of patients with rheumatic conditions (SIGN 2000, Wollheim 1999).

General management of patients with rheumatic conditions should be geared towards the following areas:

- Minimization of damage/destruction in the joints and other tissues

- Maximization of function within the boundaries of the disease, considering the patient's ability, motivation level and environment
- Matching of goals to the requirements of the particular patient.

These aims of management can be mapped closely to those already identified as aims of physiotherapy intervention.

Review point

Use your background knowledge and the information given in this chapter to work out who might be included in the healthcare team involved in the management of patients with rheumatic conditions (hint – they will not all be healthcare professionals).

Elements of general management

Pharmacological management

As explained earlier in the chapter, most patients with rheumatic conditions will need some sort of drug therapy as part of their management.

Rest

In the past it was common practice to recommend resting joints with active synovitis. More recently it has been shown that moderate, even, in some cases, fairly vigorous exercise does not exacerbate the disease. Overuse, however, especially involving repetitive motion, can cause synovitis to worsen (Bernhard 2001). For many patients the key point here is the importance of finding a balance between carrying out exercise and taking sufficient rest periods throughout the day. This is especially pertinent in those conditions where fatigue may be one of the symptoms, e.g. RA. Appropriate rest periods can improve symptoms, minimizing general fatigue and local joint discomfort. But the balance between rest and exercise is essential to avoid complications that may be caused by immobility.

Occupational therapy

Occupational therapists (OTs) offer a functional approach to the management of patients with rheumatic conditions. The OT will carry out an assessment to discover which activities are important to the patient and to highlight any particular difficulties. S/he will then explore possible solutions with the patient. The following interventions may be included in the approach to patients with rheumatic conditions:

- Practical advice on dealing with everyday problems. This may involve retraining in activities of daily living (ADL), from household and personal tasks to work and leisure activities. This may involve assessing for and providing special equipment for the home and any other relevant situations (e.g. leisure, work)
- Discussing the condition with patients, how it affects them and what they can do to help themselves
- Making and fitting splints to rest or support affected joints
- Teaching activities to improve muscle strength or joint mobility
- Teaching techniques to help the patient to manage pain levels (Arthritis Research Campaign 2002).

One area that is particularly important for patients with rheumatic conditions is that of joint protection. Both the OT and the physiotherapist may be involved with this (see later).

Problem–solving exercise 7.4

'Joint protection aims to reduce pain and stress on joints while carrying out everyday activities' (SIGN 2000). With the information you have so far about the problems encountered by patients with rheumatic conditions, try to come up with some ideas that could help a patient to protect joint surfaces and surrounding structures.

Physiotherapy

The role of the physiotherapist in assessing and treating patients with rheumatic conditions is well recognized in clinical practice (SIGN 2000). Responsibility for physical rehabilitation falls largely to the physiotherapist at all stages, although there are many areas of overlap with other health-care professionals. Physiotherapists can employ many modes of treatment but, as mentioned earlier, these need thoughtful application, monitoring and fine tuning in order to fit the particular patient. Physiotherapy management will be returned to later.

Podiatry

Podiatry is concerned with the management of foot disorders and the problems associated with general health conditions that manifest themselves in the feet and the lower limb. The main aim is to reduce pain and disability and thereby increase patient mobility. Podiatrists can undertake the following areas of work:

- Gait assessment/biomechanics
- Diagnosis and treatment of conditions of the lower limb
- Foot health education
- Prescription and manufacture of orthotics
- Footwear assessment and advice
- Working with a team to manage conditions such as RA
- Foot surgery including the use of local anaesthetics.

The management of the foot in patients with rheumatic conditions can be complex, with problems ranging from discomfort to destruction of the dynamic structure of the foot. Podiatrists are most likely to use their skills in assessment of the feet of patients with rheumatic conditions followed by the production and fitting of orthoses and advice on footwear. The importance of appropriate footwear provision for comfort, mobility and stability is well recognized in clinical practice (SIGN 2000, Stewart & Monoghan 1998).

Patient education

It appears to be accepted that patient education is beneficial in enabling patients to manage their disease and that it may also enhance compliance and co-operation with management interventions.

It is important, however, for you to consider the possible adverse effects of educational programmes. It has been suggested that, for patients with recent onset of a chronic illness, information could cause depression, feelings of helplessness and fear (Kirwan 1990). Donovan et al (1989) also suggested that confusion can occur if the content of the programme 'does not relate to the beliefs of the group or the individual'. It must be remembered that any educational input must be adapted to the current needs of the patient.

Taking these points into account, work has been done that suggests that education for patients with rheumatic conditions can be beneficial in improving outcomes of treatment. Although the mechanism is not clear, it seems that access to information and therapist contact reduce pain and disability, improve patient autonomy (self-efficacy) and reduce healthcare costs (Doherty et al 2001). There is evidence that more positive outcomes for health status and prognosis correlate with higher education and self-efficacy levels. Programmes can positively affect knowledge levels, behaviour, attitude, disability and depression. This type of arthritis patient education programme has been shown to be a useful method for enhancing self-care management techniques and improving physical and psychological health outcomes (Barlow et al 1998). Because of this evidence, therefore, it is suggested that the effectiveness of current treatments for arthritis can be enhanced through education. It is essential, however, that a common approach to this patient education is adopted by all members of the healthcare team to ensure that the patient receives a consistent message (SIGN 2000).

Problem-solving exercise 7.5

What subjects do you think could be usefully covered in an educational programme for patients with rheumatic disorders?
  In what ways do you think the information can be communicated to the patients?

An educational programme should be based on the needs and beliefs of the patient, building on his/her current level of knowledge. It is therefore important for an agenda to be agreed by both patient and the 'educator' – who is often the physiotherapist. As well as providing information and advice, the programme can help to reinforce advice provided by the healthcare team, enable the patient to achieve appropriate behavioural changes (if necessary) and offer psychological support. Programmes including a psychobehavioural component in addition to providing information appear to have better outcomes in terms of pain relief, joint protection and functional ability.

One disadvantage of this approach is that it tends to be labour-intensive (SIGN 2000). It has been shown that a single session can improve patients' knowledge and that this is sustained over a period of 6 months (Barry et al 1994). In order to change behaviour on a longer-term basis, however, there needs to be regular repetition of verbal and written information, repeat demonstration and practice of techniques with weekly review and goal setting (Wade & Rimmer 1998).

The educational elements of patients' management may be organized by a range of people and presented in a variety of ways, often depending on local policies, staffing and resources. There may be time to provide the relevant information and advice when a patient comes for treatment, but this is not always possible in a busy department. Some hospitals may have the resources to organize one or more sessions to enable the patients to learn about the condition, either as an individualized package or in a group setting. For group sessions one or a number of health professionals may be involved. This could be based at a hospital, clinic or GP practice, or the programme may be organized entirely by a self-help group run by patients and carers with input from an organization such as the Arthritis Care. This may still involve some health professionals such as rheumatologists, physiotherapists and OTs perhaps being asked to speak on particular areas of interest, to give demonstrations of equipment or run exercise sessions.

For example, some National Ankylosing Spondylitis Society (NASS) groups are run on a weekly basis by physiotherapists. These may involve exercise sessions on dry land and in a hydrotherapy pool if this is available, as well as presentations by outside speakers. Meetings can provide opportunities for questions and answers, group discussions, films and videos, lectures, practical exercise groups, distribution of literature and social interaction. This type of arrangement enables group members to support and encourage each other, which can lead to increased compliance with management (Wade & Rimmer 1998).

The advantages of a group setting are that more people can be seen at one time, wider issues may be brought up for discussion, encouragement is often given to new members and each patient realizes that he or she is not the only person with the condition and the particular problems it engenders. These groups may help patients to be less reliant on health professionals and to take more responsibility for their own management as they often take place outside the hospital setting.

There are some disadvantages to group sessions in that information is not tailored for specific patients, and some people are discouraged by seeing other individuals whose condition may be at a more advanced stage. These problems are negated if it is possible to see the patients on a one-to-one basis, i.e. it is possible to make the information pertinent to each individual and to ensure that s/he understands. There are often difficulties, however, with time constraints and this method may also make the patients focus very much on their own problems.

Other ways of providing information include literature (produced in-house or obtained from organizations such as the Arthritis Research Campaign), monthly telephone reviews, interactive computer programs (Doherty et al 2001) and recommending relevant websites for those patients who are computer literate.

The sort of information and advice that could be included in an educational programme for patients with rheumatic conditions can be seen in Box 7.2. Compare this to the suggestions you came up with in response to Problem-solving exercise 7.5. This is a basis from which to work and you can add to or subtract from it to make the programme as relevant as possible to the patient. You will note that it is presented under specific headings and then suggests the sort of questions that patients might ask in each section.

Box 7.2   Possible information/advice to be included in educational programmes for patients with rheumatic conditions

Rheumatic conditions: information and advice

Nature of condition
- What is it?
- What effects will it have on me?

Investigation
- How is it diagnosed?
- What is the meaning of the tests I've had?
- Will there be any more?

Prognosis
- Can it be cured?
- How will it affect me in the future?

Management
- Can it be treated?
- How can it be treated?
- When should treatment begin?
- What treatments should I have?
- Will I need surgery?

Drugs
- What medication should I have?
- What are the possible side effects?
- How long should I continue on the medication?

Exercise/relaxation
(techniques may be taught in the sessions)
- Should I exercise?
- What can I do to keep moving and how much?

Activities of daily living
(including aids and appliances/splints and orthotics)
- Should I continue to work?
- Should I continue with my hobbies?
- How can I carry on with my everyday activities?
- Is there any equipment that might be helpful to me?
- How can I look after my joints?

Resources available
- Is there anywhere I can go for help and advice?
- Are there any organizations I can contact by telephone and/or via their websites? (about support, equipment, footwear, weight loss, exercise groups/venues, etc.)
- Are there any local self-help groups?

Other interventions
(could include links to local counsellors who may be able to help with low mood/depression, coping skills, pain management, etc. and complementary therapists)
- Do any complementary therapies help my condition?
- Is there a diet that will help me?
- The pain is really getting me down, is there anyone I can talk to?

From SIGN 2000, Doherty et al 2001, ARC 2003a, Harvey 2003.

Review point

The three key features in relation to patient education are as follows:

- It should be consistent and undertaken by all members of the healthcare team in both primary and secondary care settings
- Patients should be provided with at least an information booklet or leaflet and if possible an individualized programme of education (SIGN 2000)
- Sustained change in behaviour requires reinforcement including repetition of information and demonstration and supported repeated practice (Wade & Rimmer 1998).

Joint protection

As mentioned earlier, joint protection is particularly important for patients with rheumatic conditions because it aims to reduce the stress on the joints while carrying out ADL. This relates closely to two of the key aims of management: minimization of joint damage and maximization of function. Not only do these techniques help to maintain function, they also enable the patient to achieve a sense of control over the disease and a positive, proactive approach (Wade & Rimmer 1998). Joint protection involves a range of strategies, including the adaptation of habitual movement patterns, use of assistive devices, energy conservation techniques, exercise and splinting (SIGN 2000). The principles of joint protection are illustrated in Box 7.3.

Joint protection involves energy conservation techniques and these are particularly important for patients with conditions such as RA, where fatigue can be one of the symptoms. Disturbed sleep can also contribute to feelings of tiredness and lack of energy. Energy conservation techniques are designed to enable patients to make maximum use of limited energy resources and include work simplification, pacing and the use of assistive equipment. Work simplification involves analysis of specific activities within the environment to ensure they are carried out in the most efficient way. Pacing is simply obtaining a balance between rest, exercise and activity. Assistive equipment can be used if the patient experiences particular functional difficulties (Wade & Rimmer 1998).

Review point

After looking at Box 7.3, you should go back and compare the points it covers with those you thought of in response to Problem-solving exercise 7.4. The areas mentioned in Box 7.3 are indicative and are designed to apply to patients with a range of conditions. They can also be applied to any problem highlighted by the patient and may involve a collaborative and creative problem-solving exercise for the patient and the therapist. A little later in the chapter these principles will be considered more specifically in relation to Mrs Stamford and this will help you to understand how they can be applied in practice.

Box 7.3   Principles of joint protection for patients with rheumatic conditions

- Use the largest and most stable joints to accomplish a task
- Spread the load of carrying and lifting over a number of joints and avoid subjecting one joint to maximum load
- Use each joint in its most stable and functional position
- Use body mechanics efficiently, e.g. use the large muscles of the lower limbs when lifting, keep objects close to the body
- Put less effort into accomplishing a task, thinking about posture and body position
- Maintain joint mobility, muscle strength and function: exercise, but where possible under low load conditions, e.g. in sitting/lying, in water, cycling, bouncing on a trampette
- Avoid maintaining joints in one position for prolonged periods (including tight grips) especially those that emphasize a position of deformity
- Change activity from one group of joints to another – avoiding undue stress on one group
- Avoid excessive activity and sustained repetitive movements
- Balance work/activity periods with rest
- Select tasks carefully
- Use splints/assistive equipment as necessary
- Respect pain as a warning sign
- Avoid stress when possible – both physical and psychological

From Brattstrom 1987, Swezey 1990b, Wade & Rimmer 1998, SIGN 2000, ARC 2003a, Doherty et al 2001.

Surgery

Surgery is another element in the continuum of treatment. The improvement in surgery for patients with rheumatic conditions has probably been one of the most significant advances in treatment and it is a well-established speciality within orthopaedics. It may be undertaken for a number of reasons but the most significant to patients is probably its use in relieving pain. Once pain is reduced, function and independence increase. Surgery can also be used to correct deformity, improve cosmesis and in some cases to prevent further joint damage or damage to the nervous system. This is in addition to any operations performed to repair structures such as tendons.

As with other aspects of treatment, a team approach is essential, with good communication systems in place between the rheumatology and orthopaedic teams. This will ensure an optimal outcome in terms of pain relief and restoration of function (West & Hall 1998).

Probably the most common operation to be carried out is arthroplasty (joint replacement), where part or all of the joint surfaces are removed and replaced with an artificial joint (see Chapter 8). Two other common types of operation are arthrodesis and osteotomy. Arthrodesis is the fusion of a badly damaged joint (or joints) that may be painful and/or unstable. It may also be used following failed joint replacements. Osteotomy, where a wedge of bone is taken out or inserted in order to realign the overall shape of the bone, can be used either to redistribute stress to a less damaged part of the joint, so relieving pain, or to correct deformity. Other operative procedures such as arthroscopy, synovectomy and debridement may be used in some cases (Dandy & Edwards 2003, West & Hall 1998). A detailed account of the various surgical procedures can be found in orthopaedic textbooks.

Splinting

Splinting can be carried out by occupational therapists, physiotherapists or orthotists. A careful assessment must be carried out for each patient for each splint required. This needs a thorough knowledge of anatomy. Generally, splints are removable, should be comfortable and must be reviewed regularly in case the patient's requirements change. Clear instructions must be provided about when to wear the splints and when to exercise as there is evidence to suggest a danger of reduced bone mass and strength and the development of soft tissue contractures with prolonged use (Arthritis Research Campaign 2002, SIGN 2000, Wade & Rimmer 1998). The indications for the use of splints are listed in Box 7.4.

Box 7.4   Indications for the use of splints

- Pain relief by resting and supporting the joint
- Resting inflamed joints by preventing movement (this also helps to relieve pain)
- Provision of support and stability – supporting one joint can facilitate more movement in others, e.g. supporting the wrist can improve hand function
- Protection and immobilization of joints, e.g. a hard collar to support the neck in a patient with an unstable atlanto-occipital joint or after surgery
- Improvement of function by holding joints in a more functional position
- Increase in range of movement and/or correction of deformities, e.g. serial splinting
- Prevention of deformity
- Aid to mobility, e.g. footwear adaptations

From RCACP 1994, Wade & Rimmer 1998.

Dietetics

Nutritional advice can be an important part in the management of patients with rheumatic conditions and enquiries about diet are among the most commonly received (SIGN 2000). Obesity aggravates pain and disability in lower limb arthritis. It is an important risk factor and an indicator for poor outcome, particularly in disorders such as OA. Weight reduction is important therefore, when weight-bearing joints are involved. Patients who are overweight should be provided with a rationale for slow but steady weight loss through alteration of dietary and eating habits (Doherty et al 2001).

Conversely, several studies have shown that patients with RA who have a low body mass index (BMI) do less well and have poorer functional status. It is not clear whether intervention regarding diet improves outcome but for general health reasons an adequate BMI should be maintained (SIGN 2000).

Some patients use special diets and/or dietary supplements in the hope that these will improve their condition. Evidence regarding the efficacy of this approach is sparse and often anecdotal or inconclusive. Some exclusion/elimination diets can be difficult to follow and if patients follow them for a protracted period they can lead to nutritional deficiencies, which could affect their health. It is important for you to be aware of these approaches, however, as you may encounter patients who are trying these alternative methods.

Self-assessment question

- **SAQ 7.7** What are the elements involved in the general management of patients with rheumatic conditions? An answer is given in the following section, but try to work this out for yourself first.

ELEMENTS OF PHYSIOTHERAPY MANAGEMENT IN PATIENTS WITH RHEUMATIC CONDITIONS

Physiotherapy intervention is generally well recognized in clinical practice as an important element in the management of patients with rheumatic conditions. Although largely related to the patient's physical rehabilitation, physiotherapy input also impacts upon the psychosocial aspects of the patient's life. As already explained, assessment is essential, providing information about the patient's physical condition and functional levels. It also helps with overall understanding of the patient so enabling the physiotherapist to design a treatment programme in collaboration with the patient.

Self-assessment question

- **SAQ 7.8** What are the aims of physiotherapy management for patients with rheumatic conditions? Why is it important for these aims to be matched to the patient's requirements and beliefs?

(Answer at end of chapter.)

Pain relief

It is important for you to realize that none of the treatments used by physiotherapists will permanently reduce pain. They may temporarily reduce it so enabling the patient to undertake exercises more actively, or they could be used after exercise to soothe any 'treatment pain'. More permanent pain relief may occur in response to other types of intervention (see below).

The main physical modalities available to the physiotherapist for pain relief are heat, cold and some electrical techniques. Evidence of their efficacy is, however, conflicting. Weight-relieving and supportive methods may also be included here, e.g. provision of walking aids and splints. Hydrotherapy is a specific method that combines heat with weight relief and ease of movement. There may also be the opportunity for the patient to benefit from less orthodox treatments such as acupuncture, reflex therapy and aromatherapy, depending on the scope of practice of the particular physiotherapist involved.

Heat

Heat has been used in different forms for many years, varying from the more superficial infrared irradiation, hot packs and wax to the deeper, more penetrating short-wave diathermy and low-power laser therapy. Many claims have been made for these methods but very few of them are supported by scientific evidence. A study carried out by Goats et al (1996) on low-intensity laser and phototherapy for RA concluded that these treatment methods have little to offer the rheumatoid patient. Swezey (1990b) states that 'heat increases molecular activity, causes vasodilation, and increases nerve conduction, and can be used to facilitate stretching and, above all relieve pain'. He goes on to point out, however, that it can also 'increase collagenase activity and potentially aggravate joint damage', which is undesirable in patients with rheumatic conditions where management is aiming to minimize joint damage. It has been reported, however, that wax baths relieved pain and stiffness in patients with RA of the hands with no apparent detrimental effects on the disease process (Ayling & Marks 2000). Exercise combined with wax baths is recommended for the beneficial short-term effects for patients with arthritic hands (Robinson et al 2002). Brosseau et al (2002), in a review of the available literature, conclude that low-level laser therapy could be considered for short-term relief of pain and morning stiffness in RA.

It appears that superficial, moist heat is probably of most use for its short-term pain relieving effect. This can help to reduce muscle spasm, enabling the patient to perform exercises more comfortably. Superficial methods of heating are also easier for patients to duplicate at home by the use of hot water bottles, heat pads and warm baths or showers.

Cold

Cold is also used by the physiotherapist, but again for short-term palliative pain relief (Robinson et al 2002). In contrast to heat, cold slows down the metabolism and reduces the speed of nerve conduction. Ice treatment should precede exercise and again patients can duplicate the method at home.

Elderly patients particularly often prefer heat to cold as it is more soothing and comforting.

Electrical techniques

There are several stimulating electrical modalities available to the physiotherapist; probably the most commonly used are interferential and transcutaneous electrical nerve stimulation (TENS). Claims have been made that these have longer-lasting analgesic effects due to the release of endorphins by the body in response to the stimulation, but evidence is conflicting (SIGN 2000). If a patient finds this method of treatment particularly helpful, TENS machines are often available to borrow. This means they can be taken home and used over a longer period. It is also possible to buy them commercially. These modalities have not, however, been found to be very successful in peripheral joint pain control (Swezey 1990b), although a recent study reported some success in reducing pain in patients experiencing mild to moderate symptoms of OA (Lone et al 2003). With regard to other types of electrical modality, there is limited evidence showing symptomatic benefit from ultrasound (SIGN 2000).

Exercise

It has been suggested that exercise is perhaps the best form of treatment for patients with rheumatic conditions. The physiotherapist's role here is extremely important in advising on the correct levels of exercise and rest for each individual. The necessity and reasons for exercise seem fairly well agreed upon. It helps to maintain or increase joint range, muscle strength and flexibility as well as providing general conditioning. Traditionally, patients have been excluded from vigorous activity because of their particular problems and, as mentioned earlier, physicians have tended to advise curtailment of exercise of this sort. It has been shown, however, that people with arthritis have poor physical fitness involving reduced muscle strength, endurance and aerobic capacity and tend to have more problems due to inactivity (Ike et al 1989, Minor et al 1989, SIGN 2000, Ven den Ende 2002).

Evidence indicates the efficacy of exercise for patients with arthritis (Bernhard 2001, Harvey 2003). It is emphasized, however, that the patients need to be well motivated and that the exercise should be supervised and of low to moderate intensity. Supervision, certainly in the initial stages, is important. Patients need to be advised that if they experience increased joint pain that does not subside within 2 hours or if it causes pain and swelling and/or persistent muscle soreness that increase overnight, the exercise is probably excessive and indicates a need for reduction in intensity. The intensity should also be reduced if the patient experiences significant fatigue.

It is important to note, however, that some patients may need to undertake activities that challenge pain behaviour. Fear of pain can lead to increased levels of disability. If levels of activity are not maintained, there is the potential for a self-reinforcing cycle to occur involving pain, limitation of movement, loss of function and lowering of mood. Physical management that exposes patients to pain triggering activities is more effective than that which protects them from it (Harvey 2003).

The patient should be encouraged to undertake leisure activities if possible to improve function but also for other reasons, such as enjoyment and social interaction. These activities might include walking, dancing, swimming or golfing. Physical activity has a favourable effect on anxiety states and stress, so this may be another positive factor for those patients with chronic disease.

In general the nature of the exercise will depend on the acuteness of joint symptoms at the time, and so treatment must be altered accordingly. This could be done, for example, by showing isometric methods of strengthening and reducing repetition rates during an acute period.

You may be involved in designing a dynamic exercise programme for your patients with rheumatic disorders. It may be helpful to look at relevant websites, particularly those that include input from individuals with rheumatic conditions. On the Arthritis Research Campaign website, for example, there is a section where handy hints and tips are posted by people with arthritis. This type of site can provide both you and your patients with ideas, e.g. using lightweight walking poles if the patient is a keen walker; using a mini trampoline for low-impact exercise; going to aqua aerobic sessions at a local pool; improving posture using the Alexander technique, yoga or Pilates, and so on.

Hydrotherapy

This is an ancient and popular form of treatment, which in the broadest sense involves the external application of water for therapeutic purposes. This usually means the patients attending a warm hydrotherapy pool for exercise and relaxation.

Movement through water provides much of the resistance and progression is achieved by working through from the easy exercise to the most difficult. The advantage here is the self-regulating nature of the exercise in that the harder the patients work the more resistance is experienced, but this will never be more than they can manage. The water allows an almost infinite range of resistance for patients at any stage of a condition. This is an advantage for patients with rheumatic conditions. See Chapter 11 for more information.

APPLICATION OF MANAGEMENT PRINCIPLES TO CASE STUDY

The preceding section should have helped to give you an overview of the principles that you can use to decide on appropriate interventions with your

patients experiencing problems due to arthritis. Before we go on to review some common conditions other than OA that you may come across in clinical practice, let us return to Mrs Stamford to consider how these principles could be applied more specifically in her case. Remember that these are suggestions relating to a hypothetical situation, and you must use your problem-solving and decision-making skills to decide what would be the best approach for each patient you deal with.

As a reminder, this lady has pain and swelling in the left knee, stiffness, reduced range of movement (with some deformity), muscle wasting and weakness; all of which have led to a decrease in function. She identifies her main problem as not being able to walk far enough to carry out her everyday activities.

Problem–solving exercise 7.6

Using the information provided earlier, jot down your suggestions for the management of this patient.

It is unlikely that you will see Mrs Stamford on a regular basis for a number of weeks. It is more likely that, after an initial assessment, you will have a discussion with her to agree the overall management; demonstrate and supervise her practice of a dynamic home exercise programme and provide advice on joint care and ADL. You may set up a system of regular reviews in order to both monitor her progress and to ensure that she does not feel that she has been abandoned. Working with the patient in this way is often appropriate as long as opportunities are provided to contact the physiotherapist if there are any concerns or problems. This system does depend on the patient being willing to comply with this self-care model of management. If this is not possible, then it is important for the physiotherapist to agree a certain number of treatments with the patient and then to make it clear that discharge will occur after completion of the last visit.

As with many patients with OA, pain presents as a major factor. Considering the information already given, it is unlikely that any of the treatment modalities available to you will alleviate this other than as a temporary measure. There are ways, however, in which you may enable the patient to modify her behaviour, which in turn can help to reduce the pain in the longer term.

It is important to briefly explain the pathology of OA to the patient (if this has not been done before) and to discuss how this has affected her activities. This will mean that the patient is better able to understand the suggestions that are made regarding treatment. It will also contribute to the process of identifying realistic expectations for intervention. Many patients are reassured by being given information, particularly if it helps them to understand the low probability of a 'crippling outcome' (Hutton 1995).

We will assume that this patient has been prescribed some appropriate anti-inflammatory and/or pain-relieving drugs by her GP. This will do much to alleviate the pain and reduce swelling but it is vital that you also teach the patient how to reduce pain as much as possible herself.

Some of the pain may be due to muscle weakness and deformity in and around the knee, which is altering the joint biomechanics. It will be important to teach the patient exercises she can carry out at home to increase strength and range of movement. In order to make this easier you can also advise her to apply superficial heat or an ice pack to the area (whichever she prefers) either before or after the exercises. Provision of an exercise sheet will act as a reminder. This could be already available in the department or you may need to make one up with specific exercises for the patient. A software package such as PhysioTools can be helpful here. In the case of Mrs Stamford the exercises would particularly include work for the quadriceps, hamstrings and probably the glutei. These can be taught in a variety of starting positions.

If the flexion deformity in the left knee has a bony end feel (i.e. fixed flexion deformity) then you will not be able to improve it. If there is a soft end feel, however, but the joint is stiff, you may be able to mobilize it further into range. The patient must be encouraged to maintain this with her home exercises. You will not be able to improve the varus deformity but the strengthening exercises may help to prevent further angulation. Unfortunately,

contractures have a tendency to recur as enthusiasm for maintenance exercises may not be long-lived – depending on the patient.

As discussed earlier, weight bearing increases pain in OA joints. Walking aids help to reduce the compressive forces applied to the joint surfaces and so reduce the pain. Mrs Stamford already has a stick but you should check it for height and safety and then instruct her in correct usage, i.e. particularly to use it in the right hand to deflect weight on to the unaffected leg (Hutton 1995). This can be combined with any necessary gait re-education.

Advice on the careful use of her joints will also be an important factor here and may be of considerable help in alleviating pain from over- or incorrect use. This relates back to the earlier information on joint protection. There are a number of points that may be helpful for this patient.

Reduction of stress through the joints by weight relief

If Mrs Stamford is overweight you should tactfully encourage weight loss, which will help function and reduce loading on the left knee. If appropriate you could refer her to a dietitian or provide information on local organizations that may help with her weight loss regimen. She should also be advised not to carry heavy weights and could perhaps use a shopping trolley, wheeled suitcases and so on, which again reduce joint loading.

Climbing any step (e.g. stairs, getting onto buses, kerbs) increases the compressive force in the knee joint to 4.25 times that of body weight (Adler 1985). You can therefore advise Mrs Stamford to lead with her unaffected leg on the way up and the affected one on the way down, so putting the stress on the non-painful limb. At home it is sensible to try and limit the number of times she goes up and down stairs each day. For example, perhaps going up to the toilet and then performing several tasks such as making the bed, fetching clean laundry from the airing cupboard and so on. She should also use bannisters, her stick, lifts and escalators whenever available. Check her footwear and emphasize the benefits of having a cushioned sole or insole to prevent jarring. If she has particular problems with her feet you might feel it necessary to refer her to a podiatrist or orthotist.

Seating

When rising from the sitting position the forces through the knee joint are again increased. If the arms are used to help push up then the corresponding forces are much less. This is much easier if the armchair/dining chair used by the patient has arms. It is also helpful to increase the height of seats by putting blocks under the legs of the chair or extra cushions, or newspapers under the cushions. Some patients are able to purchase a high seat chair or may find an ejector cushion/chair (spring loaded or motorized) helpful.

Toileting and bathing

A raised toilet seat can be provided if necessary – probably in liaison with social services or the OT department. It may be possible to fit rails in the bathroom/toilet if this patient finds getting up from the toilet and getting in and out of the bath particularly difficult. It is also possible to obtain a frame that combines a seat and arms to place on the toilet.

In the bath it may be helpful to use a bath board and seat or a mechanical bath seat that can help lower the patient into and raise her out of the bath tub. If she uses the shower over the bath, this can be used in combination with a bath board. If the patient has a walk-in shower there may be room to place a plastic seat inside the cubicle so that the patient does not need to stand while washing. A rail may be necessary to enable her to sit and stand with ease. Non-slip mats are also essential.

Beds

As with chairs, the height of beds can be increased if necessary. Firm mattresses are easier to turn over on and to stand up from. Duvets are lighter than sheets and blankets and enable the patient to make the bed more easily.

Standing and kneeling

Mrs Stamford should avoid standing for long periods. There may be activities that she can carry out just as easily in sitting or possibly perched on a high stool (e.g. ironing, preparing food, washing up). Kneeling should be discouraged and the use of long-handled tools suggested to enable her to reach items. If the patient insists on kneeling, a thick foam pad or knee pads could be used (Adler 1985).

Walking

Walking distance is a problem for this patient. She should be encouraged to continue to take walks but to plan them so that they involve calling on a friend or sitting on a seat halfway so that she can rest before going on. Improved use of her stick will help as should the increased strength in the surrounding muscles, any decrease in pain and reduction in her weight. She should start with walking a short distance and then gradually increase this as long as there is no major aggravation of her symptoms.

Mrs Stamford may not find all these ideas easy to accept at first, especially if it means changing long-standing behaviour patterns. But it is hoped that, by providing clear explanations and discussing the issues with her, you would be able to persuade her to try them. Changes in the home may require visits from community therapists if this service is available. This gives the opportunity to tailor advice very specifically to the patient's own circumstances. Carers or friends may also be present and their help could be enlisted to encourage the patient to try out the new methods of carrying out everyday tasks. If the patient is able to comply with the management plan you have devised together, she should find that the pain does decrease and she is able to carry out her ADL more easily.

Let us return briefly to the list of goals we identified earlier in the chapter:

1. Reduction of pain
2. Maintenance of, or increase in (if possible), range and ease of movement
3. Maintenance of, or increase in (if possible), muscle strength
4. Correction of current or prevention of the occurrence of any further deformity
5. Maximization of functional potential and maintenance of, or increase in, exercise tolerance
6. Provision of education, advice and support for the patient with regard to her condition
7. Encouragement for the patient to take on responsibility for self-care and self-management.

Matching intervention to goals

Let us assume that Mrs Stamford is a compliant patient who takes careful note of all your advice and acts upon it. The following section shows how the management plan applies to the earlier goals:

1. Pain relief:
   - Drug treatment
   - Application of heat or ice
   - Reduced loading of the joint by careful use, walking aid, weight loss, change of behaviour, improved muscle strength
2. Maintenance of, or increase in (if possible), range and ease of movement:
   - Regular exercise
   - Pain relief due to above factors
3. Maintenance of, or increase in (if possible), muscle strength:
   - Regular exercise
   - Gradual increase in activity level
4. Correction of current or prevention of the occurrence of any further deformity:
   - As for point 3, especially the mobilizing exercises to correct deformity and the strengthening to prevent further deformity occurring
   - Good positioning of the knee (i.e. not holding it in flexion at rest) and stretching
5. Maximization of functional potential and maintenance of, or increase in, exercise tolerance:
   - Able to do more as pain decreases and strength/mobility increases
   - Changes in methods of carrying out ADL
   - Provision of aids
   - Improved use of stick, gait re-education
6. Provision of education, advice and support for the patient with regard to her condition:
   - Information about OA and how it has affected patient's abilities
   - Advice on exercise and ADL
   - Availability of physiotherapist over the telephone for further support if necessary
   - Follow up appointment for reassessment
   - Provision of literature from department and possibly leaflets and videos from the Arthritis Research Campaign or other relevant organizations as an adjunct to treatment
7. Encouragement for the patient to take on responsibility for self-care and self-management:
   - Overall approach to management of patient but with contact when necessary to prevent patient feeling isolated or unsupported.

The interaction of these goals and interventions may vary from patient to patient, depending on their attitude to health, the particular home environment and the severity of the condition, but this gives an example from which you can extrapolate. You may need to use all or only some of the ideas suggested and, once you are more used to dealing with this type of patient, you will develop your own approach. Remember, your problem solving abilities in any particular area improve with experience but you also need to have a good knowledge base from which to work. In this way you move from being a novice through the experienced beginner stage and on towards the expert end of the continuum. You can see an example of a more complex OA case study (Mr Nicholls) in Chapter 8.

RHEUMATOID ARTHRITIS

Rheumatoid arthritis is a chronic, inflammatory condition mainly affecting the synovial joints. It is manifested by an erosive, symmetrical polyarthritis but it also has variable systemic features. Patients with RA vary widely in both the symptoms they experience and their severity (Kill 2002, Lloyd 1998, Pipitone & Choy 2003).

It is approximately 200 years since RA was first described. There is still uncertainty as to whether it is a 'disease of antiquity' (Bellamy 1991), i.e. some sort of inherent weakness in the human make-up, or whether it is a disease of only the last two centuries due to some infection or combination of environmental factors. It is possible that RA is a recent entity not seen in Europe until the end of the 18th century, but there is also some evidence that it may have been described by Hippocrates and other early writers. The latter is very difficult to substantiate, however. RA was not clearly defined until 1958 and there are still some differences of opinion regarding its classification.

Rheumatoid arthritis is one of mankind's most significant diseases because of its relatively high incidence throughout the world. Patients are usually affected during their most productive years and may require considerable time away from work during exacerbations. It also occurs at a critical time for the patient in terms of family and other activities. It is notable because of its chronicity, its potentially disabling effects and the associated reduction in life expectancy, which can be up to 7 years. Some of the morbidity and mortality, however, is related to the treatment of RA rather than to the disease itself (Kill 2002).

Data on incidence (i.e. the number of new cases of a disease occurring in a defined population within a defined period) and prevalence (i.e. the frequency of a disease in a defined population) of RA does vary somewhat. This may be due to some problems encountered in the classification and therefore the diagnosis of the condition. But using the American Rheumatology Association 1987 revised criteria for the classification of RA (Table 7.2) the prevalence is consistently around 1% of the adult population in every part of the world (Kill 2002, Lloyd 1998, Pipitone & Choy 2003). This figure increases to 6% in males over the age of 75 and 16% in females over the age of 65 (Lloyd 1998).

There is a marked sex difference overall and it is generally agreed that women are affected up to three times more frequently than men. This female predominance may become less prominent in patients over 65 (Bhardwaj & Paget 1992, Dandy & Edwards 2003, Hazes & Silman 1990, Kill 2002, Lloyd 1998). It has been postulated that there may be some hormonal influence in the pathogenesis and course of certain rheumatic and autoimmune diseases, one of which is RA. This would seem to be supported by the beneficial effects that many women with RA report during pregnancy (Yaron 1995). Female predominance may suggest that antibodies are also important in pathogenesis (Edwards 2002).

Table 7.2 The American College of Rheumatology revised criteria for the classification of rheumatoid arthritis (Pipitone & Choy 2003)

Criterion	Definition
1. Morning stiffness	Lasting at least an hour before maximal improvement
2. Arthritis of three or more joint areas	At least three joint areas simultaneously have had soft tissue swelling or fluid (not bony overgrowth alone). The 14 possible areas are right or left PIP, MCP, wrist, elbow, knee, ankle and MTP joints
3. Arthritis of hand joints	At least one area swollen (as defined above) in a wrist, MCP or PIP joint
4. Symmetric arthritis	Simultaneous involvement of the same joint areas (as defined in 2) on both sides of the body (bilateral involvement of PIPs, MCPs or MTPs is acceptable without absolute symmetry)
5. Presence of rheumatoid nodules	Subcutaneous nodules over bony prominences or extensor surfaces or in juxta-articular regions, as observed by a physician
6. Positive rheumatoid factor	Demonstration of abnormal amounts of serum rheumatoid factor by a method for which the result has been positive in <5% of normal control subjects
7. Radiographic changes	Changes typical of rheumatoid arthritis on posteroanterior hand and wrist radiographs, which must include erosions or unequivocal bony decalcification localized in or most marked adjacent to the involved joint (OA changes alone do not qualify)

For classification purposes, a patient shall be said to have RA if they satisfy at least four of the seven criteria. Criteria 1–4 must have been present for al least 6 weeks.
MCP: metacarpophalangeal joint; MTP: metatarsophalangeal joint; PIP: proximal interphalangeal joint.

The onset of the condition is usually in young adults between the ages of 15 and 35 but it can affect those both younger and older (Dandy & Edwards 2003). Epidemiological studies suggest that a monozygotic twin of an affected individual has a 25% greater chance of sharing the disease than the general population and some familial clustering has been noted (Edwards 2002).

There is some evidence to suggest that there may be a declining trend in incidence, especially in the female population, plus an indication that the severity of the condition could be decreasing. But the latter may only be due to better prevention of joint damage and abnormalities by early treatment and rehabilitation (Hazes & Silman 1990).

Aetiology

A great deal of work has been carried out on RA but, although the clinical features and treatment are now better defined, the specific cause is still unknown and there is much to be learned regarding the pathogenesis of the disease. As mentioned at the beginning of the chapter, there could be several factors interacting that are implicated in the onset of RA. Research has shown that immunologic mechanisms are of importance both in the initiation and perpetuation of the disease. The key clues to pathogenesis appear to be rheumatoid factor (RF), major histocompatibility complex (MHC) class II and tumour necrosis factor-α (TNFα).

Multiple genetic elements appear to contribute to the risk of developing RA. In monozygotic twins the relative risk of developing RA is 12–62 times higher than in unrelated individuals. In dizygotic twins or siblings this risk reduces to 2–17 times more likely to develop the condition. This significant difference indicates a genetic basis for the aetiology of RA (Weyand 2000). In the 1970s advances were made in relating MHCs located on the 6th chromosome to the epidemiology of certain diseases. In RA the primary association appears to be with the DR4 locus, at least in certain populations. Over 70% of white patients with RA will have the DR4 haplotype as opposed to less than 30% of controls. In comparison 46% of black patients with RA have DR4 present in contrast to 14% of the normal population. This does seem to be an indication of susceptibility to the disease and there also appears to

be a link between more aggressive disease states and the presence of DR4. It must be remembered, however, that 30% of patients with RA are not DR4-positive as well as there being people who do not have RA but do have the DR4 haplotype (Bhardwaj & Paget 1992, Dandy & Edwards 2003, Edwards 2002).

As to the initiating factors, the stimuli that can activate the immune response in a susceptible host are possibly multiple and ubiquitous. Smoking has, however, now emerged as a clear external risk (Edwards 2002). Other initiating theories include the possibilities of infectious agents, i.e. a virus or bacteria, as aetiological pathogens of RA. The Epstein–Barr virus, which belongs to the herpes family of DNA viruses, has been implicated in the pathogenesis of RA for a number of years, but the actual relationship has not been determined. Lentiviruses, parvoviruses, rubella virus and mycobacteria are also suspected but a specific link has not been identified (Bhardwaj & Paget 1992, Lloyd 1998). Environmental factors are often seen as 'triggers' that determine disease onset. Monozygotic twins, however, rarely acquire RA at the same time. This may indicate that the trigger concept is misconceived (Edwards 2002).

The slow development of many human autoimmune responses is still a mystery. As discussed above, it is commonly assumed that the non-genetic factors in aetiology are environmental. It is possible, however, that the remainder of the causation might be random, i.e. due to chance. This idea is familiar in the causation of cancer but is often overlooked in autoimmune disease. The lack of a link to external factors, such as that identified in some other conditions (e.g. Reiter's syndrome), again indicates a random element in RA, as does the rise in incidence with age. Another feature of this pathogenesis is the time frame for RA. Changes in immunoglobulins can occur many years before any symptoms become evident. The immune response can take years to evolve in RA whereas in the usual model of immune dynamics this process takes around 20 days. It is, therefore, possible that, aside from the genetic component, the disease arises through a sequence of infrequent chance events with earlier events facilitating later ones. At present, however, these postulated random events have not been identified. One possibility is 'physiological immunoglobulin gene mutation leading to a new antibody species' (Edwards 2002).

Course

Onset is slow and insidious in 60–70% of patients and the initial symptoms can be either systemic or articular. Some patients experience fatigue or diffuse musculoskeletal pain followed later by joint involvement, but morning stiffness may be the first symptom. Articular symptoms classically start peripherally and spread proximally. In 10–15% onset is acute, tending to begin in the joints with severe muscle pain. This group is the most difficult to classify as there are many possible differential diagnoses. Some 15–30% of patients exhibit an intermediate onset where symptoms develop over days or weeks and the systemic effects are the most noticeable. Occasionally patients will present with acute arthritis of one or two joints that resolves completely over a short period but may occur again and evolve into RA (Lloyd 1998).

Self-assessment question

- **SAQ 7.9** Briefly review the factors involved in the aetiology of RA. (See above.)

Rheumatoid arthritis is a multidimensional disease with a highly variable course from patient to patient (Kalden & Smolen 2000). Achieving a state of stable remission leaving little or no abnormality is the most desirable outcome. It is, however, very difficult to predict which patients may go into remission, although some studies have shown that it may be more likely in seronegative patients and those with fewer active joints (Eberhardt & Fex 1998).

Remission can be defined according to the American Rheumatism Association (ARA) criteria seen in Box 7.5. Two main patterns of disease are described; the 'classic' course is intermittent, relapse followed by complete or partial remission. This gives a slow but steady progression of damage to articular and periarticular structures and gradual increase in disability. There is, however, great

---

Box 7.5   American Rheumatology Association remission criteria for rheumatoid arthritis (Eberhardt & Fex 1998)

Five or more of the following criteria must be fulfilled for at least two consecutive months:

- Duration of morning stiffness not exceeding 15 minutes
- No fatigue
- No joint pain (by history)
- No joint tenderness or pain on motion
- No soft tissue swelling in joints or tendon sheaths
- Erythrocyte sedimentation rate <30 mm after 1 hour for a female or <20 mm after 1 hour for a male

---

variability in patterns of progression from patient to patient (Scott 2000). The second pattern is the chronic persistent course with relentless progression, either rapid or slow, with no remission and many complications. The disease pattern can have prognostic implications but evidence here is conflicting (Eberhardt & Fex 1998, Rasker & Cosh 1989).

Key issues in the course of RA are joint damage and functional disability. These increase steadily over the 10–25 year course of the disease. Joint damage accounts for approximately 25% of the disability in established RA. Avoiding or reducing joint damage in both early and late stages of the condition is, however, likely to maintain better functional levels (Scott 2000, Scott et al 2000). The goals of treatment are, therefore, symptom control, reduction of joint damage and disability and maintenance or improvement of quality of life. According to current research it is evident that the most effective way to achieve this is to treat patients with DMARDs as early as possible after diagnosis (SIGN 2000).

Prognosis

In all chronic diseases, a number of factors predict poor outcome. These include the severity of the disease, late presentation, multiple health problems, poverty and old age. More specifically in RA the indicators of poor outcome are:

- Many active joints
- High erythrocyte sedimentation rate (ESR) or C-reactive protein (CRP) at outset
- Positive rheumatoid factor
- Early radiological erosions
- Poorer scores of function at outset (e.g. using the Health Assessment Questionnaire)
- Adverse socioeconomic circumstances and lower educational level (SIGN 2000).

Prognosis for patients with RA varies considerably and early prediction of outcome is not reliable (Eberhardt & Fex 1998). The prognostic indicators identifying patients who are at risk of poor outcome would enable the healthcare team to intervene at an early stage in the disease process to prevent worsening of the disease and to limit joint damage. It is unfortunate, however, that features indicating poor prognosis (number of joints affected, acute phase response CRP levels) are not in evidence at the initial diagnosis. The most consistent prognostic factor seems to be rheumatoid factor positivity. As well as predicting a poor prognosis overall, seropositive patients tend to have more severe joint damage and greater functional disability (Scott 2000).

Generally prognosis in RA is not good, but it is a dynamic process when placed within the settings of patient response, changing therapy and alteration in the natural course of the disease. As mentioned earlier, there does appear to be a direct correlation between RA and decreased life expectancy. In general, women tend to have more chronic and disabling disease than men (Bhardwaj & Paget 1992, Rasker & Cosh 1989).

There are varying opinions on whether treatment is effective in altering prognosis. Harris (1990) states that there is little evidence that present treatment alters outcome, although he concentrates mainly on drug therapy, whereas Wolfe (1990) is of the opinion that outcome can be improved by treatment. He looks at a wider spectrum of management, including orthopaedic surgery, DMARDs, patient education and self-management as well as other types of therapy including occupational and physiotherapy. More recent work on the identification of prognostic factors to detect early RA, early arthritis clinics, early referral to specialist care and the consistent, sequential use of DMARDs

indicates that long-term disease outcomes can be improved with treatment (Kalden & Smolen 2000, Scott 2000).

Psychosocial impact

The socioeconomic impact of functional disability in chronic diseases such as RA is significant (Kalden & Smolen 2000). The costs incurred in delayed treatment can also be considerable. These include:

- Personal costs
  - Lost work opportunities
  - Decreased leisure activities
  - Stress on relationships
- Costs to society
  - Loss of working skills of individuals with RA
  - Loss of contributions to the home
  - The burden of economic cost for care (SIGN 2000).

It is clear, therefore, that RA imposes a substantial economic burden on both patients and society, quantified in terms of direct and indirect costs. Direct costs are those for which actual payments are made, such as treatment and hospitalization, whereas indirect costs result from the loss of resources, especially loss of productivity. Hospital admissions make up the largest proportion of direct costs. The functional status of patients is the most important factor in determining cost. Patients with poor function need more services and support than those with mild impairment (Guillemin 2000, Pipitone & Choy 2003).

It is estimated that for almost 50% of patients with RA the maximum duration of time that they are able to work after diagnosis is around 10 years (Guillemin 2000). Those performing light work fare the best and are still often able to continue for the full 10 years after diagnosis, whereas individuals carrying out jobs involving heavy labour are often work-disabled. Work type and the physical demands are related to the patient's ability to continue. Many patients do, however, stop work in the first year after the onset of RA (SIGN 2000). The problems encountered by 'homemakers' are more difficult to quantify as there is no control group. They do, however, report decreased ability to carry out their usual activities (Wolfe 1990). Because of individuals with RA being unable to work or needing to reduce or change the work that they do, family income can be reduced by an average of 35% over the course of the illness (Guillemin 2000). Early intervention through retraining and liaison with the patient's employer will enable the patient to remain in work for as long as practical, so minimizing the economic impact of the disease (SIGN 2000).

Loss or modification of employment will inevitably have an effect on livelihood and quality of life. This emphasizes that not only do patients with RA have to manage the physical issues resulting from the disease but they also have to deal with its impact in terms of significant financial, social and psychological costs. More information on the psychological impact of chronic disease can be found at the end of the chapter.

Review point

Take a few moments to review the possible patterns of onset and progression of RA.

Self-assessment questions

- SAQ 7.10
  a. Name the factors that indicate poor outcome in chronic disease.
  b. What factors indicate the possible prognosis of RA?
  c. Briefly explain the factors that may have a positive effect on disease outcome. (See above.)

Pathological changes in rheumatoid arthritis

Rheumatoid arthritis is a chronic, inflammatory, systemic disease characterized by joint pain and swelling, joint destruction and pannus formation. The pannus consists of a hypertrophic synovial membrane. T cells, B cells and CD68$^+$ macrophage-like cells, mast cells and endothelial cells are all present in the synovium and contribute to the inflammatory processes. The T cells are the key element of the adaptive immune response in RA.

T cells recognize antigen on the surface of antigen presenting cells and so the latter are involved in regulating T-cell function.

Stage 1

Antigen presenting cells are the first to be involved in the human immune response. They ingest, process and present foreign protein antigens to T lymphocytes. The processed antigen binds to glycoproteins and is then recognized by helper T-cell receptors. A cellular immune response is then initiated. This is the early stage of RA, where no symptoms occur.

Stages 2 and 3

These are similar to Stage 1; the main difference is in severity of the reactions. Antibody–antigen complexes activate the cascade of reactions known as the complement system and this causes substances to be released into the synovial fluid that influence the behaviour of certain cells. The inflammatory reaction begins with the induction of vascular exudation by vasoactive substances leading to congestion and oedema of the synovial lining, followed by effusion into the joint space (Bhardwaj & Paget 1992, Lloyd 1998). Cytokines such as interleukins 2, 3 and 4 and interferon gamma produced by immunocytes, macrophages and fibroblasts amplify and perpetuate the inflammation which becomes self-sustaining (Harris 1990). They also cause proliferation in the cells of the synovium within the joints and tendon sheaths. The hypertrophied synovium is sustained by increased capillary growth (angiogenesis). Clotting cascades are activated, which cause fibrin to be deposited on the synovial membrane and articular cartilage. Lysosomal enzymes are released, which begin to degrade cartilage, any menisci present and ligaments.

These stages become gradually symptomatic and the products of inflammation then drive the proliferative response into stage 4 of the disease (Harris 1990).

Stage 4

In this stage, irreversible destruction of cartilage occurs. The synovium is normally a single layer of cells but increases to a thickness of five or seven cells. Synovial surface area increases enormously because of the formation of villi as the pannus is formed. Proteinases are released that are capable of destroying many of the proteins making up the matrix of articular cartilage and bone. Pannus replaces bone at the joint margins and erosions appear. Prostaglandins are released, which increase osteoclast activity, and minerals are resorbed from the underlying bone (osteolysis), which is then further degraded by collagenases and proteinases (Bhardwaj & Paget 1992, Harris 1990, Lloyd 1998).

Articular cartilage is also replaced by the pannus, which is subsequently transformed into fibrous tissue. This can go on to cause decreased movement in the joint and in some cases leads eventually to fibrous ankylosis.

Very little gross destruction of cartilage is necessary before normal function is reduced to the point that progressive disintegration occurs in response to everyday activities involving the weight-bearing joints (Harris 1990). Proliferation and destruction also occur in the capsule, ligaments and tendons. This can cause an altered use pattern and the structures may become very lax or rupture, so affecting the stability of the joint (Harris 1990).

Stage 5

This is a continuation of the irreversible destructive changes in the joint. There may be subluxation of the joint surfaces plus muscle atrophy and fibrosis, leading to a significant decrease in functional ability. There may also be secondary OA changes by this time.

Try the following problem-solving exercise before you go on to read the next section.

Problem-solving exercise 7.7

Using the information provided try to work out:

a. the symptoms that a patient with rheumatoid arthritis might describe to you
b. the clinical signs you would expect to find on examination of this patient. (See below.)

Clinical features of rheumatoid arthritis

Rheumatoid arthritis affects all parts of the body and not just the joints – it is an autoimmune disease affecting connective tissue, which is present in all areas. It has, therefore, a very broad spectrum of clinical presentations.

Case study 7.2: Mrs White (1)

This 60-year-old lady has been admitted for bilateral total hip replacements. She was diagnosed with RA 6 years ago. Within 12 months the disease had affected the small joints of her hands, her neck, shoulders and elbows. As the condition progressed her hips and knees started to be problematic; the knees getting worse as the hips deteriorated. Her feet and ankles have been symptom-free but are now starting to be affected and to cause more functional difficulty.

Currently her hands are sore but her hips are proving to be the most problematic.

Mrs White feels that her condition has deteriorated quite rapidly over the last 6 months. She lives at home with her husband and son, sleeping downstairs as she has for the last 3 years. There is a shower and toilet downstairs. Her husband is self-employed and helps with most things. She was able to mobilize with a walking frame until approximately 2 months ago.

Until 5 years ago she worked in a chemists shop dispensing medicines but had to leave because of her symptoms and functional problems.

Problem-solving exercise 7.8

Review your answers to the previous exercise and now briefly relate them to this case study. Do you think that all the symptoms and clinical signs you listed would be relevant to this lady?

Make a list of headings that you would use when assessing this patient and think about why physiotherapists need to investigate these areas.

The headings and some of the reasons for investigating these areas are discussed in the following section. It is important for you to try this exercise for yourself before you go on with your reading, however, in order to check your understanding.

Approach to the assessment of Mrs White

Make a note of the time of day you make your assessment; this could be very important for your reassessment as many patients have variation in symptoms throughout the day. For example, if you carried out your initial assessment early in the morning but then reassessed the patient at mid-day, you could get very different responses because at the later time her morning stiffness would have eased.

Subjective assessment

When interviewing this patient you would need to ask about a range of issues:

1. Demographic details and history of present condition

- The time since diagnosis, how quickly the disease had progressed and how she is at present (are her symptoms staying the same, getting worse or better?)
- Which other joints are affected apart from her hips, as this will impact on your intervention and her ability to comply with any treatment?
- What are her main problems as she perceives them and what does she have most difficulty with functionally?
- How long does her morning stiffness last?
- Does she have any systemic symptoms that might impact upon your ideas for management? (e.g. has the RA affected her heart or does she fatigue easily?)
- Has she had any physiotherapy before and how has she responded?

2. General health and past medical history

It is important to get an overall picture of Mrs White's pattern of health and well being as this could affect your ideas about possible interventions and her ability to comply with management. There are a number of established questionnaires that may be available in your department that can be used to investigate these issues. (You will need to access Mrs White's medical notes to find out the results of relevant tests such as ESR, presence of RF or anaemia and to see if there is any information of note regarding her past medical history.)

3. Present medication and drug history

This is important as it could influence your intervention. It is essential that you keep a check on Mrs White's medication. This is particularly important if it changes during the period she is having physiotherapy or if she had recently commenced taking a DMARD at your initial assessment. Both of these situations could give a false impression of the effectiveness of physical treatments.

Self-assessment question

- **SAQ 7.11** Why might you get a false impression of the effectiveness of your intervention if Mrs White's drugs were changed part way through your treatment programme or if she had recently started to take a DMARD?

---

4. Splints

- Does she have any?
- If so, does she wear them regularly?
- On which joints?
- If the patient is not wearing splints currently but has done so in the past, have they been helpful (again find out which joints were involved)?

5. Social history

This can cover a wide range of areas. It is important to focus on the patient's living arrangements, however, in order to assess how well she is managing at home and whether referral to the OT and/or social services may be appropriate.

- What is her accommodation like?
- Who if anyone, is available to help at home?
- Leisure activities; what she enjoys doing and any activities she has had to give up recently?

Objective assessment

1. General observation

For example:

- Appearance and gait
- How does she get up and down from chairs?
- What is her bed mobility like?
- How does she manage getting on and off the bed?
- How does she manage with dressing/undressing (if you have the opportunity to observe or assist with this activity)?

2. Joints involved

Observe, examine, palpate.

- In each case is there:
  - Pain?
  - Swelling?
  - Tenderness?
  - Decreased range of movement?
  - Decreased muscle power in adjacent muscle groups?
  - Instability?
  - Deformity?
- Is there spasm in the muscles?
- Are tendons affected?
- Can you access Mrs White's X-rays?

3. Extra-articular manifestations

- Has she any rheumatoid nodules?
- What is the condition of her skin: thin, papery, any ulcers?
- Are there any areas of reduced or altered sensation?

4. Functional assessment

This would need to be tailored specifically for Mrs White in relation to her particular problems.

Now we will continue with more information about this patient.

Case study 7.2: Mrs White (2)

Subjective assessment

You already have information on the diagnosis, onset, rate of progression, the present state of Mrs White's condition and the joints affected, as well as her social situation.

The main problems that she identifies are pain, stiffness and loss of function in all the affected joints, particularly over the last 6 months. She describes herself as having good and bad days. At present she experiences some pain at rest and finds that it increases in intensity on movement or if she stays in one position for too long. It is eased by painkillers (every 4 hours). She wakes two or three times every night and has marked morning stiffness (1½ hours).

Functionally she is able to do less, needing help with all ADLs, and she can no longer walk with her ordinary walking frame because of pain in her hips and not being able to take weight through her hands.

From the notes you find that she is anaemic but that this is being treated. Fatigue is a problem, particularly in the afternoon and evening. Apart from this, her general health is satisfactory.

Drugs – penicillamine, NSAID (naproxen), paracetamol/co-didramol as necessary, an antacid and vitamin B_{12} supplement. She has never taken steroids.

Mrs White has had previous physical treatment involving hydrotherapy and land-based physiotherapy. She felt that these helped her to retain function for a longer period.

Objective assessment

Generally this lady looks very thin and quite pale. She has great difficulty moving about the bed and is unable to walk more than a few steps around the bed.

Muscle strength is reduced in all groups – grade 3+ to 4.

Joints: all the affected joints have a reduced range of movement; both hip and knee flexion is limited by pain, particularly on the left side. Mrs White was unable to lie in supine and so the tests had to be performed in long sitting. It was not possible to test hip extension as she was unable to get into position. Her knees and shoulders were warmer to the touch than the other joints.

Swelling was obvious in her knees, elbows, wrists and fingers.

Areas of pain and tenderness can be seen on the body charts in Figure 7.8.

Self-assessment question

- SAQ 7.12 Briefly review the five stages in the pathological development of RA, with particular reference to the changes occurring in the joints and whether these are symptomatic or not.

Review of the clinical features of RA

Characteristically the patient is a woman aged between 20 and 50 years with a symmetrical

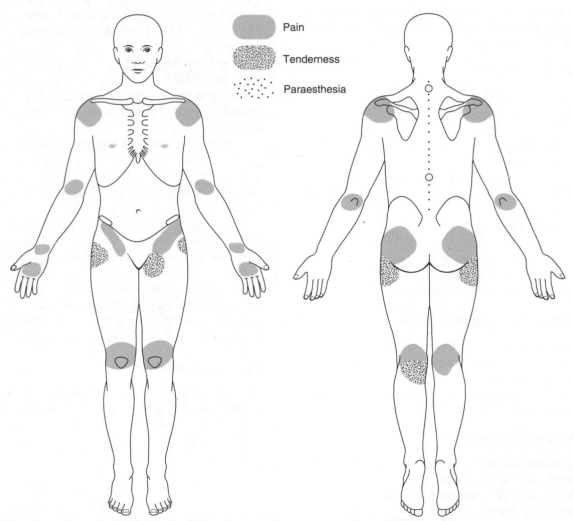

Figure 7.8   Body charts showing areas of pain and tenderness in the patient Mrs White.

polyarthritis usually involving the small joints of the hands and feet. She may complain of fatigue and will experience significant morning stiffness. Blood tests show an elevation in ESR; anaemia and rheumatoid factor may be present. There however, are many other ways in which this disease can present (Bhardwaj & Paget 1992).

Early in the course of the disease, symptoms can be either articular or systemic. There may only be prodromal symptoms at first, i.e. fatigue, weight loss, diffuse musculoskeletal pain with low-grade fever. The fatigue is often accompanied by morning stiffness, which is very characteristic of inflammatory joint disease and diagnostically significant if it lasts for an hour or more. The onset of joint disease varies – this has already been covered in the section on course and prognosis.

Joint symptoms are usually symmetrical and, as mentioned earlier, often begin in the small joints of the hands and feet. Hips and ankles are rarely affected in the early stages. When the pathological changes are confined to the synovial membrane, capsule and tendon sheaths, the patient complains of pain, swelling, tenderness and stiffness of a number of joints. Initially there will be pain on movement but with increasing disease activity there is pain at rest. Movement is guarded and there is a subjective feeling of stiffness and decreased range of movement.

In the finger joints the swelling produces a spindle shape. The fingers may be warm and tender and feel 'boggy' and difficult to move. Effusion is commonly found in the knees and swelling of bursae and tendons occurs, especially related to the wrists, dorsa of hands and feet. There may be swelling at the hip joint but this is very difficult to assess because of the large muscle mass in the area. If swelling is visible, it is seen in the groin or femoral triangle. There can be trochanteric bursitis with tenderness directly over the greater trochanter.

As the joints become more painful and stiff there will be atrophy of muscle tissue due to altered use patterns. The muscles are often tender and reduced in strength. These factors lead to an overall decrease in functional activity. In the case of the lower limbs mobility will be inhibited and because of the changes occurring at each joint there will be an altered gait pattern. Knowledge of the normal biomechanics of the joints, the changes due

to the disease process and the requirements for normal mobility is necessary in order to design an appropriate rehabilitation programme.

Morning stiffness remains a prominent symptom throughout and can be used as a guide to the activity of the disease and to gauge responses to therapy.

Joint deformities are not usually present early on and X-ray will only show soft tissue swelling and osteoporosis around the joints with no erosions. Radiographic changes occur at a steady rate throughout the course of the disease.

The outstanding complaints are of joint pain, stiffness and loss of function.

In the later stages of the disease, with cartilage destruction, necrosis and fibrosis of synovial membrane, contracture or stretching of the joint capsule and ligaments, and granulation tissue invading tendons and sheaths, there tends to be increasing and irreversible impairment of function. There may be limitation of movement in some joints but there may also be subluxation and instability in others.

There are some characteristic deformities associated with RA. Ulnar deviation at the metacarpophalangeal joints is common but causes surprisingly little functional disability. Deformities of the fingers may be more problematic. 'Swan neck' deformity (Fig. 7.9) is hyperextension of the proximal interphalangeal (IP) joints and fixed flexion of the distal IP joints. The 'boutonnière' (or buttonhole) deformity (Fig. 7.10) is due to protrusion of the proximal IP joint through the extensor expansion, producing fixed flexion, with extension of the distal IP joint. The latter two deformities markedly affect the patient's ability to grip.

Of the 20% of patients whose initial joint involvement is in the foot, problems for 80% of these begin in the forefoot. Common deformities are hallux valgus, dropped metatarsal heads and possibly hammer and claw toes. With hind foot involvement

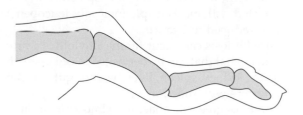

Figure 7.9 'Swan neck' deformity.

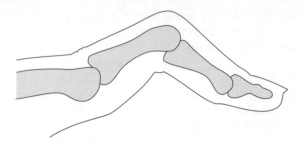

Figure 7.10   'Boutonnière' or 'button-hole' deformity.

there will be excessive pronation, subjecting the foot to extreme stress on weight bearing.

At the knees there may be fixed flexion deformity and valgus or less commonly varus. The typical RA knee deformity has been described as one of flexion, subluxation, valgus and external rotation. The valgus deformity is often combined with an eversion deformity at the subtalar joint with increased pronation of the forefoot. There may be deformities at other joints depending on the amount of destruction, bony erosion and the effects of the disease on the capsule and other soft tissue structures that normally play important roles in joint stability.

The following clinical manifestations also occur to varying degrees in RA patients:

- Subcutaneous rheumatoid nodules over pressure points in 20% of patients. Nodules can also be found in the lungs, pleura, heart, pericardium and the eye
- Vasculitis with all layers of the vessel wall infiltrated by lymphocytes, proliferation of the intima and possible disruption of the elastic lamina. This can lead to occlusion, ulceration or occasionally thrombosis
- The skin becomes atrophic, thin and papery
- Peripheral neuropathy may occur, and rarely, if there is subluxation of the cervical spine, cord compression
- The lymph nodes and the spleen may be affected with marked splenomegaly, leucopenia and reduced resistance
- Amyloidosis can occur rarely: amyloid is a protein crystal that can be deposited in organs such as the kidney, spleen, liver, heart or gut and can interfere with function
- Some degree of anaemia almost invariably accompanies RA

- X-rays and magnetic resonance imaging (MRI) scans show soft tissue swelling, osteoporosis, narrowing or loss of joint space, erosions and any deformities
- On laboratory tests many RA patients have a raised ESR. A normal ESR does not, however, preclude the presence of active disease
- In approximately 80% of patients rheumatoid factor is found in the serum. This is a standard test in the diagnosis of the condition and if RF is present it indicates a less favourable prognosis (Bhardwaj & Paget 1992, Eberhardt & Fex 2000, Kill 2002, Lloyd 1998, Scott 2000, Wollheim 1999).

Problem-solving exercise 7.9

Using the information on management of patients with rheumatic disorders from earlier in the chapter and the findings from the assessment of Mrs White, formulate

a. a problem list
b. goals of treatment
c. a treatment plan for this lady.

Take into account her physical, social and psychological wellbeing. (Bear in mind that she has been admitted for hip replacement – but don't spend too much time on immediate postoperative management as this is covered in Chapter 8. You may make the assumption that her drug regimen is adequate and stable.)

After you have attempted this, you can check your ideas in the following section.

An approach to the physiotherapy treatment of Mrs White

This section provides some ideas of possible problems, goals and treatment ideas that you might identify in your initial contact with Mrs White. It is important for you to remember, however, that these will differ for each patient that you see and you will need to make modifications depending on the specific circumstances. This is not a 'recipe' for you to follow but a template for you to adapt and build on.

1. Problem list

- Pain in all joints affected especially hips and knees
- Reduced range of movement in all affected joints
- Reduced muscle strength
- Reduced mobility both in bed and during loco-motion (no longer able to get around with walking frame)
- Reduced function.

The above problems will impact upon Mrs White's everyday activities and probably on the amount of interaction she has with others. This could cause her to feel despondent, which may consequently affect both her ability and her motivation to social-ize. It is possible, therefore, for some patients to enter into a descending spiral where pain and other physical problems cause difficulties in the social and psychological areas of their lives. This may increase negative feelings and could consequently magnify the patient's pain experience by focusing more attention on physical problems. The magni-tude of these effects will depend on your patient's outlook and the support she obtains from family and friends. As a physiotherapist you are not expected to be able to assess the patient's mental state. During your assessment, however, you should be able to get an idea of how the patient is feeling and how self-motivated she is.

2. Goals of treatment

- To reduce pain – this may or may not be a goal for the physiotherapist involved with RA patients. In this situation the pain from Mrs White's hips will be reduced by the surgery once the operative soreness fades. Her other joints will continue to be painful, however, and so you may be able to inter-vene here with some local treatment and advice
- To maintain or increase range of movement in affected joints within the limits of the disease and the patient's tolerance level
- To maintain or increase muscle strength in affected muscle groups within the limits of the disease and the patient's tolerance level
- To improve bed mobility if possible while on bed rest and then to help the patient to mobilize post-surgery
- To enable the patient to undertake as wide a range of functional activities as possible, particularly

locomotion (these must be decided upon in dis-cussion with Mrs White and appropriate mem-bers of the healthcare team).

3. Treatment plan

This could be dictated to a certain extent by the regimen within the particular hospital. It could, however, include the following:

- Pre- and postoperative care as necessary, e.g. regarding respiratory function and bed exercises.

- Pain relief – if one or two of the non operated joints was/were particularly problematic you could use ice or superficial heat for temporary pain relief before the patient carried out her exercises. Most of the pain should, however, be managed by the drug therapy.

  Because of Mrs White's widespread problems, she would appear to be an ideal candidate for hydrotherapy, which does have a pain-relieving aspect. This pain relief would, however, only be temporary, while the patient was in the pool. You would need to ensure that the benefits of pool treatment were not cancelled out by the increase of her fatigue to a debilitating level. Some patients do find that this is a problem after immersion in warm water.

  Pain relief may also be achieved by the use of appliances such as splints and walking aids. The pain in Mrs White's upper limbs would need to be considered here.

- Range of movement and muscle strengthening will be addressed by an exercise regimen. This could include passive or active assisted move-ments initially, building up to active and then resisted work as appropriate. Static muscle work could be used to begin with if movement was particularly difficult. Bed mobility could be addressed at the same time as this is something the patient has problems with (as noted on initial assessment).

- Once the patient is out of bed, mobility usually involves the use of a walking aid. A gutter frame may be helpful with Mrs White as this will divert the strain from her hands and wrists. You should work with Mrs White on her gait – both the quality of her walking and the distance she covers each time need to be addressed. As progress occurs you may change the walking aid as appropriate: for example, you might move on to gutter crutches. The rate of progression with mobility may be dictated either by the surgeon (it may be a set number of days before the patient is allowed out of bed after hip replacement), or it may depend on the patient's own abilities.

It would be usual to check Mrs White's safety on the stairs (this sometimes needs more practice) before she could go home.

- Advice/education – this should be an integral part of your treatment. Mrs White will need information about do's and don't's following hip replacement, which could be provided verbally, in written form or a combination of both. With regard to advice about other issues, this will vary from patient to patient. Mrs White has a 6-year history of RA and so she may already know a significant amount about the condition and the possible self-help strategies such as joint protection. This is not always the case, however, and you may need to spend some time with her and possibly with her husband going over important points. This should be carried out in conjunction with, and with input from, relevant members of the healthcare team.

Review point

When you go on to consider the Problem-solving exercise regarding Mr Nicholls in Chapter 8 (p. 259), you will note a number of similarities between that and Mrs White's management. This should help to reinforce the idea that, although patients may have different conditions, often the problems they have and the possible interventions you could use are very similar. This book does not aim to cover all eventualities; we want to enable you to realize, however, that as long as you remember the principles of treatment you will be able to apply them to a wide range of situations. It is important to carefully consider your patients as individuals and to investigate

their problems fully during the assessment period, both from your perspective and from theirs. Decide on your intervention by collaborating with the patient; so in each instance you tailor physiotherapy management specifically for the individual.

Additional treatment modalities

Some patients have reported finding relief from symptoms with alternative therapies. These include modalities such as homeopathy, acupuncture, aromatherapy and reflex therapy.

There is a suggestion of some connection between RA and hypersensitivity to environmental toxins, especially food and food-related products. It has been proved, however, that no food has anything to do with causing arthritis and no food is effective in curing it. Some observations do suggest that, for selected patients, dietary manipulation may be beneficial. Some patients have identified strong relationships between eating certain foods and a flare of symptoms. In this case it would seem sensible to avoid these foods.

It has been found that cow's milk may induce or exacerbate symptoms in some patients and a controlled fast can help to alleviate this. Fasting has been shown to be of benefit but the resultant weight loss can be a problem if the patient already has a low BMI (SIGN 2000). There is some evidence to suggest that dietary fish oil supplements could help to alleviate the symptoms of RA. Subjects showed a significant reduction in the number of tender joints and in duration of morning stiffness after 3 months of therapy. There was, however, no effect on disease activity or progression. Practically, this approach is problematic because of the large amounts of fish oil required, the difficulty in taking it and its expense (SIGN 2000). It should also be noted that this oil can prolong bleeding time and inhibit platelet aggregation. This could be dangerous if the patient was taking an anticoagulant such as aspirin (Bhardwaj & Paget 1992). Evidence of the beneficial effect of other oils on disease activity in RA, such as evening primrose and blackcurrant seed, is uncertain (SIGN 2000).

Conclusion

Approximately 70% of patients with RA will experience chronic disability with remission and exacerbation. Total clinical remission is a very rare event and therefore most patients will require intervention from the healthcare team. Drug therapy is essential and at present is the only method that has been shown to retard disease activity; in many cases this is only a temporary reduction in the rate of progression.

The physiotherapist's role is one of enabling patients to improve their functional abilities within the limits of the disease. This may involve combinations of active treatment, advice, education, splinting and provision of, or advice about aids and appliances. Consultation with other members of the healthcare team, especially the OT, is often necessary, particularly with regard to aids and appliances.

Currently, the overall functional status of patients with RA is maintained by medication, physical interventions, education, emotional support and surgery where indicated. This is the limit of management until the aetiology and pathogenesis of the disease is understood more clearly.

ANKYLOSING SPONDYLITIS

Ankylosing spondylitis (AS) is another example of a common rheumatic disorder to be considered in this chapter. As you read through this section, try to think about the similarities and differences between this disease and the two you have already learned about.

Ankylosing spondylitis belongs to a group of disorders, known as the seronegative spondyloarthropathies, that share key clinical features and an association with the human leukocyte antigen (HLA)-B27 found on chromosome 6. The combined prevalence of these disorders in the general population is estimated to be approximately 1% (Packham & Bowness 2001). These conditions predominantly affect the joints of the spine and no rheumatoid factor is found in the serum. Characteristic clinical features can be seen in Box 7.6.

Ankylosis means 'bony fusion' and spondylitis is inflammation of the spine. AS is the commonest of the spondyloarthritides, with a prevalence

---

Box 7.6   Characteristic clinical features of the seronegative spondyloarthropathies

- Predominantly axial joint involvement including sacroiliitis
- Peripheral arthritis – often asymmetrical
- Negative rheumatoid factor
- Absence of extra-articular features of rheumatoid arthritis
- Presence of other extra-articular features characteristic of the group, e.g. iritis, ulcerative colitis and cardiac involvement
- Enthesitis – inflammation at the site of tendon and ligament insertions
- Familial clustering
- Association with HLA-B27
- Male predominance

Adapted from Caldron 1995, Inman 1992, Packham & Bowness 2001, Rai & Struthers 1994.

---

of 0.2–0.86% in the adult caucasian population (Packham & Bowness 2001). It is a chronic, progressive inflammatory arthritis predominantly affecting the axial skeleton, but it also has some systemic effects (Dziedzic 1998). Peripheral joint involvement, however, is also a significant feature most commonly associated with the hips and shoulders (Bhardwaj & Paget 1992, Dandy & Edwards 2003). It affects both synovial and cartilaginous joints as well as the sites of insertion of both tendons and ligaments (enthesopathy). The inflammation is followed by partial or complete fusion of the joints mentioned above.

Ankylosing spondylitis is a significant cause of disability in young men (0.4% in men, 0.05% in women). The condition is more common in males than females but this sex-linked ratio becomes less marked as the age of onset increases (for onset at less than 16 years the male:female ratio is 6:1, and for onset at 30 years, it is 2:1). It is estimated that there are approximately 70 000 cases of AS in the UK but there are probably large numbers of subclinical, undiagnosed cases within the population. AS still tends to be considered a predominantly male condition, however, and so many of these undiagnosed cases are likely to be female. Women are believed to experience a milder, atypical disease process that may go unrecognized for long periods, although speed of diagnosis in females is improving (Dziedzic 1998).

Aetiology

There is a marked familial incidence in AS, but other factors probably determine onset in predisposed individuals. Of the spondyloarthropathies the association with HLA-B27 is greatest in AS – it is present in over 95% of patients (Packham & Bowness 2001, Rai & Struthers 1994) as compared to only 10% of healthy controls (Dziedzic 1998). Family and twin studies have shown that predisposition to AS is largely genetically determined (Packham & Bowness 2001). It is important to note, however, that not everyone with the HLA-B27 genetic marker will develop AS. Fewer than 10% of the population who are HLA-B27-positive develop AS, suggesting that other genes may also be involved in the aetiology of the condition (Arthritis Research Campaign 2003b, Brophy et al 2003). As a consequence of these factors, therefore, part of the management for patients with AS may involve genetic counselling (Rai & Struthers 1994).

As with other rheumatic conditions, it is thought that an environmental trigger may initiate the development of the disease in predisposed individuals. The specific mechanism is unknown but there is evidence to suggest that there could be a link with bowel or urogenital infections as in Reiter's syndrome (Brophy et al 2003, Packham & Bowness 2001).

Diagnosis of ankylosing spondylitis

For an individual to be diagnosed as having AS, s/he must have the following:

- Sacroiliitis on X-ray or MRI
- Limited movement of the lower back in frontal and sagittal planes
- Inflammatory back pain for more than 3 months, improved by exercise and unrelieved by rest
- Morning stiffness in the back lasting in excess of one hour
- Restricted chest expansion (Brophy et al 2003, Dziedzic 1998).

A rapid response to anti-inflammatory drugs, family history of AS and painless effusions in a large joint may also be indicative (Dandy & Edwards 2003). Until recently, AS could only be diagnosed by X-ray, which was a disadvantage as many patients have symptoms prior to the development of X-ray changes. Recent improvements in imaging, such as MRI scans, mean that AS can be diagnosed much earlier (Brophy et al 2003).

Course and prognosis

The onset of AS usually occurs in a young adult (15–30 years) who complains of gradually increasing back pain and stiffness. The course is variable but generally prolonged, with many patients maintaining good or adequate function. A small percentage may experience a more progressive and disabling manifestation of the disease. It is not unusual for diagnosis to be delayed where the presentation is one of chronic, mechanical low back pain (Dziedzic 1998, Rai & Struthers 1994).

The disease runs a progressive cyclical course with each exacerbation leaving an increase in the amount of residual damage and disability. In a small percentage of patients the eventual outcome may be total fusion of the joints, particularly in the spine and thorax, with a consequent reduction in functional ability. Many patients, however, never reach this stage and overall functional outcome is good.

It used to be believed that AS would burn out when the patient reached the fifth decade. More recent work, however, provides no evidence for this view. Progression and severity appear to depend on the disease activity at initial diagnosis, i.e. the prognosis of those patients with more active disease is poor. There is also a correlation with age, with older patients experiencing more severe disease activity (Kennedy et al 1993).

Ankylosing spondylitis does not in itself cause a reduction in life expectancy but there may be associated problems. These are usually due to the extra-articular manifestations affecting the heart and/or lungs. There may also be secondary amyloidosis, which can cause premature death (Dziedzic 1998, Viitanen & Suni 1995). If the thorax is so fused as to seriously reduce chest expansion there may be some extra risks involved with surgery, particularly for those patients with marked deformity. In the majority of cases, however, with treatment and advice including family education and awareness of the condition, the prognosis is good (Rai & Struthers 1994).

Pathological changes in ankylosing spondylitis

Ankylosing spondylitis is an inflammatory arthritis affecting the synovium, capsule and ligaments around the joints, as well as the insertions of tendons into bone. The inflammation is known as an enthesopathy and is particularly obvious around the spine and pelvis. This process also involves an imbalance in bone production and reabsorption. The increased levels of cytokines found in patients with AS have an effect on bone mineral absorption. There is increased bone turnover, with more being absorbed than laid down, leading to osteoporosis early on in the disease process (Brophy et al 2003).

During the inflammatory stage, bone is eroded at its junction with the soft tissue structures that attach to it. A healing process then occurs, which involves extra bone being laid down, so causing protuberances to appear that increase in size with each episode. If this continues it can eventually cause bridging between the bones involved. In the spine the inflammation occurs where the annulus fibrosus joins the margin of the vertebral body, and the bony overgrowth that results is referred to as a syndesmophyte. Ligamentous calcification can occur in the posterior and anterior longitudinal ligaments and the inferior and superior interspinous ligaments so making the spine more rigid. When the syndesmophytes of adjacent vertebrae join, the spine takes on a particular appearance on X-ray and is referred to as a 'bamboo spine' (Fig. 7.11). By this time the spine is fused, as are the sacroiliac joints. Similar ankylosis occurs in the symphysis pubis, costovertebral and manubriosternal joints.

Up to 50% of AS patients have clinically significant hip involvement, which is often bilateral. In severe cases, findings here can include protrusion deformities and/or completely ankylosed hips (Ranawat et al 1992). If hip disease has not appeared within the first 10 years of the patient

experiencing the symptoms of AS then this is unlikely to occur. The shoulders, hands, knees and feet can also be affected (Arthritis Research Campaign 2003b, Brophy et al 2003,).

The ESR is sometimes raised early on or during a period of active disease but conversely there is sometimes a normal ESR during this time (Rai & Struthers 1994).

The earliest X-ray changes are seen in the sacroiliac joints.

Problem–solving exercise 7.10

With reference to the clinical reasoning processes you have used previously in the chapter and considering the information provided, compile a list of the possible clinical features you would expect to see in a patient with ankylosing spondylitis. (See below.)

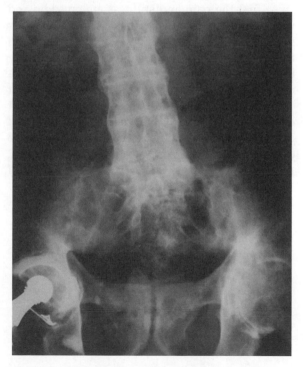

Figure 7.11   X-ray appearance of a 'bamboo spine' in a patient with ankylosing spondylitis. (With permission from Caldron 1995.)

Self-assessment question

- SAQ 7.13 What are the characteristic features of the seronegative spondyloarthropathies? (Clue: there are nine).

Clinical features of ankylosing spondylitis

The onset of AS is insidious in most cases and, as mentioned earlier, it often begins with low back pain and stiffness. Patients are generally seen after several months of symptoms for which an inciting event cannot be recalled. The pain, which is usually described as severe aching, can also radiate to the buttock and posterior aspect of the thigh or knee, it can be uni- or bilateral and may alternate from side to side. A small number of patients may not have back pain at all but could present with pain in the hip or knee. This can add to the difficulty in diagnosis. Figure 7.12 shows the typical areas where patients with AS may feel pain.

At first the pain and stiffness are episodic and worse after immobility. A total of 65% of patients with AS complain of fatigue as a major symptom from time to time. These patients are more likely to be women and those with severe manifestations of the disease. This is a complicated symptom that could be linked to the inflammatory process but it could also be due to the chronic discomfort, which disturbs normal sleep patterns. Patients may also experience weight loss and low-grade pyrexia. As mentioned earlier, most patients complain of morning stiffness but this can be variable (Arthritis Research Campaign 2003b, Brophy et al 2001, Viitanen & Suni 1995).

As the disease begins to affect more joints, the pain will spread to encompass these – they may include the thoracic and cervical spine, the manubriosternal and costochondral joints, hips, knees, shoulders and heels. The last is due to enthesopathy at the tendo calcaneus (pain at the back of the heel) and possibly the plantar ligaments (pain on weight bearing in the morning – plantar fasciitis). Some patients also complain of anterior chest pain precipitated by laughing or coughing. This is due to the disease affecting the insertions of the intercostal muscles and may extend around the thorax. Muscle spasm may accompany the pain in any of the above areas.

Later in the course of AS the patient will complain of more constant pain and stiffness. This is still worse after immobility and improves with exercise. There will also be a noticeable decrease in spinal mobility in multiple planes (Packham & Bowness 2001) and a decrease in chest expansion. Some patients may find that the stiff lower back becomes painless and does not interfere with physical activity, particularly if the upper regions of the spine and the peripheral joints are not affected. Many patients, however, experience active disease in a range of joints. This causes widespread pain and stiffness that can have a significant effect on functional ability. Patients may also experience tenderness, particularly in the axial joints – the spine, the sacroiliac, manubriosternal and costovertebral joints and the symphysis pubis. Sitting may be uncomfortable because of tenderness at the ischial tuberosities.

In progressive disease the patient will have noticeable deformities, which often include the following:

- Increased thoracic kyphosis
- Poking chin
  (If the above deformities are severe, they can cause problems with intubation during surgery)
- Flattened lumbar lordosis with posterior pelvic tilt
- Slightly flexed hips and knees (this can become fixed with habitual change in posture).

The above postural changes are often grouped together and called the 'question mark' deformity,

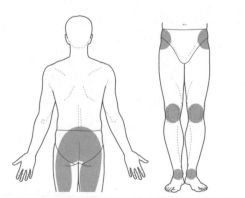

Figure 7.12   Pain distribution in ankylosing spondylitis.

as this can be the appearance of the patient when viewed from the side (Fig. 7.13). This characteristic stooping posture and stiff spine lead to muscle shortening and further loss of movement. There will also be abnormal loading in and around the joints, which can lead to secondary problems including degenerative changes. Loss of muscle strength is common and this may be due to reduced activity levels, limited movement or some structural change in the muscle cells (Viitanen & Suni 1995).

The nine most significant physical problems as rated by patients with AS can be seen in Box 7.7.

> **Self-assessment question**
>
> - **SAQ 7.14** Using your knowledge of anatomy, work out which muscle groups may become shortened and tight because of the changes in posture that occur in ankylosing spondylitis.

Extra-articular features

Some patients experience extra-articular features that are associated with AS.

- *Iritis* is inflammation of the iris causing pain and light sensitivity. Onset is usually sudden, it can last between a few weeks and 2 months and it

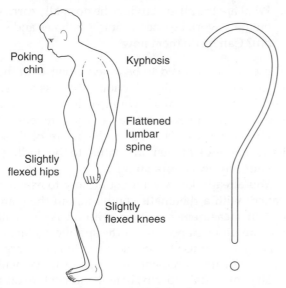

Figure 7.13 'Question mark' deformity.

> **Box 7.7** The nine most significant physical problems as rated by patients with ankylosing spondylitis (Dziedzic 1998)
>
> - Difficulty sleeping on the stomach
> - Stiffness on waking
> - Standing for long periods
> - Prolonged sitting
> - Bending
> - Being a spectator rather than participating in activities
> - Pain increasing with higher levels of stress
> - Tiredness on waking
> - Limitation of leisure activities

often recurs. This does need treatment with topical corticosteroids and the patient often needs to wear sunglasses because of acute light sensitivity that causes pain. If you notice, therefore, that one of your patients has developed a red eye it is important to advise him/her to go to the GP.

- There does seem to be some link with *psoriasis*. Drugs, stress reduction and not smoking or drinking heavily can be effective in treating this condition.

- *Inflammation of the gut* and spondyloarthritis are closely linked and some patients may have Crohn's disease or ulcerative colitis. Up to 50% of individuals with AS, however, may show evidence of gut inflammation but will be asymptomatic (Brophy et al 2003).

- Rare complications include problems with the *heart, lungs* or *nervous system*.

- *Psychosocial factors* can be an issue for these patients. One-third of people with AS report high levels of depression. More women are affected than men. There may be issues to manage with regard to relationships (particularly in relation to body image and sexual problems), work and social activities. Problems in controlling the disease and failure to develop personal strategies may initiate the onset of learned helplessness where the patient feels that there is little point in trying anything (Dziedzic 1998). This will inevitably compound the individual's difficulties.

Case study 7.3: Mr Smith

Mr Smith is attending the outpatient department with a suspected diagnosis of AS. He is a 29-year-old carpenter, married with two young children and living in a sixth-floor flat.
He has been unable to work for the last 2 weeks and has spent most of that time on bedrest.
His symptoms have improved somewhat after starting on NSAIDs and this is his first visit to a physiotherapy department.

Problem-solving exercise 7.11

Decide how you would assess this patient. If you wish, go back to the earlier section about OA to refresh your memory about assessment, but keep in mind how this patient differs from the scenarios you have dealt with so far.

Assessment

It is not intended that this section should repeat all the information provided earlier in the chapter. By this time it should be fairly clear that you can use very similar questioning and examination techniques for all the patients that have been presented. The overall structure of the assessment is the same; you need to make sure, however, that the structure you choose to adopt is flexible enough to be personalized for each patient that you see. Decide which sections you need to keep and which can be left out or looked at in less detail. As mentioned in the last Problem-solving exercise, for general assessment guidelines go back to the section on OA.

As an autonomous practitioner you need to carry out a thorough examination in order to satisfy yourself as to whether or not the patient's diagnosis matches your findings. As you know, AS can sometimes appear to be chronic low back pain; you need, therefore, to be clear on the presenting features of the condition so that you can distinguish between the two.

Self-assessment question

• SAQ 7.15 What are the diagnostic features of ankylosing spondylitis?

In this case, your assessment should address a number of issues that are different from those you considered in the earlier case studies. These are particularly related to Mr Smith's functional and psychosocial status. In order to ensure that you examine these issues, you may find it useful to ask questions about some of the following points:

• At the time of assessment what is Mr Smith's function like?
• Does he feel that he is getting better, getting worse or staying the same?
• Is he able to manage his ADL?
• Can he get up all six flights of stairs to his flat?
• If not, why not? Is it too painful, does he get tired or breathless?
• If he has morning stiffness, how long does it take to wear off?
• Can he drive? (if this question is relevant)
• Is he the main breadwinner for the family?
• How will the disease affect his ability to carry out his job?
• Exactly what activities does his job involve?
• What are the other activities he normally carries out (any work he does at home, hobbies and so on)? Can he do them now?

These questions need to be asked along with the usual ones about pain behaviour, stiffness and so on. This patient is much younger than the others you have considered and has a very different set of circumstances. You need to be aware of these issues and look at them in relation to the findings of your physical examination.

You already know a lot about how to assess a patient with a rheumatic condition, but there are certain measurements taken with an AS patient that are different because of the specific problems experienced. It used to be the norm to take a large number of measurements of range of movement in all joints, vital capacity, height and posture on a regular basis to assess both the disease progression

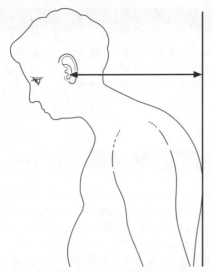

Figure 7.14   Measurement of tragus to wall.

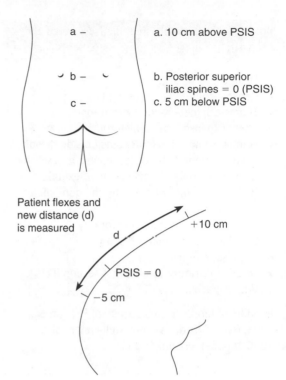

a. 10 cm above PSIS

b. Posterior superior
   iliac spines = 0 (PSIS)

c. 5 cm below PSIS

Patient flexes and
new distance (d)
is measured

+10 cm

d

PSIS = 0

−5 cm

Figure 7.15   Modified Schober's test of lumbar flexion.

and the effects of exercise. Recent work at the Royal National Hospital for Rheumatic Diseases in the UK has, however, streamlined this approach to a smaller number of measures (the Bath AS Metrology Index – BASMI), which appear to give the same information about disease activity. Of the 20 measurements, five were found to most closely coincide with the X-rays and laboratory results that are used to indicate disease status (Mallorie et al 1995). The five measures are:

- cervical rotation
- tragus to wall distance (Fig. 7.14)
- lateral flexion
- modified Schober's test of lumbar flexion (Fig. 7.15)
- intermalleolar distance.

This makes for a much speedier assessment and gives a baseline from which to measure any changes in the patient's condition. The team in Bath have designed a range of outcome measures for AS that can be used to focus on various areas: function, metrology, disease activity, a global score of the effect of the disease on the patient and radiology. Most of these are based on visual analogue scales and the aim of producing these was to make the measurement of outcome in AS simple, reproducible, fast and sensitive to change (Calin 2002).

If you find that one of your patients has a problem with a particular joint or area not included in the outcome measures mentioned above, you could of course use any others that you felt appropriate. Other possible measurements can be seen in Box 7.8.

Remember that these measures are just suggestions and it would not be necessary to use them all for every AS patient.

Management

The main approaches to management of patients with AS include:

- Patient education
- Family education
- Genetic counselling
- Pain relief
- Physiotherapy
- Occupational therapy
- Possible surgery (Calin 2000).

> **Box 7.8   Possible physical measurements for use with ankylosing spondylitis patients**
>
> - Height
> - Cervical spine – all movements
> - Thoracic spine – flexion/extension
> - Chest expansion at xiphisternum
> - Lumbar spine – flexion/extension/side flexion
> - Finger to floor distance (unreliable by itself for lumbar flexion as it includes hip flexion)
> - Hip – all movements (with goniometer), Thomas test
> - Knee – check for flexion deformity
> - Shoulder – particularly flexion
> - Exercise tolerance
> - Forced expiratory volume in 1 second (FEV_1)
> - Vital capacity
>
> (Modified from Chartered Society of Physiotherapy 1993, Rai & Struthers 1994, Helliwell et al 1996, Viitanen & Suni 1995.)

The key point to note is that the pain and stiffness experienced by patients with AS improve with exercise. This is extremely important and the patient must be helped to understand that activity is a major part of the management of the condition. Although exercise plays a large part in the treatment of many rheumatic conditions, in AS it is a major consideration.

As discussed earlier in the chapter, drug therapy plays an important part in the management of all patients with rheumatic conditions and this is also the case with AS. Drug treatment usually consists of analgesics, muscle relaxants and NSAIDs, which are taken to reduce inflammation (Dziedzic 1998). This in turn reduces pain and stiffness, allowing the patient to be generally more active and to undertake an exercise programme. DMARDs such as those helpful in RA are less effective in AS. Occasionally, sulfasalazine may be prescribed. This is usually for those individuals with major peripheral joint involvement and significant systemic disease; it has virtually no effect on spinal symptoms. Low-dose amitriptyline can ease pain and stiffness and also improves sleep patterns, so reducing fatigue (Calin 2000).

> **Self-assessment question**
>
> - **SAQ 7.16** What are the main five objective measures that can be used to record the progress of a patient with AS?

> **Problem-solving exercise 7.12**
>
> During your assessment you found that Mr Smith has low back pain referring into his buttocks and posterior thigh region. Movements of his whole spine are restricted and painful but he has no fixed deformity at present. He complains of discomfort in both hips and shoulders and on examination you find that there is reduced range of movement in these joints (especially flexion and abduction). Mr Smith explains that he feels very stiff in the morning; the stiffness decreases, however, if he is able to get up and move around a little during the day. Generally he feels rather fatigued and gets breathless on light exercise.
>
> Devise a plan of physiotherapy treatment for Mr Smith. Include any advice you might give him about ADL. Note any points where input from other members of the healthcare team might be useful.
>
> (As usual, you can read the next section for some ideas on this – but try it yourself first.)

A plan of treatment for Mr Smith

The plan of physiotherapy for Mr Smith will mainly involve exercise and stretches, for the following reasons:

- to generally maintain muscle strength and improve it if necessary. It may also be necessary, however, to target specific muscle groups that are in danger of becoming weak, e.g. back extensors, shoulder and hip abductors
- to maintain or improve muscle length and joint range of movement (especially in the spine, hips and shoulders)
- to improve exercise tolerance.

Both hydrotherapy and land-based regimens are used regularly in the management of AS. Active participation is very important in maintaining function in this condition. If pain can be controlled by drug therapy and/or physiotherapeutic methods, there are few reasons that preclude a patient with AS carrying out effective training that can be as intensive as s/he can tolerate. A patient experiencing very active disease with involvement of peripheral joints or another serious illness may need to carry out a modified exercise programme (Viitanen & Suni 1995).

Advice on activities of daily living

In order for Mr Smith's management to be optimally effective he needs to take responsibility for his own health and wellbeing. This may include the development of strategies to avoid becoming overtired and prioritization of his activities to ensure that he does not take on too many commitments.

If the disease is in a very active phase, then some rest may be indicated. This might involve time away from work or even a short period of hospitalization. Rest does not mean immobility, however, as this could increase the stiffness in Mr Smith's spine. It is important that he continues to exercise and to practise good posture. Prone lying is helpful in maintaining extension in the hips and back but it is not always an easy position for patients to adopt. Initially Mr Smith may need to place a pillow under his chest for support. He should be encouraged to stay in prone for 20 minutes at a time but he may have to work up to this (Arthritis Research Campaign 2003b). The bed should be firm without sagging to avoid any tendency for increasing spinal curvature. You could advise Mr Smith to put a board between his mattress and the bed frame if his bed is too soft. This will help to maintain good posture.

A high chair with a firm seat and upright back is often found to be better for the posture but may not be as comfortable as an easy chair. Sitting in low, soft chairs will result in bad posture and increased pain. You should advise Mr Smith to keep his head against the back of the chair (or a small cushion if necessary) to reduce the risk of developing a poking chin. This can be particularly important if he spends any time using a computer, where the unconscious tendency is to protract the head forward on the neck.

The same attention to posture should be given when travelling by car. It is important for Mr Smith to stop the car periodically to allow him to get out and stretch, as pain and stiffness can distract attention. It is essential that he does not spend protracted amounts of time in one position, especially any that involve flexion of hips and back. Reversing into parking spaces or garages may be difficult if the patient's neck is very stiff; special mirrors can be fitted to the car to help with this activity. As stiff joints are more easily damaged, it is important for head supports to be used effectively to avoid the risk of neck injury.

It is important to remain physically active. You should inform the patient of the risks of taking part in contact sports such as rugby or basketball. When the joints are more rigid, as in AS, damage can occur more easily. Swimming is an excellent form of exercise because it works the whole body without jarring and it can be used to improve cardiovascular and respiratory endurance. Respiratory exercises are very important for some patients with thoracic cage joint involvement as they can help to maintain vital capacity.

Individuals with AS are often able to continue working in a wide range of employment settings ranging from sedentary (e.g. office workers and computer programmers) to manual (e.g. carpenters and builders). There will be some issues to address but difficulties may be dealt with in two ways, first by the individual with AS developing personal strategies to manage his/her work tasks and second by the employer making reasonable adjustments to enable the employee with a disability to carry out his/her employment role effectively. This is a duty placed upon the employer (in the UK) by the Disability Discrimination Act 1995.

If it became impossible for Mr Smith to continue his work as a carpenter he could contact the local disability services team (via the Jobcentre), who can arrange work assessment and retraining. It is important for you, as a member of the health-care team, to be aware of these schemes so that you can include the information in your advice to patients if appropriate.

Sexual activity may be painful for patients with AS because of inflammation in the sacroiliac joints and the lower back. Lack of mobility in the hip joints can also cause problems. If fatigue is a significant problem this can reduce the desire for sex. These factors can cause stress to the individual and may have an effect on relationships. Drug therapy can help the pain and alternative positions can be used for sexual intercourse. This is an area where education may be necessary and in some cases counselling for both partners may be appropriate (Arthritis Research Campaign 2003b).

You could also provide the following advice to Mr Smith if it seemed appropriate:

- Do not use a revolving chair if you work at a desk – this will stop you rotating the spine. This lack of turning will lead to you being unable to turn.
- Get up to change the channel on the TV, don't use the remote control!
- A hot bath may help to relieve morning stiffness and it could ease aches and pains. You could do some exercises in or after the bath.
- Avoid working at a flat-topped desk or table as this means you are bending your head forward. Try to arrange some sort of inclined surface.
- When working in a standing position, try to raise the task up so you are not bending forward.
- Check posture regularly and correct it as much as possible. You can use a wall to stand against – try to get the back of your head, hips and heels touching it.
- Include some exercise/activity in your daily routine. This could either be a particular type of activity – e.g. regularly taking part in a sport, doing yoga or Pilates, aerobics, swimming, exercising with a large GymBall – or it may involve increasing general activity levels, e.g. by walking instead of driving, going upstairs instead of using the lift, cycling to work and so on.

Other members of the healthcare team

The members of the healthcare team involved with Mr Smith's management will vary depending on his specific requirements. His GP will definitely be involved and the OT may have an input, especially if Mr Smith needs any aids or appliances, e.g. modified mirrors to enable him to continue to drive. Mr Smith may wish to attend the local

National Ankylosing Spondylitis Society group if there is one in the area. It is important, therefore, for you to have details of meetings and contact names/numbers available to pass on to the patient as necessary.

As noted earlier, depression can be a consequence of AS for a significant number of patients. Your interaction with Mr Smith and any contact he has with a self-help group will provide some psychological and emotional support. It is, however, essential for you to be able to refer him to other health professionals (e.g. a counsellor) as appropriate if he reports that he is finding his situation too difficult to manage and needs more support. Patients with AS may not need intervention from a large healthcare team as they tend to be more functionally able than those with severe RA or OA. If you do come across patients who are severely affected, however, then more members of the team would be involved, e.g. the orthopaedic surgeon if a joint replacement was necessary.

Conclusion

Ankylosing spondylitis patients show definite improvement when they have effective drug therapy plus an exercise regimen. Different approaches to management have been investigated, e.g. 2–3 weeks as an inpatient with daily land-based exercise and hydrotherapy, outpatient treatment (land-based and/or hydrotherapy) and home exercises, or home exercises alone. Other individuals attend groups run by the National Ankylosing Spondylitis Society, which is a self-help group with input from health professionals. Improvement has been reported in patients who have had AS for many years with marked decrease in range of movement and significant deformity. In many cases there is little objective measurable improvement in terms of increased movement and so on; the improvement is, however, usually of functional significance to the patient.

The available research evidence regarding the efficacy of exercise in AS is patchy because of the differences and shortcomings of the methodologies. The main message that comes through from virtually all the studies, however, is that patients must maintain the exercise level themselves, incorporating it into their lifestyle, otherwise any improvement seen with treatment (whatever approach is used) is not maintained. The exercise should also be as intensive as the patients can tolerate in order to keep any improvement to a maximum (Helliwell et al 1996, Viitanen & Suni 1995).

You should consider these points whenever you are treating patients with AS as it may be your input that helps to motivate them to continue with their exercises. You could even become involved in running sessions in the pool and on dry land at a NASS group.

As with all the rheumatic diseases, you must make every effort to encourage patients to take on the responsibility for their own management with support and input from health professionals when necessary.

ARTHRITIS IN CHILDREN

It is important for you to realize that arthritis can affect individuals at any stage of their life cycle. In order to illustrate this we will briefly introduce you to juvenile idiopathic arthritis in order that you can consider some of the issues relating to the management of children with chronic disease.

Physiotherapists come into contact with children in many areas of practice, which can include primary care settings, health centres, outpatient departments and hospital wards as well as nurseries and schools. These children range in age from babies born prematurely through to adolescents, with all the concomitant developmental and psychosocial changes that occur as they grow up. This is in addition to any physical, mental, developmental, learning or emotional issues they may have to manage. The most important point for you to remember whenever treating children is that they are not just small adults; they are developing human beings (APCP 1995), with issues that need to be addressed at all stages. It is essential to see the child first and the child with problems second (Eckersley 1993).

A key consideration in the management of children with arthritis is that members of the healthcare team are not just dealing with the child but with parents and possibly, the rest of the family, as well as other carers such as teachers. As mentioned earlier, these carers must be part of the healthcare team. If any intervention is to be successful, the child must be seen in the context of the family, which has a key role in this team. It is essential that everyone works together with agreed management plans. If this consistent approach is not taken, the child and the parents may become confused and find it difficult to comply with any intervention. There must be a balance between the needs of the child and the needs of the family. It is important to remember that whatever problems a child has, he or she has 'special needs for fun, play and love' and parents and other professionals are partners with the physiotherapist in this enterprise (APCP 1995).

Working with children

When working with children it is essential that you consider the needs of both the parents and the child and that you are able to communicate effectively. A majority of the knowledge and skills that you employ when treating children are the same as those you make use of in other settings. This relates to the overall philosophy of this book – where the 'condition' the patient has is almost a secondary consideration; the important aspect is to focus on the individual and his/her needs and expectations. You must assess the child and then use the same problem-solving and decision-making skills you employ with any other category of patient (based on your existing knowledge and skills base) in order to plan the intervention. Techniques must be appropriate for use with infants and children and may need to be modified. You will need to:

- acquire and refine a variety of handling skills that are specifically for use in the treatment of children
- have knowledge of normal child development to facilitate recognition of any deviation from this
- have knowledge of specific childhood pathologies and their common signs and symptoms
- be familiar with the theories and philosophies of different approaches to the treatment of children
- have an understanding of any statutory obligations
- have an awareness of social, environmental and cultural variables that influence family structure, dynamics and motivation.

One major difference, however, between managing a child with arthritis and managing an adult is that for the child the regular therapy sessions are often carried out by another person, such as a parent, rather than by the physiotherapist.

Self-assessment question

- **SAQ 7.17** What skills and knowledge are needed by the physiotherapist to work successfully with children and their carers?

Assessment

Many of the general features covered in the earlier assessment chapter will be of relevance when dealing with children. There are, however, some areas that will need to be modified, and there may be specific tests or techniques that need to be carried out.

Self-assessment question

- **SAQ 7.18** Review the role of assessment within the overall physiotherapy management of a patient (i.e. why is assessment essential?).

Review point

Before reading this section, use your previous knowledge and experience to consider any similarities and differences in your approach to assessing patients in the following categories:

a. a 70-year-old adult
b. a 20-year-old adult
c. a 14-year-old adolescent
d. a 5-year-old child.

It is essential that assessment of children at any age is a holistic and ongoing process. This is particularly important in younger children, where many developmental changes are occurring at the same time as any intervention. This approach to assessment is necessary in order to ensure that any treatment outcomes are successful. (It should be noted that this principle applies to varying degrees in the assessment of all patients.) Many children referred to the physiotherapist have ongoing problems that require ongoing intervention over a long period (APCP 1995). Knowledge of the changes in performance that occur as a result of growth and development, therefore, becomes even more important.

Accurate and appropriate assessment is necessary to enable the following processes to take place:

- Development of initial plan of intervention
- Prioritization with regard to future therapy
- Monitoring of any changes and progress
- Evaluation of effectiveness of treatment
- Evaluation of outcomes.

Physiotherapy assessment

Environment

The environment in which the assessment takes place is an important factor, as it can affect how well the child performs. If possible, the surroundings should be familiar and comfortable to help the child to feel as secure as possible, but should also be appropriate for the assessment process. If the room and contents are familiar to the child before the assessment, it will mean that there is less distraction. If these points are considered, any behaviour, responses to different stimuli and ability to perform activities that you observe will more closely mirror the 'normal situation'. Your first contact with the child and family may be in the home, unless specific equipment is necessary or there is a need to attend a specialist clinic. This is the most familiar situation in which the assessment can take place – but you must be aware of any distractions. There may also be other situations where assessment could take place, such as nursery or school.

It is not absolutely necessary to see previous medical records before the initial contact. This avoids preconceptions and may mean that observations are more objective. The key issue is to regard the child as a whole.

Developmental assessment

Depending on the situation and the age of the child, you may have to carry out some form of developmental check along with the more specific examination. Many schedules are available to guide these checks and can be found in a range of paediatric textbooks. Schedules of this type usually give the age of the child and a range of activities/abilities expected at that stage. The child attending for assessment can then be observed, compared and monitored against this body of knowledge considered to be 'the norm'. The available schedules give a guide for this, but you will benefit from possessing a good background knowledge of child development in order to be able to quickly and effectively identify any problems.

Subjective assessment

Discussion with parents or carers is essential in the subjective assessment. This should also continue throughout any intervention you suggest. It is important to find out how much the parents know and understand about the child's condition. During any discussion it should also be possible to obtain some indication of how well they are managing and whether they have any support from relatives, friends and other professionals. It is essential to build up as good a relationship as possible with the parents, particularly if they will be carrying out any part of the physiotherapy intervention. If they understand the underlying reasons for any techniques or exercises, they will be able to help in a more informed way. Overall compliance may also be improved.

In babies and younger children, any background information will have to be obtained from the parents or carers. It may also be useful to investigate family history and any past medical history of note. Some of the data may be obtained from medical notes but it is useful to check them with the child's parents/carers for accuracy. An older child or teenager may be able to provide you with all the information, or it may be a joint procedure.

Objective assessment

Depending on the age of the child, you will obtain objective data in various different ways. In an older child or teenager, the physical assessment may be very similar to that of an adult patient. In younger children, however, the objective assessment may involve a mixture of observation of free play, physical examination and the use of a series of specific tasks or activities, plus questioning of the parent or carer (APCP 1995).

Any test techniques used must be modified especially when assessing children younger than 6 years old. For infants and toddlers much information has to be obtained by observation and palpation while they are involved in age-appropriate developmental/functional activities. When looking at neonates and infants, their state of alertness is important because, if they are sleepy, it is not possible to elicit optimal performance. Most activity, particularly in the muscles, is observed when the child is alert, hungry and/or crying. Because of these differences in behaviour it may be necessary to repeat observations at various times of the day. The child's level of alertness should be recorded. It may be possible to look at the more passive elements early in the assessment, followed by observation of spontaneous movements before any handling occurs. Then tactile and/or auditory stimuli can be used to arouse more active responses. Some resistance can be given to normal activities such as crawling to give an idea of muscle strength. For accurate assessment, it is very important that a physiotherapist can distinguish between active and reflex movements (Hinderer & Hinderer 1993).

For older children, between the ages of 2 and 5 years, more functional tests can be carried out. This is suggested as they probably will not co-operate with the usual assessment procedures.

Children of school age and older are usually more able to participate in standard testing procedures. It is important that you explain each test carefully and, if possible, that the child understands what each one is for. This helps to ensure that effort is maximal; although it is essential to remember how easily young children can be distracted. It may be necessary to demonstrate certain movements or positions. Any commands given should be short, clear and, above all, consistent, to avoid confusion. As with any assessment, issues such as comfort, posture and correct positioning need to be addressed. If any equipment is used, further simple explanation is necessary to reassure the child and to allay any fear or anxiety that could affect performance (Hinderer & Hinderer 1993).

Gait

In children with rheumatic problems, it is important to be particularly aware of their method of locomotion. Children become increasingly skilled in locomotion as they develop, and move through a recognized progression from rolling through crawling to walking (although some children have interim stages such as bottom shuffling or 'walking like a bear' on hands and feet).

If a child has a rheumatic condition then some of the prerequisites for normal gait may be affected. Reduced general mobility may mean a reduction in muscle strength and general debilitation, which would have a major effect on locomotion.

You need to be familiar with the normal gait cycle in children and any differences there may be due to each stage of development. It will probably be necessary to look at the child's walking on a number of occasions, and for fairly long periods, to obtain a full picture of any problems. The most useful observations usually occur when the child is unaware that an assessment is taking place. As well as looking at the quality of the gait, you should make a note of the distance the child is able to walk and whether s/he complains of any pain or discomfort. If the child has a walking aid, you should assess gait both with and without it if possible. A useful strategy may be to use video to record walking and other activities, to allow repeat viewing, so reducing stress on the child and parents. Other tests could be carried out if you have access to a gait laboratory, but this will depend upon facilities and the compliance of the child.

General assessment point

The Association of Paediatric Chartered Physiotherapists recommends that the following points are recorded in writing as evidence of a full assessment:

- Child's history and relevant developmental milestones
- History of presenting problem
- Family history
- Child's abilities and inabilities, physical and functional, appropriate to age
- Child's own perception of any difficulties
- Parental anxieties
- Family interaction
- Social conditions (APCP 1995).

Physiotherapy intervention

Once you have completed your assessment, the next step is to identify areas suitable for intervention and to plan an appropriate treatment programme, bearing in mind the needs and expectations of the family and the child. They need to be kept informed at all times regarding the proposed intervention and encouraged to be involved and to make active choices. The treatment should be offered rather than imposed. It is important to ensure that you modify any information in order that the child as well as the parents/carers can understand it. Depending on the age and ability of the child, possible ways of modification may be:

- by simple understandable explanation
- by demonstration
- through story telling using visual and/or verbal methods
- by the use of toys
- through games.

Self-assessment question

- SAQ 7.19 Review the main points that should be recorded as evidence of a full paediatric assessment.

Some family issues

Parents do encounter a wide range of problems in obtaining a child's co-operation with home physiotherapy programmes. Management of children with special needs of any sort, either temporary or in the long term, can be complex and so support from the healthcare team is vital. Caring for a chronically ill or disabled child can place considerable demands upon particular family members and/or on the family as a unit, and the therapy itself can disrupt family life. There is a fine balance to be struck between the demands on the parents of any therapy programme and the demands of siblings, partners, work, social commitments and so on. It is also important to remember that no two family situations are exactly alike and so there is no convenient blueprint of management. This is where problem-solving and clinical-decision making skills are so important for the physiotherapist.

You must carefully assess the ability and willingness of parents to take on the responsibility for home supervision of any therapy. It is vital that they believe that the advice you give to them regarding their child's care will be of benefit, otherwise compliance will be low. You should negotiate realistic and developmentally appropriate goals and a management programme with the child, or the child and the family. These should be based on the child's lifestyle and should be relevant and achievable but flexible enough to be modified on monitoring and review. It is important to be aware of family circumstances when organizing visits and treatment sessions; for example, appointment times should be flexible and arranged to suit parents/carers wherever possible, and alternative venues could be considered where access is difficult (APCP 1995).

You may have a role in helping the parents to develop any skills that may be necessary, e.g. hands-on techniques or the use of certain equipment, and you need to monitor and evaluate these throughout the management period. Here you are acting as an educator and so must be able to modify your communication in order to ensure that any instructions are easily understood.

With regard to interaction with the child during any contact, the APCP (1995) highlights the importance of encouraging confidence and self-worth by using the following strategies:

- Highlight the child's assets rather than difficulties
- Handle the child's behaviour consistently
- Reward the child for effort made rather than final result (this alludes to the fact that children are not encouraged by excessive praise of something they have not done well)
- Show appreciation of achievements, however small

- Make every effort to boost the child's confidence
- Allow the child responsibility during the therapy sessions.

Self-assessment question

- **SAQ 7.20** In what ways can you modify information about proposed management to make it understandable for the child?

Areas of conflict and management strategies

In many cases there will be some conflict between parents and child, or sometimes between the parents themselves. In a long-term condition such as JIA, for example, the child must usually perform daily exercises and wear splints. It is not always easy to convince the child that these things are necessary, particularly if some parts of the process are painful or difficult. Children often do not understand the reason behind exercises and this means they will be reluctant to perform them (Puddefoot et al 1997). This can cause distress if the parent has to battle with the child each time treatment time arrives, and resentment of the 'therapist' role can build up if it causes alienation between them. Distress can also be increased if parents are very anxious to follow a professional's instructions and resort to threat or punishment in order to gain the child's co-operation.

There might be an issue if partners do not support each other in relation to the child's therapy. Occasionally one parent might insist on taking the whole responsibility for the child's treatment programme, which could cause problems, with the other partner feeling isolated. Conversely, one parent might consciously or unconsciously opt out of the therapy sessions, which would shift the responsibility on to the other. This could again result in alienation between child and the 'therapist' parent, as well as giving mixed messages to the child about the importance of the treatment. Either of these scenarios would cause dissonance between the parents and add extra stress to what may be an already difficult situation. The child could well sense this and become more anxious.

The issues may be different for older children who are able to understand the importance and relevance of their therapy. Just because they are able to appreciate these points, it may still be difficult to motivate them to do their exercises, as extra pressures come to bear, such as homework and social life. There are other factors involved as these children move into adolescence. They are finding their own identities and becoming more independent, while at the same time trying to come to terms with the implications of having a chronic orthopaedic condition. This can lead to feelings of anxiety, guilt, anger or depression as well as to a realization of being different from their peers.

In the young child, external enforcers may be useful as incentives to encourage co-operation with the treatment programme. These could include star charts, prizes or certificates of bravery as appropriate (Hartley 1993). This should be done in conjunction with explanations suitable to the child's level of understanding and support for the parents.

Adolescents tend to become less compliant if parents try to use reasoning, threats or persuasion to gain co-operation with the therapy programme. As restrictions on social activity increase, so compliance decreases. Compliant adolescents have a greater sense of autonomy and self-esteem than those who are non compliant (Litt et al 1982).

You should provide support for the parents in these situations whenever it is possible or appropriate.

RHEUMATIC CONDITIONS IN CHILDHOOD

Musculoskeletal pain and other problems are common in childhood, occurring in 4–30% of children and encompassing a wide range of conditions and injuries (Gardner-Medwin 2001).

One child in 1000 will have some form of arthritis during childhood years. These are chronic conditions with variable aetiologies, most of which are uncertain or unknown. Generally the child will complain of pain and there is swelling in the joints with reduction in range of motion. There may also be systemic features such as a rash, a raised temperature and/or fatigue.

The outcome of these rheumatic conditions depends very much on how the children are managed by the healthcare team. As with the majority of rheumatic conditions, drug therapy is a key element of intervention. The physiotherapist has an important role in working with children and their carers, particularly in providing education and advice about strategies to enable successful management of ADL within the limits of the disease. There are usually some periods of active physiotherapy treatment, which may involve hydrotherapy and land-based exercises and/or splinting, but much of the management will be carried out by the parents.

Juvenile idiopathic arthritis

Juvenile idiopathic arthritis is the most common of the autoimmune musculoskeletal conditions in children (Manners 2002). JIA is the relatively new term unifying the existing classifications for inflammatory arthritis in children. This diagnosis is only made after exclusion of other specific causes of arthritis. A number of other conditions can mimic JIA and present problems in initial diagnosis:

- acute lymphoblastic leukaemia
- non accidental injury
- some systemic diseases especially inflammatory bowel disease
- Kawasaki's disease (in the younger child)
- rheumatic fever
- septic arthritis (Gardner-Medwin 2001).

The aetiology of JIA is unknown. There is believed to be some genetic predisposition linked to HLA and there may be a trigger factor related to onset (Gardner-Medwin 2001, Manners 2002). The incidence of the condition is 5–18 per 100 000 children and the prevalence varies from 30 to 150 cases per 100 000, which is similar to childhood diabetes (Gardner-Medwin 2001). The pathogenic mechanisms are becoming better understood, with links to the role of cytokines, which are inflammatory substances found in the synovial fluid. As with RA, there is some evidence that activated T cells are important elements in pathogenesis of the condition (Manners 2002). The classification of JIA is illustrated in Table 7.3.

Oligoarticular JIA is the most common type of arthritis, accounting for approximately 50% of cases. Up to four joints, mainly in the lower limbs, can be affected. For most children no further joints become involved and prognosis is generally good.

Table 7.3   The new classification of juvenile idiopathic arthritis with clinical criteria and the adult equivalents

Characteristic	Juvenile idiopathic arthritis	Clinical features as defined by ILAR classification	Adult equivalent
Age at onset	<16 years		
Minimum duration of arthritis	6 weeks		
Subtypes	Systemic arthritis	Arthritis with/preceded by daily fever for at least 2 weeks and one/more of: evanescent, non-fixed erythematous rash, generalized lymphadenopathy, hepato/splenomegaly and serositis	Adult Still's disease
	Oligoarthritis	Arthritis of 1–4 joints during the first 6 months	
	– Persistent	Affects no more than 4 joints throughout the disease course	
	– Extended	Affects more than 4 joints after the first 6 months	
	Polyarthritis (RF-negative)	Affects 5 or more joints in first 6 months of disease	
	Polyarthritis (RF-positive)	Affects 5 or more joints in first 6 months of disease. Tests for rheumatoid factor are positive on two occasions at least 2 months apart	Rheumatoid arthritis
	Enthesitis-related arthritis	Arthritis and enthesitis, or arthritis or enthesitis with at least two of: sacroiliac tenderness and/or inflammatory spinal pain; HLA-B27-positive, family history in a first- or second-degree relative of medically confirmed HLA-B27-associated disease	Ankylosing spondylitis
	Psoriatic arthritis	Arthritis and psoriasis, or arthritis and at least two of: dactylitis, nail abnormalities, family history of psoriasis in at least one first-degree relative	Psoriatic arthritis
	Other	Arthritis of unknown cause persisting for at least 6 weeks that either does not fulfil criteria for any categories or fulfils criteria for more than one category	

Adapted from Gardner-Medwin 2001.
ILAR = International League of Associations for Rheumatology.

This form of JIA may be associated with inflammation of the eyes known as uveitis: 10–30% of children diagnosed with JIA may experience chronic anterior uveitis. This can result in loss of vision, most commonly in the youngest children, but prognosis is good if it is identified and treated early. All children with JIA should be examined by an ophthalmologist with follow up every 3–6 months. This should be continued until the child is old enough to recognize painless change in vision or until there has been 7 years of follow up with no eye disease (Gardner-Medwin 2001, Institute of Child Health 2002).

Polyarticular JIA accounts for approximately 20% of cases and affects more than five joints. Any joint can be involved (Institute of Child Health 2002). In these children it is most important to exclude reactive arthritis, rheumatic fever and other systemic or inflammatory disease (Gardner-Medwin 2001).

Systemic JIA accounts for 10% of cases and often affects most of the joints. Initial symptoms include a high temperature, which presents as a daily spiking fever, and a rash that is salmon-pink in colour and may only appear fleetingly at the height of the fever. This is characteristically in the evening and appears on the trunk, upper inner thighs and axillae. Children with this form of JIA are generally unwell and severely lacking in energy (Gardner-Medwin 2001, Institute of Child Health 2002). As well as the fever and rash, those children with systemic onset may also present with lymphadenopathy, hepatomegaly, splenomegaly, pericarditis and other general symptoms of inflammation, with little or no joint manifestation. In order for a definite diagnosis to be made, however, they do have to exhibit the required signs of arthritis eventually. The systemic features are often in evidence for some time before joints are affected.

While 50% of the children with systemic onset recover almost completely, the rest go on to develop polyarticular symptoms, with resulting disability. These are the individuals in most danger of life-threatening complications and general growth problems.

Growth and nutrition

Arthritis has a major impact on the growing skeleton. Persistent inflammation markedly reduces growth and bone mass and this can be exacerbated by immobility and the use of steroids as part of drug management. Growth hormone has been used in an attempt to prevent some of these changes but with limited success. Up to 50% of children with JIA may have protein energy malnutrition related to increased expenditure of energy (Gardner-Medwin 2001). The promotion of a balanced diet is, therefore, essential and referral to a dietitian may be helpful.

Prognosis

The majority of children go into permanent remission and have no serious disability. About 70% are probably in remission 10 years after onset. Mild disability persists in approximately 45% of those assessed after the age of eighteen. The overall prognosis, therefore, is considered to be good. Between 10% and 30%, however, do have severe residual problems, the worst functional outcome being in those with major involvement of the hip.

Recently, there have been developments in the understanding of the pathogenesis of JIA, with parallel developments in improved treatment options. This means that there has been an increase in the number of children recovering from JIA and entering adulthood as independent individuals. Nevertheless, a percentage of adults with JIA do have significant levels of disability, which is related to active disease over prolonged periods. This emphasizes the importance of ensuring good

transition from paediatric to high-quality adult rheumatology care (Manners 2002, Packham & Hall 2002).

Case study 7.4: Rosie

Rosie is 2 years old. Her mum and dad became concerned when she was reluctant to use her hands and to join in games when she was at play group. She also started to limp and was not keen to walk, when previously she had always been energetic and enjoyed running around. In the previous few weeks they noticed a rash appearing in the late afternoon on her back, tummy, thighs and under her arms, which then faded. This seemed to be linked to a spiking fever, which then returned to normal. At these times she seemed rather poorly and did complain of tummy ache. For the rest of the day, and during the night these symptoms were absent.

Sometimes she was uncharacteristically badly behaved or withdrawn, unusually tired later in the day, and her movements appeared to be stiff when she first got up in the morning.

On examination by her GP, Rosie was found to have some swelling in the metacarpophalangeal joints of both hands, both wrists and both knees. Although there was no apparent tenderness, her range of movement was decreased.

A tentative diagnosis of systemic-onset JIA was made. This was confirmed at a visit to the rheumatology clinic. The decision was made to admit Rosie to the rheumatology ward for a short period for thorough assessment and to begin drug treatment. She was started on intravenous steroids to tackle the systemic symptoms.

Problem–solving exercise 7.13

a. Which members of the healthcare team would be involved in Rosie's management?
b. You are Rosie's physiotherapist and are going to see her for the first time. After obtaining subjective information from the notes and from

talking to her parents, what areas would you include in your objective assessment?

c. What useful information do you think any professional member of the healthcare team should be able to ascertain from observing Rosie with her parents?

After you have considered these questions, read the following section for the approach to the second and third questions.

Objective assessment of Rosie

The points made earlier in the chapter, in the section on assessment of children, should be carefully considered here, particularly as Rosie is so young.

Observation

You should make sure that Rosie is undressed sufficiently to allow you to clearly observe the affected and unaffected areas. Swelling may be quite obvious in the hands, wrists and knees. You should also look at her movements and general activities, as they may give you more information than specific tests about limitations due to pain and stiffness.

Palpation

You may use gentle palpation to test for any tenderness around the joints. Pain is rarely complained of but this may be due to the natural tendency of young children to complain less of pain than adults. They also seem to find it difficult to localize pain to a specific area. Some of Rosie's joints may feel warmer than normal.

Movements

You may be able to perform passive range of movement if Rosie is willing, but active movements may need to be observed when she is playing or moving around. It may be very difficult to use a goniometer to measure range of movement unless Rosie is particularly tractable. With knee involvement, it is important for you to consider

leg length, as there may be flexion deformities. Her hands may show reduction in flexion and radial deviation at the metacarpophalangeal joints. You might also find some ulnar deviation at the wrists. As Rosie is only a short time from onset, there may not have been time for these deformities to occur. It would still be important for you to note the range and position of these joints to give you a baseline against which to monitor progress.

Muscle testing

It will probably be impossible for you to do specific muscle tests with a child as young as Rosie. So again, functional activities can be used to estimate these. It is an important area to look at as muscle atrophy occurs quickly in children with JIA.

Functional activities

These may involve going up and down stairs, getting up from the floor and walking on tip toe, as well as dressing and play activities.

Observation of Rosie with her parents

Observation is an important skill for any health professional. It is important to watch Rosie and her parents as they come into the room or treatment area. From facial expression and movement, it may be possible to get an idea of how Rosie is feeling. Is she being allowed to walk in or is one of her parents carrying her? Do they allow her to take her own clothes off or insist on doing it for her? (Given her age she may need some help with the latter activity anyway.)

If Rosie's parents are being extremely protective, it may make it more difficult for you to carry out an assessment. This may change, however, when you have had the opportunity to explain what the assessment is all about. Watching Rosie with her parents may also give you some idea as to how they might manage the home programme.

If both parents are present, you may get some feeling about who is going to take on the responsibility for Rosie's treatment. Will it be an equal partnership or is one parent much more dominant?

These and other, similar issues are extremely important for the physiotherapist to consider. They may enable you to modify your approach in order to facilitate a successful implementation of the treatment programme.

Management

As with the adult types of rheumatic disease investigated earlier, JIA requires a team approach to management. The primary aim is to preserve joint function and vision by controlling the inflammatory process. As the child develops, however, management must address ongoing needs related to ADL, school, physical and mental growth and the transitional needs of adolescents. This can be supported by a central programme of management for the child, parents, school and involved professionals.

The team must be experienced in the field. Ideally a rheumatologist and a paediatrician (and/or a paediatric rheumatologist) should be involved plus a physiotherapist, OT, nurse specialist, ophthalmologist, social worker, growth clinic, orthotist, orthopaedic surgeon and GP as necessary/appropriate. It is also essential to remember that the child and the parents must be part of this team approach and should be consulted and included in discussions when decisions are being made.

Drug therapy

The majority of children with JIA benefit from the use of NSAIDs, which provide basic symptomatic relief (Manners 2002). They are perhaps more commonly used in those children with oligoarthritis (Gardner-Medwin 2001). It is now more common for non-aspirin NSAIDs to be used as they are easier to administer and some are approved specifically for use with children. Unfortunately they can take a long time to have their maximal effect – 2 weeks

to 3 months. They are well tolerated, but all the usual side effects have been observed.

The use of DMARDs is rather more contentious, although these drugs do appear to be more commonly used now. The first-choice agent is methotrexate and it is the most widely employed in the management of polyarticular disease. Evidence suggests that it is the most effective and well tolerated, leading to its earlier use in increasing numbers of children. Sulfasalazine is used in some children, usually in enthesitis-related arthritis. It is difficult for smaller children to take, however, as it does not come in liquid form. For those children who do not respond to single DMARDs, combination therapy has been tried to some effect. If these drugs are prescribed they need to be carefully monitored by the rheumatology clinic (as described earlier in the chapter) (Gardner-Medwin 2001, Manners 2002).

Corticosteroids may be used as intra-articular injections in the case of persistent active arthritis, particularly in individuals with polyarticular onset. These may be administered to multiple joints and so are usually performed under a light general anaesthetic (Gardner-Medwin 2001). Following the injections the joints may need to be rested in a splint for 24–48 hours.

Systemic steroids are used particularly in the case of systemic onset JIA. They do, however, have marked side effects, such as osteoporosis, water retention and growth retardation. If their use is deemed to be unavoidable, then the dose should be tapered down at the earliest opportunity.

There are a number of biological agents available for the treatment of inflammatory rheumatic conditions. These are sometimes used in severe JIA where conventional remittive agents have failed. They work against inflammatory substances such as TNFα. These agents, such as Etanercept, Infliximab and Anakinra, are presently undergoing trials in both children and adults (Manners 2002).

Physiotherapy

The most central aims of physiotherapy are to protect the joints, prevent deformity and maximize function (these should be the aims of the whole healthcare team once the inflammation is reduced by the drug therapy). The overall philosophy should be to encourage the child's parents to assume and maintain responsibility for the physiotherapy programme as soon as possible. Care can then be transferred home, with monitoring and updates of advice occurring at regular clinic visits (Hartley 1993).

The overall programme of physiotherapy involves the provision of information about JIA and advice on its management to the parents and/or carers of the child. Specific exercises need to be taught for the affected joints and a daily general exercise regimen involving active exercises and stretching should be provided that addresses the rest of the body. These need to be introduced as early as possible and have a number of uses:

- maintenance/improvement of mobility
- maintenance/improvement of exercise tolerance
- maintenance/improvement of muscle strength
- monitoring of joint range, allowing early detection of any problems with other joints, or regression in those joints already affected.

A certain amount of activity regulation may be necessary in older children. Younger children often regulate their own activity depending on the state of their disease. Teenagers, however, may perceive that they need to 'keep up' with their peers and be tempted to do too much, thus exacerbating their symptoms. Some external structure may relieve this situation, helping the child to avoid getting overtired and putting too much stress on the joints. Increased levels of rest may be necessary at times but bedrest is not appropriate. Certain positions and activities may be discouraged in the interest of joint protection:

- high-impact activities such as jumping/road running
- use of pillows holding the neck in flexion
- supporting total body weight on non-weight-bearing joints, for example press ups, cartwheels, chin-ups and so on
- activities/positions that put stress across the joints, such as skiing or sitting cross legged.

Hydrotherapy is an ideal form of therapy for children with JIA as long as they are happy and confident in water. This can lead on to swimming, which is a good all-round exercise and is suitable as it does not involve weight bearing and avoids overstressing the joints.

In many cases part of the management of JIA involves wearing splints. These are provided in order to support and maintain joints in a good position. The most commonly used are either resting splints, usually worn at night, or functional splints, which support a joint during activity.

Self assessment question

- **SAQ 7.22** Rosie's physiotherapy management will be supervised at home by mum and dad, and this may involve exercises, splinting and the application of temporary pain-relieving modalities (heat or cold) as necessary. Thinking back over the information given in the chapter, review the areas you might need to discuss with her parents in order to facilitate this process (remember – she is only 2 years old). (A suggested approach to this is outlined below. As usual, you should attempt to consider the issues yourself before going on to read this.)

You will need to discuss many issues with parents who are about to take on responsibility for the home programme of their child with JIA. The content and direction of the discussion will vary greatly, depending upon the situation, the resources available, the existing support networks and the personalities involved.

It is vital for the parents to have adequate information. You must ensure that they understand the purpose of any exercises, activities, hands-on techniques and/or splinting that you recommend. They must recognize the importance of and be prepared to carry out the treatment daily, on a regular basis.

The main aims of physiotherapy intervention (particularly during active disease phases) are to protect the joints, avoid muscle weakness and loss in range of movement, so preventing deformity.

The programme that you design must cause the minimum possible disruption to Rosie's family life/routine. This is where discussion with the parents is essential. It is also important to be aware of any home programmes designed by other members of the healthcare team so that you can avoid unnecessary duplication. A more preferable team approach would be to formulate a combined programme rather than doing this in isolation.

It is well known that compliance with therapeutic home programmes is fairly poor for a number of very valid reasons. If you and your colleagues try to incorporate the following characteristics into the design of the programme, it may help to improve compliance levels. The programme should be:

- as simple as possible
- the most efficient in time and effort
- the least painful
- the least expensive
- designed to achieve individual goals that are relevant, achievable, realistic and developmentally/age appropriate
- regularly monitored and modified as necessary in discussion with parents and child.

Compliance may also be enhanced if you can show Rosie's parents a simple method of checking her range of motion at home.

You could suggest that Rosie's parents try to make the exercise programme part of her daily routine. It is extremely important to explain that a number of the exercises (particularly the stretches) will cause some discomfort. This does not mean, however, that they are damaging her joints or muscles. It is quite likely that a child as young as Rosie may cry during some of the exercises. Her parents should be reassured that this is not a contraindication to treatment. This situation can be very difficult for them to accept as they may already feel guilt associated with Rosie having a chronic illness. Reassurance is, therefore, of paramount importance.

Rosie should be involved in the treatment as much as possible. Strategies such as counting up to 10 for the stretches may help her to feel more in control. As mentioned in the earlier text, sometimes external enforcers are useful, such as star charts and certificates of bravery.

This section has given you some suggestions with regard to discussion with parents prior to starting a therapeutic home programme. As you gain more experience and discuss options with other physiotherapists who are experts in the field, you will gradually develop a larger background database to use in these situations.

Surgery

This is generally only used in very severe cases of JIA but would be considered if joint deformity has occurred despite drug and physical therapy. Procedures that may be undertaken include soft tissue release (most commonly of hip or knee), or joint replacement. The reason to perform surgery is focused more on regaining function than on pain relief.

THE IMPACT OF CHRONIC PROGRESSIVE DISEASE

When you are involved in the management of patients with chronic progressive diseases, it is imperative that you take the psychological and social implications into account alongside the purely physical effects. When a patient presents with an illness, both the health professional and the patient have to 'make sense' of the disease. The meanings that the disease has for each will, however, be very different. For the health professional the diagnosis, symptoms and treatment are often the initial considerations, but for the patient the main focus is more likely to be on the impact it has on his/her life. Awareness of this difference in approach is important when devising a treatment plan and when deciding what may need to be covered in a patient education programme. Overall it should help to improve communication between the patient and members of the healthcare team as well as improving compliance with treatment.

Responses to treatment depend on the patient. Different people have different personal strategies, motivation levels and values regarding aspects of life that they consider to be important. There can also be variation in one patient at different times if we take into account the phasic nature of many of the rheumatic disorders. Patients need to try to be flexible, therefore, if they are to manage variation in pain, functional ability and possibly progressive deformity.

Major problems can occur if patients perceive that the disease is controlling their lives instead of them controlling it. Stress and anxiety levels increase and it is difficult to know whether this is a cause or an effect of the condition. Patients make attributions for their overall disease and may even make separate attributions for exacerbations and remissions. It has been found that the presence of psychological stress is most often cited as the reason for an exacerbation in RA patients. The second most popular reason for an increase in symptoms was given as excessive physical activity. Patients who gave this as a reason, however, reported that they felt less helpless when they were more active. This may be because activity levels can be altered easily by the patients so enabling them to believe that they have some control over the disease (Selly 1990).

Points to consider

Self-concept

This relates to the way that we perceive ourselves and our relationship to or with the environment. Patients with a chronic progressive disease often revise their own self-concept and it is axiomatic that this will have an effect on the personal strategies they employ in managing their condition and their response to treatment. Interestingly, however, it has been shown that people will only seek as much help as is compatible with maintaining their self-concept (Skevington 1990).

Self-image

This involves several facets. First, there is the physical image, which may be positive or negative. The media are constantly reinforcing so-called 'acceptable' images and many people feel that they should conform to these. This will of course be affected when a person has a chronic progressive disease, particularly if there is reduction in functional ability and/or any deformity. Second, there is the public image of people with arthritis, particularly related to altered appearance. These two areas of self-image may cause isolation or withdrawal. Closely connected to this is the third facet of self-image, which concerns sexual identity. A person with arthritis may feel that it is more difficult or impossible to form relationships, or the consequences of the disease could affect established relationships.

Disease process

The possibility of eventual deformities is very important to patients. These may be difficult to conceal if they affect the gait or particularly the hands, which are used for expression and non-verbal communication. Perceptions also differ, with one patient's 'mild' deformity being perceived as 'severe' by another patient who has the same degree of change. This relates to the patient's coping strategies (Newman 1990).

As a result of the disease process, individuals with rheumatic conditions may have to rely on carers to select clothes, put on their make up and do their hair. This can become an issue if the carer has different ideas about appearance and image.

Treatments involved in the management of rheumatic conditions can affect appearance, e.g. water retention due to steroids. There could be scarring from surgery and some patients may need to wear obtrusive splints or orthoses if they are to carry out their ADL effectively.

Perceptions

People with chronic progressive disease also have to deal with common public perceptions. Some people perceive that a person with arthritis will be 'old, gnarled and twisted' and may be surprised when they meet a person with a rheumatic condition who is none of these. Others have more realistic expectations and will not expect any change in appearance or will avoid prejudging the situation. Some individuals will perceive that people with rheumatic conditions are disabled and some will not.

Role changes

Chronic progressive disease does force very far-reaching role changes, both within society and with other people.

Employment

People with arthritis may have to get up extremely early to allow their morning stiffness to wear off before going to work. In conditions where fatigue is an issue, this will only compound the problem. Generally the person has decreased energy and needs more time to do things. Because of these problems, therefore, the evenings and weekends are often used for rest, which means that individuals have fewer opportunities for leisure and social activities.

A variable condition (i.e. one with exacerbations and remissions) will mean variable performance, possibly with time away from work and, depending on the situation, fear of dismissal. If the person is already unemployed it is more difficult to get a job and career opportunities are reduced. With less work or the loss of a job, finances will be decreased, and there will be less purpose and structure to the person's life and decreased independence. If the patient is a housewife there may be problems managing the home.

Family

If an individual develops a rheumatic condition it can affect the whole family. Employment issues may impinge here especially if the patient is the main breadwinner.

Partners may begin to feel isolated if they have to sleep in separate rooms or beds because of pain and/or sleeplessness. The person with the disease may have less energy and be unable or unwilling to go out very much. There could also be decreased physical contact either because it is painful or because the partner is afraid of causing pain.

Individual and family plans will be affected. Partners and other family members may have feelings of guilt or other emotions that they find difficult to understand. This can increase stress levels and reduce effective communication, so causing a cycle that is very hard to break without some external help, such as relationship counselling. Increase in stress is a key issue for those with rheumatic disease as it may cause exacerbation of symptoms.

Community

As a result of the disease process and consequent possible changes in employment and family situations, the individual may perceive a change in his/her role in the wider community setting. This could reduce opportunities for taking part in social and leisure activities.

There are also issues around the different concepts of 'disability' in varying cultural settings.

Stages of life

The disease process will have different effects depending on when in the person's life it starts. Think back to the case studies earlier in the chapter and consider the differences due to age at onset.

Review point

When you come into contact with patients with rheumatic conditions remember to consider the ways in which these issues could affect your approach and their responses.

SUMMARY

This chapter provides an overview of the issues involved in the management of rheumatic conditions, including background information on a number of common conditions, assessment, identification of problems and treatment planning. It has also addressed pharmacological management, the roles of the healthcare team and the implications of chronic progressive disease for the physiotherapist and the patient.

As stated at the beginning of the chapter, the physiotherapy interventions used with patients with rheumatic conditions are often quite routine – but it is the decision-making process of when and where to use them that is the most important. It is not possible to cover every eventuality; it is hoped, however, that you now would feel more confident in your ability to deal with patients with any rheumatic condition. One of the most important points to remember is that there is no cure for these diseases and the patients are not going to 'get better'. Your role is to help them to develop personal strategies in order to function more effectively within the limits of the condition. In order to carry out this role you will use a wide range of knowledge and techniques, in partnership with other members of the healthcare team.

On reading this summary, do you feel that you have grasped the above points? If not, perhaps you should go back and re-read any appropriate parts of the chapter before moving on.

ANSWER TO QUESTIONS AND EXERCISES

Self-assessment question 7.1

See information in text.

Self-assessment question 7.2 (page 164)

- **SAQ 7.2** An NSAID will suppress the classical features of inflammation – what are these features?

  Answer: The classical features of inflammation are: redness, heat, swelling, pain and loss of function.

Self-assessment questions 7.3–7.5

See information in text.

Problem-solving exercise 7.1 (page 172)

- With the information that has been provided so far try to work out the clinical features you might expect to find when assessing a patient with OA.

  Answer:
  - Joint pain
  - Stiffness
  - Enlargement of joint size
  - Limitation of movement
  - Loss of function.

Problem-solving exercises 7.2–7.6

Refer to text.

Self-assessment questions 7.6 and 7.7

See information in text.

Self-assessment question 7.8 (page 186)

- **SAQ 7.8** What are the aims of physiotherapy management for patients with rheumatic conditions?
  See information in text.

  Why is it important for these aims to be matched to the patient's requirements and beliefs?

  Answer: If patients do not perceive that the aims of physiotherapy treatment are relevant to their particular situation and environment then they may be less willing to participate and less compliant. This is

particularly important when we are expecting patients to take on responsibility for their own management. Your success in dealing with patients will depend to a certain extent on how effectively you identify their problems (this is related to assessment and your modification of it as necessary) and then how appropriately you intervene.

Self-assessment questions 7.9 and 7.10

See information in text.

Problem-solving exercise 7.7 (page 197)

See following section in text.

Problem-solving exercise 7.8 (page 197)

- Review your answers to the previous exercise and now briefly relate them to this case study. Do you think that all of the symptoms and clinical signs you listed would be relevant to this lady?

  Answer: Compare with your response to Problem-solving exercise 7.7.
- Make a list of headings that you would use when assessing this patient and think about why physiotherapists need to investigate these areas.
  See information in text.

Self-assessment questions 7.11 and 7.12

See information in text.

Problem-solving exercise 7.9

See following section in text.

Problem-solving exercise 7.10

See information in text.

Self-assessment question 7.13

See information in text.

Self-assessment question 7.14 (page 209)

- **SAQ 7.14** Using your knowledge of anatomy, work out which muscle groups may become shortened and tight because of the changes in posture that occur in ankylosing spondylitis.

  Answer: Because of the typical overall flexed position of the patient with AS, it is the flexor groups of muscles which become shortened and tight because of changes in posture (and possibly because of physiological changes in the muscle itself). This means that physiotherapy intervention often involves a large element of stretching as well as strengthening of the antagonists. The patient needs to be given advice and to be reminded about positioning and posture.

Although the flexor groups are the obvious muscles to stretch, the exercise regimen always includes more general stretching (often of adductor and rotator groups) to combat reduced range of movement.

Problem-solving exercises 7.11 and 7.12

See information in text.

Self-assessment questions 7.15–7.20

See information in text.

Problem-solving exercise 7.13

For (a), see information in text; for (b) and (c), see following section of text.

Self-assessment question 7.21

See information in text.

Self-assessment question 7.22

See following section of text.

References

Adler S 1985 Self care in the management of the degenerative knee joint. Physiotherapy 71: 58–60

APCP 1995 Association of Paediatric Chartered Physiotherapists Standards of Practice. Chartered Society of Physiotherapy, London

Arthritis Research Campaign 2002 Occupational therapy and arthritis: an information sheet. Available on line at: www. arc.org.uk/about_arth/infosheets (accessed January 2004)

Arthritis Research Campaign 2003a News and features: Benefits of exercise/healthy lifestyle. Available on line at: www.arc.org.uk/newsviews/hints/exercise.htm (accessed January 2004)

Arthritis Research Campaign 2003b Ankylosing spondylitis: an information booklet. Available on line at: www.arc.org.uk/about_arth/booklets (accessed January 2004)

Ayling J, Marks R 2000 Efficacy of paraffin wax baths for rheumatoid arthritic hands. Physiotherapy 86: 190–201

Barlow JH, Turner AP, Wright CC 1998 Long term outcomes of an arthritis self-management programme. British Journal of Rheumatology 37: 1315–1319

Barry MA, Purser J, Hazelman R et al 1994 Effect of energy conservation and joint protection education in rheumatoid arthritis. British Journal of Rheumatology 33: 1171–1174

Bellamy N 1991 Prognosis in rheumatoid arthritis. Journal of Rheumatology 18: 1277–1279

Bernhard GC 2001 Exercise recommendations for common rheumatic disorders. Available on line at: www.rheuma21st.com/archives/cutting_edge_Exercise_Recommendations.html. Accessed 26/9/03

Bhardwaj N, Paget SA 1992 Rheumatoid arthritis. In: Paget SA, Fields TR (eds) Rheumatic disorders. Butterworth Heinemann, Boston, MA, ch 3

Bland JH 1993 Mechanisms of adaptation in the jint. In: Crosbie J, McConnell J (eds) Key issues in musculoskeletal physiotherapy. Butterworth Heinemann, Oxford, ch 4

Brattstrom M 1987 Joint protection and rehabilitation in chronic rheumatic disorders. Wolfe Medical, London

Brophy S, Pavy S, Roussou T et al 2003 Ankylosing spondylitis research. Available on line at: www.asresearch.co.uk (accessed January 2004)

Brosseau L, Welch V, Wells G et al 2002 Low level laser therapy (classes I, II and III) for treating rheumatoid arthritis (Cochrane Review). In: The Cochrane Library, issue 4. Update Software, Oxford

Butler R 1990 Monitoring drug therapy in rheumatoid arthritis: efficacy. Reports on rheumatic diseases (series 2) 15. Arthritis and Rheumatism Council, London

Caldron PH 1995 Screening for rheumatic disease. In: Boissanault WG (ed) Examination in physical therapy practice – screening for medical disease, 2nd edn. Churchill Livingstone, New York, ch 11

Calin A 2000 Ankylosing spondylitis. Available on line at: www.24dr.com/reference/library/musculo/ankylosing_spondylitis/ankspond.htm (Accessed January 2004)

Calin A 2002 Defining outcome in ankylosing spondylitis. Where have we been, where are we and where do we go from here? Joint Bone Spine 69: 101–104

Cawston T, Rowan D 1998 Mechanisms of cartilage breakdown and repair. Reports on rheumatic diseases. Topical reviews 15. Arthritis Research Campaign, Chesterfield, Derbyshire

Chartered Society of Physiotherapy 1993 Standards of physiotherapy practice for the management of people with ankylosing spondylitis. CSP, London

Christian CL 1992 Introduction and differential diagnosis of rheumatic disorders. In: Paget SA, Fields TR (eds) Summaries in clinical practice: rheumatic disorders. Andover Medical Publishers, Boston, MA, ch 1, p 1–6

Cott CA, Finch E, Gasner D et al 1995 The movement continuum theory of physical therapy. Physiotherapy Canada 47: 87–95

Dandy DJ, Edwards DJ 2003 Essential orthopaedics and trauma, 4th edn. Churchill Livingstone, Edinburgh

Doherty M, Lanyon P, Hosie G 2001 Osteoarthritis of the knee and hip. In: Practice: practical advice on management of rheumatic disease 8. Arthritis Research Campaign, Chesterfield, Derbyshire

Donovan JL, Blake DR, Fleming WG 1989 The patient is not a blank sheet: lay beliefs and their relevance to patient education. British Journal of Rheumatology 28: 58–61

Dziedzic K 1998 Ankylosing spondylitis. In: David C, Lloyd J (eds) Rheumatological physiotherapy. Mosby, London, ch 10

Eberhardt K, Fex E 1998 Clinical course and remission rate in patients with early rheumatoid arthritis: relationship to outcome after 5 years. British Journal of Rheumatology 37: 1324–1329

Eckersley PM (ed) 1993 Elements of paediatric physiotherapy. Churchill Livingstone, Edinburgh

Edwards JCW 2002 Pathogenesis of rheumatoid arthritis. Topical reviews: an overview of current research and practice in rheumatic disease 8. Arthritis Research Campaign, Chesterfield, Derbyshire

Furst DE 1990 Rheumatoid arthritis – practical use of medications. Postgraduate Medicine 87: 79–92

Gardner-Medwin J (2001) Current developments in juvenile arthritis. Topical reviews: an overview of current research and practice in rheumatic disease 5. Arthritis Research Campaign, Chesterfield, Derbyshire

Glynn L 2003 Grass isn't greener. Disability Now (October): 7

Goats GC, Hunter JA, Flett E, Sterling A 1996 Low intensity laser and phototherapy for rheumatoid arthritis. Physiotherapy 82: 311–320

Golding DN 1991 Local corticosteroid injections. Reports on Rheumatic Diseases (Series 2) 19. Arthritis and Rheumatism Council, London

Guillemin F 2000 Functional disability and quality-of-life assessment in clinical practice. Rheumatology 39 (suppl 1): 17–23

Harris ED 1990 Rheumatoid arthritis: pathophysiology and implications for therapy. New England Journal of Medicine 322: 1277–1289

Hartley J 1993 A survey to identify problems with home exercises and splint wear in children with juvenile chronic arthritis. Unpublished project, University of East London, London

Harvey AR 2003 Preventing and managing chronic disability in the rheumatic diseases. In: Practice: practical advice on management of rheumatic disease 11. Arthritis Research Campaign, Chesterfield, Derbyshire

Hazes JMW, Silman AJ 1990 Review of UK data on the rheumatic diseases 2, rheumatoid arthritis. British Journal of Rheumatology 29: 310–312

Helliwell PS, Abbott CA, Chamberlain MA 1996 A randomised trial of three different physiotherapy regimes in ankylosing spondylitis. Physiotherapy 82: 85–90

Hinderer KA, Hinderer SR 1993 Muscle strength development and assessment in children and adolescents. In: Harms-Ringdahl K (ed) Muscle strength. Churchill Livingstone, Edinburgh, ch 7

Hutton CW 1995 Osteoarthritis – clinical features and management. Reports on rheumatic diseases (series 3) 5. Arthritis and Rheumatism Council for Research, Chesterfield, Derbyshire

Ike RW, Lampman RM, Castor CW 1989 Arthritis and aerobic exercise: a review. Physician and Sports Medicine 17: 128–137

Inman RD 1992 Reiter's syndrome and reactive arthritis. In: Paget SA, Fields TR (eds) Rheumatic disorders. Butterworth Heinemann, Boston, MA, ch 6

Institute of Child Health 2002 Juvenile idiopathic arthritis factsheet. Available on line at: www.ich.ucl.ac.uk/fact-sheets/diseases_conditions/juvenile_idiopathic_arthritis/ (Accessed January 2004)

Kalden JR, Smolen JS 2000 Editorial. Rheumatology 39(suppl 1): 1–2

Kaufmann LD, Sokoloff L 1992 Osteoarthritis. In: Paget SA, Fields TR (eds) Rheumatic disorders. Butterworth Heinemann, Boston, MA, ch 5

Kennedy G, Edmunds L, Calin A 1993 The natural history of ankylosing spondylitis. Does it burn out? Journal of Rheumatology 20: 688–692

Kill D 2002 Rheumatoid arthritis. Clinical Research Focus 13 (1)

Kirwan JR 1990 Patient education in rheumatoid arthritis. Current Opinion in Rheumatology 2: 336–339

Litt IF, Cuskey WR, Rosenberg BA 1982 Role of self esteem and autonomy in determining medication compliance among adolescents with juvenile chronic arthritis. Pediatrics 69: 15–17

Lloyd J 1998 Rheumatoid arthritis. In: David C, Lloyd J (eds) Rheumatological physiotherapy. Mosby, London, ch 8, p 65

Lone AR, Wafai ZA, Buth BA et al 2003 Analgesic efficacy of transcutaneous electrical nerve stimulation compared with diclofenac sodium in osteoarthritis of the knee. Physiotherapy 89: 478–485

McKenna F 2000 The relevance of Cox-2 specificity. In: Practice: practical advice on management of rheumatic disease 1. Arthritis Research Campaign, Chesterfield, Derbyshire

McLellan DL 1991 The UK experience of rehabilitation. In: The national concept of rehabilitation (Conference Proceedings). Disablement Service Authority and the Royal College of Physicians, London, p 13–29

Magliano M, Morris V 2002 Use of analgesics in rheumatology. Topical reviews: an overview of current research and practice in rheumatic disease 7. Arthritis Research Campaign, Chesterfield, Derbyshire

Mallorie PA, Whitelock HC, Garrett SL et al 1995 Defining spinal mobility in ankylosing spondylitis (AS): the Bath AS Metrology Index (BASMI). Proceedings of the 12th International Congress of the World Confederation for Physical Therapy. American Physical Therapy Association paper PL-RR-0886-T

Manners PJ 2002 State of the art: juvenile idiopathic arthritis. APLAR Journal of Rheumatology 5: 29–34

Minor MA, Hewett JE Webel RR et al 1989 Efficacy of physical conditioning exercise in patients with rheumatoid arthritis and osteoarthritis. Arthritis and Rheumatism 32: 1396–1405

Newman S 1990 Coping with rheumatoid arthritis. In: Selly S, Kirwan J (eds) Arthritis and the psyche. ARC Conference Proceedings 9. Arthritis and Rheumatism Council, London

Nuki G 2002 Osteoarthritis: risk factors and pathogenesis. Topical reviews: an overview of current research and practice in rheumatic disease. ARC, Chesterfield

Packham JC, Bowness P 2001 Seronegative spondyloarthropathies. Topical reviews: an overview of current research and practice in rheumatic disease 4. Arthritis Research Campaign, Chesterfield, Derbyshire

Packham JC, Hall MA 2002 Long-term follow up of 246 adults with juvenile idiopathic arthritis: functional outcome. Rheumatology 41: 1428–1435

Pipitone N, Choy EHS 2003 Treatment of rheumatoid arthritis. Topical reviews: an overview of current research and practice in rheumatic disease 10. Arthritis Research Campaign, Chesterfield, Derbyshire

Puddefoot T, Hillard H, Burl M 1997 Effect of verbal feedback on the physical performance of children. Physiotherapy 83: 76–81

Rai A, Struthers GR 1994 Ankylosing spondylitis. Reports on rheumatic diseases (series 3) 3. Arthritis and Rheumatism Council for Research, Chesterfield, Derbyshire

Ranawat CS, Maynard MJ, Flynn WF 1992 Total hip replacement arthroplasty in patients with inflammatory arthritis. In: Paget SA, Fields TR (eds) Rheumatic disorders. Butterworth Heinemann, Boston, MA, ch 14

Rasker JJ, Cosh JA 1989 Course and prognosis of early rheumatoid arthritis. Scandinavian Journal of Rheumatology 79(suppl): 45–56

Ray A, Cowie R 2002 What should be done for the patient with neck pain (X-rays show cervical spondylosis)? In: Practice: practical advice on management of rheumatic disease 7. Arthritis Research Campaign, Chesterfield, Derbyshire

Rheumatic Care Association of Chartered Physiotherapists 1994 Guidelines of good practice for the management of people with rheumatic diseases. Chartered Society of Physiotherapy, London

Robinson V, Brosseau L, Casimiro L et al 2002 Thermotherapy for treating rheumatoid arthritis (Cochrane Review). In: The Cochrane Library, issue 4. Update Software, Oxford

Scott DL 2000 Prognostic factors in early rheumatoid arthritis. Rheumatology 39(suppl 1): 24–29

Scott DL, Pugner K, Kaarela K et al 2000 The links between joint damage and disability in rheumatoid arthritis. Rheumatology 39: 122–132

Selly S 1990 Patients' views on the causes of arthritis. In: Selly S, Kirwan J (eds) Arthritis and the psyche. ARC Conference Proceedings 9. Arthritis and Rheumatism Council, London

SIGN 2000 Management of early rheumatoid arthritis. A national clinical guideline. Scottish Intercollegiate Guidelines Network. Royal College of Physicians, Edinburgh

Skevington S 1990 Psychological consequences of chronic pain. In: Selly S, Kirwan J (eds) Arthritis and the psyche. ARC Conference Proceedings 9. Arthritis and Rheumatism Council, London

Sterling LP 1990 Rheumatoid arthritis: current concepts and management, part 1. American Pharmacy 30: 47–52

Stewart J, Monoghan M 1998 The foot in rheumatology. In: David C, Lloyd J (eds) Rheumatological physiotherapy. Mosby, London, ch 18, p191

Swezey RL 1990a Rehabilitation in arthritis and allied conditions. In: Kottke FJ, Lehmann JF (eds) Krusken's handbook of physical medicine and rehabilitation, 4th edn. WB Saunders, Philadelphia, PA, p 679–716

Swezey RL 1990b Rheumatoid arthritis: the role of the kinder and gentler therapies. Journal of Rheumatology 17(suppl): 8–13

Turner-Stokes L 1993 Treatment and control of chronic arthritic and back pain. Reports on rheumatic diseases (series 2) 23. Arthritis and Rheumatism Council for Research, Chesterfield, Derbyshire

University of Southampton 2002 Disease management: pain. Available on line at: www.jointzone.org.uk/ (accessed 24/10/03)

Ven den Ende CHM, Vliet Vlieland TPM, Munneke M, Hazes JMW 2002 Dynamic exercise therapy for treating rheumatoid arthritis (Cochrane Review). In: The Cochrane Library, Issue 4. Oxford: Update Software

Viitanen JV, Suni J 1995 Management principles of physiotherapy in ankylosing spondylitis – which treatments are effective? Physiotherapy 81: 322–329

Wade M, Rimmer S 1998 Joint protection, advice and splinting. In: David C, Lloyd J (eds) Rheumatological physiotherapy. Mosby, London, ch 6, p 45

West K, Hall E 1998 Surgery for rheumatic problems. In: David C, Lloyd J (eds) Rheumatological physiotherapy. Mosby, London, ch 7, p 55

Weyand CM 2000 New insights into the pathogenesis of rheumatoid arthritis. Rheumatology 39(suppl 1): 3–8

White CE, Cooper RG 2002 Prescribing and monitoring of disease-modifying anti-rheumatic drugs (DMARDs) for inflammatory arthritis. In: Practice: practical advice on management of rheumatic disease 8. Arthritis Research Campaign, Chesterfield, Derbyshire

Wolfe F 1990 50 years of antirheumatic therapy: the prognosis of rheumatoid arthritis. Journal of Rheumatology 17(suppl): 24–32

Wollheim FA 1999 A changing world: how should we treat RA today and where are we moving? Available on line at: www.rheuma21st.com/archives/cutting_edge_ra.html (Accessed 26/9/03)

Yaron M 1995 Hormonal problems and rheumatic diseases. Reports on rheumatic diseases (series 3) 6. Arthritis and Rheumatism Council for Research, Chesterfield, Derbyshire

Chapter 8

Total joint replacements

Fiona Coutts

OBJECTIVES

By end of this chapter you should:

- Have an overview of the types of joint replacement for the lower limb and when they are used.
- Understand the assessment issues for a patient before and after joint replacement.
- Recognize how to problem solve for patient treatment and assessment, irrespective of the type of joint replacement in situ.
- Have a brief view of the problems with upper limb replacements.

KEY WORDS

Joint replacement, classification, management, complications, physiotherapy management.

Prerequisites

Re-read the chapters on assessment (Chapter 3) and fractures (Chapter 5); Dandy D, Edwards D 2003 Essential orthopaedics and trauma, 4th edn. Churchill Livingstone, Edinburgh, ch 24, p 373.

INTRODUCTION: OVERVIEW OF JOINT REPLACEMENTS

Joint replacements are now a very common surgical event and many are undertaken each year in the

UK. The first totally successful joint replacement in a human subject took place in 1959, although many previous attempts had succeeded for varying lengths of time. The hip was the first joint to be successfully replaced, and internal prosthetics for the metacarpophalangeal (MCP), wrist, elbow, shoulder, knee and ankle joints were all developed after this.

A full joint replacement, or total arthroplasty, replaces both sides of the joint, e.g. both the acetabulum and the head of the femur. Partial joint replacement (hemiarthroplasty) restores the aspect of the joint that is damaged; the commonest surfaces to be replaced are the head of the femur and the femoral or tibial compartments in the medial compartment of the knee. All partial replacements may be upgraded to a full replacement at a future date if necessary.

Another classification of joint replacement is by the degree of control offered by the joint, i.e. constrained, semi-constrained and unconstrained. Constrained indicates that there is a link between the two components and that all anatomical movements of the artificial joint are restricted to a greater or lesser extent. In a semi-constrained joint some movement, although restricted, is allowed in all planes and an unconstrained joint permits free movement in all anatomical planes. Examples of these will be discussed under particular joints.

Commonly the replacement prosthetic parts are made out of inert metals such as stainless steel or chrome-cobalt molybdenum alloys and high-density polyethylene. These components have been shown to produce low friction motion at the joint so decreasing the chance of abrasion or damage (wear) to the internal joint surfaces, aiding longevity of the joint. Only the finger joints use silicone elastomer with polypropylene reinforcement to achieve the best combination of available movement and wear capacity.

The over-riding issue through the years is the survival of the replacement, i.e. the length of time the patient may expect the joint to last for given 'normal' use. As all replacements joints are only a good 'reproduction', they cannot totally emulate the wear of the natural joint. The artificial joint has a friction coefficient approximately six times higher than a natural joint and thus loosening is inevitable, but the aim is to try to delay this as long as possible. Loosening, deep infection, fracture

and dislocation remain the main complications of joint replacement surgery (Rothman & Hozack 1988). The successful survival of a joint replacement relies on all members of the team understanding the underlying biomechanical principles of the 'normal' joint and its replacement, the limitations of the materials used, and the surgical procedure undertaken. More importantly, the patient must understand why these are issues, so that the rehabilitation programme can be modified to protect the joint.

It is the advancement of the understanding of these issues that has lengthened the average survival of a replacement hip joint to 25 years (National Audit Office 2003) and a knee joint to 15 years. However not all joints will last this length of time because of poor insertion, loosening, dislocation or fracture (Fender et al 1999).

This chapter will explore the issues outlined above and discuss the rehabilitation programmes for patients who have undergone hip and knee replacements. Ankle replacements will not be discussed, as they are not routine surgical events.

Firstly the indications for joint replacement, complications and general rehabilitation points will be discussed briefly. Lastly, upper limb replacements will be discussed briefly.

Indications for joint replacement

The commonest reasons why a patient undergoes a joint replacement are pain and loss of function (National Audit Office 2000). It is therefore not surprising that the major weight-bearing joints (hip and knee) are the most common joints to be replaced. The repetitive high loads and torsional stresses taken across these joints predispose them to wear and tear (osteoarthrosis) and the signs and symptoms outlined in Chapter 6. In patients with multiple joint pathology, e.g. rheumatoid arthritis, replacement of damaged joints includes the metacarpophalangeal joints (MCPs), elbow and shoulders as well as the more routine hips and knees, providing pain-free movement post-surgery, with some improvement in function. The functional gains post-surgery are not as good as with single joint involvement (Kirwan et al 1994) but as a result joint survival is usually better because the demands made on the new joints are far less.

Pettine et al (1991) compared the outcome of total hip replacements between an over-80-year-old group and a more normal representative group aged 64–67 years. The outcomes did not differ significantly and the authors advocated that elective hip replacement surgery should be offered to the over-80s. It is now quite commonplace for total hip replacements to be undertaken for people in their 80s and 90s (National Audit Office 2003) but it is also becoming more common to see patients having joint replacements at a younger age than the recommended 60+ (Dandy & Edwards 2003).

Although osteoarthrosis and rheumatoid arthritis are the commonest pathologies associated with joint replacement, post-traumatic joint stiffness or avascular necrosis (see Chapter 5) would also predispose the patient to pain and loss of function at specific joints. A partial or total joint replacement may be indicated even in the younger patient if the joint destruction is irreversible. Obviously, a younger person with a single joint pathology should be counselled before the surgery takes place about the potential problems of overuse and loosening.

In younger patients a total hip replacement can be prescribed if there is joint destruction following congenital dislocation of the hip. The outcome again will not be the same as for conventional total hip arthroplasty because there is likely to be severe weakness of the abductors.

A hip replacement may also be performed several years after a hip arthrodesis (surgical fusion of the hip joint). Arthrodesis is sometimes performed in younger patients if the hip has been severely damaged and joint destruction is irreparable. The patient is left with no hip movement and uses compensatory lumbar spine and knee motion. Over time this overuse can cause trauma and pain to these joints and therefore a hip replacement can be an option in later years (Kilgus et al 1990). The outcome of these examples would be very different, for obvious reasons (Joshi et al 2002). Chapter 5 outlines the rehabilitation of a patient following a subcapital fracture. The functional achievements following an arthroplasty for post-traumatic joint stiffness depends on the range of motion gained in theatre and the length of time since, and extent of, the initial damage.

The commonest example of the use of a hemiarthroplasty is the replacement of the head of the femur following a subcapital fracture. If the blood supply to the head of the femur has been traumatically interrupted then avascular necrosis will ensue and internal fixation of the fracture alone will not prevent bone death. Hence a hemiarthroplasty of the head of femur may be undertaken if the acetabulum is free of obvious signs of degeneration. Austin–Moore or Thompson hemiarthroplasties for the hip are the commonest examples used in the UK, the difference being that the Austin–Moore does not have to be cemented in place (Fig. 8.1). Similarly the head of the humerus can also be replaced with a hemiarthroplasty.

Fixation

The incidence of loosening of the prosthetic components is dependent on the skill of the surgeon, the surgical technique and the type of fixation to the underlying bone. Initially all joint replacements were inserted with a bond of polymethylmethacrylate (PMMA) cement, which held the prosthetic component tight to the bone.

Acrylic cement can sustain compressive stress well but cannot control shear or torsional stress, so

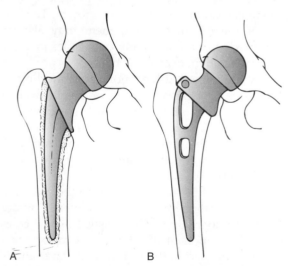

Figure 8.1 Hip prosthesis for fracture of femoral neck. A: Thompson prosthesis secured with cement. B: Austin–Moore prosthesis with no cement. (Adapted with permission from Dandy & Edwards 2003.)

that repeated rotational movement across the bone–cement interface results in a splitting of the cement and release of cement particles. These particles may then cause bone destruction and, along with the initial damage to the cement, loosening of the prosthetic component will occur. Care during the operative procedure to clean and dry the prepared bone surface before application of cement will reduce the incidence of loosening but biomechanically loosening is inevitable at some stage because cement is stiffer than bone. Thus the bone–cement and cement–prosthesis interfaces become the weakest points under excessive loads. The more obese or active the patient is, the greater the loads and risk of loosening. Also, a greater surface area of cement will create more problems, particularly for long-stem implants, e.g. the femoral component of a hip arthroplasty.

Over the last 15 years alternative types of fixation have been tried to achieve a lower loosening rate. Bioingrowth relies on the natural growth of bone around or through the prosthetic implant and no cement is used; attachment is achieved by new bone growth at the bone–prosthesis interface. Bone growth is enhanced by the tightness of the 'press fit' of the component, and the resulting trauma and compression to the bone stimulates new growth (Rothman & Hozack 1988). Additionally, a coating of hydroxyapatite on the prosthetic component is used to stimulate bone growth. The surface of the prosthetic component may also be contoured with bumps, grooves or holes to allow easier attachment of the new bone.

Hip replacement using a non-cement technique necessitates a period of non- or partial weight bearing to allow stabilization of the component. The length of time of reduced weight bearing depends on the type of joint being replaced, the expectations of the patients and the rate of bone growth.

The cementless technique is often the preferred choice of fixation in 'younger' patients (under 65 years) undergoing arthroplasty. In some cases only one component of a total joint replacement may be cemented in (hybrid design). An example of this is when the acetabular component of a total hip replacement is cemented in, allowing the femoral component with its greater surface area and higher rotational forces to attach via new bone growth and hopefully reducing the risk of loosening.

If loosening has occurred an uncemented joint can be revised to a cemented joint (Rothman & Hozack 1988).

General rehabilitation issues

A prosthetic replacement will normally ensure relief of pain and return of function following surgery but this is dependent on the presurgery range of motion, the strength of surrounding musculature and the laxity of the joint.

The replacement guarantees to remove the bony destruction caused by the underlying pathology and the release of tight soft tissues or the repair of damaged ones will help to re-align the new joint. However, it is only the rehabilitation programme that enables the patient to achieve full return of function, strength and stability to the joint (Fernandez Galinski et al 1996). This point is often forgotten when the patient awakes pain-free and more mobile. At this stage there is little evidence to show whether the lack of a rehabilitation programme is detrimental to the biomechanical complications of the joint, particularly loosening. There is research evidence to show that patients do have problems for quite a while post-surgery and do not reach return of full functional ability (Andriacchi & Hurwitz 1997, Kirwan et al 1994, Murray et al 1976).

Hydrotherapy is an excellent treatment for a patient following joint replacement surgery, particularly the hip, knee and shoulder, once the wound is healed and there are no signs of infection. Some hospitals may allow patients in the pool at an earlier stage so long as the wound is covered. Then, use of a gymnastic ball in supine lying and sitting will encourage control around the new joint and can help to promote proprioceptive feedback. The gym ball can also be for upper limb work so long as the arm is controlled either by the patient or by the therapy staff.

Assessment

The importance of assessment cannot be forgotten both pre- and postoperatively in joint replacement surgery. Specific issues will be mentioned in individual sections but it is important to remember that a full clinical examination is not necessary for a preoperative assessment of a total joint replacement, because joint stability, range of motion, muscle power, proprioception will all change postoperatively. Therefore the therapist should concentrate on respiratory function, specific joint range of motion, muscle power and general function ability – walking (distance travelled and aid used), sitting to standing, stair climbing, bending forward, dressing tasks, upper limb function, etc.

Acknowledging and recording the altered patterns used preoperatively to perform or compensate for these functions will help the physiotherapist to build a postoperative rehabilitation programme to the specific needs of the patient. For example, if a patient has been overusing the lumbar spine to gain sufficient forward flexion to put on shoes or socks, back pain may be a problem. There will need to be a specific strengthening programme for the hip flexors and extensors to achieve the hip motion required to reduce the compensatory spinal movements, or the patient will continue with their new 'learned' pattern. Patients are different and how they compensate for loss of motion/strength/proprioception will be individual, although the overall loss of function may be the same.

Leg length discrepancies are not uncommon prior to lower limb joint replacement particularly the hip because of bone erosion and pathology. Measurement of leg length discrepancy preoperatively will help the physiotherapist to evaluate the change in biomechanics as these will still remain a problem post-surgery, despite surgical correction. Noting the preoperative use of walking aids will help plan the postoperative walking aid requirements, especially if the patient has upper limb problems.

Self–assessment question

- **SAQ 8.1** How would you measure apparent and true leg length discrepancies?

(Answer at end of chapter.)

Unsure of the answer? Read Chapter 10 of *Clinical Orthopaedic Examination* (McRae 1997).

The Harris hip score (HHS) is widely used to assess hip function (e.g. Kili et al 2003, Pettine et al 1991, Söderman & Malchau 2001b). It was designed by Harris (1969) to report levels of pain, function, deformity, range of motion and walking ability, by giving an overall numerical value to hip function. The Harris hip score is detailed in Table 8.1: the lower the score the worse the hip pathology is.

The other commonly used scale is the Oxford hip score, which again uses sections on hip pain and disability to get an overall numerical value for hip function (Hajat et al 2002). The score generated (12–60) indicates the level of symptoms, higher scores indicating greater problems.

There are a number of general scales used in the literature that are not hip-specific, e.g. Western Ontario McMaster's Osteoarthritis Index (WOMAC), which is used to give a self-administered indication of disability (Nilsdottir & Lohmander 2002, Söderman et al 2001c); this scale is not disease specific. An alternative score used in the UK is the Nottingham Health Profile (NHP), which is widely used to give an indication of general health (Franzen et al 1997).

Outcomes from the NHP and HHS scores have been found to be comparable (Garellick et al 1998), so linking specific hip scores to a general health scale. In a large study of 2604 THR patients, Söderman et al (2001a) found good correlation between SF-36, NHP, the WOMAC and the HHS, and these authors suggested that all these forms could be used to assess the outcome following THR as all related well to clinical outcome. However the pain scale in the HHS was the best indicator of clinical outcome when assessed against clinical and X-ray failure (Söderman et al 2001c). Söderman et al (2001a) also recommended that, for completeness, a general health form and specific hip scale should be used.

There are also a number of knee scales that can be used to assess movement, function and stability, and once again the WOMAC or NHP can be used as a general disability scale. The Arthritis Impact Scale (AIMS) includes general well being and psychological issues as well as functional impairment.

Post–operation assessment

After the surgery the assessment will concentrate on achievement of functional goals, muscle

Table 8.1   The Harris Hip Score (Harris 1969)

1. Pain

	Score
A. None, or ignores it	44
B. Slight, occasional, no compromise in activities	40
C. Mild pain, no effect on activities, rarely moderate pain with unusual activity, may take aspirin	30
D. Moderate pain, tolerable but makes concessions to pain. Some limitation of ordinary activity or work. May require occasional medicine stronger than aspirin	20
E. Marked pain, serious limitation of activities	10
F. Totally disabled, crippled, pain in bed, bedridden	0

	Category	Score
Sitting	A. Any chair one hour	5
	B. High chair half hour	3
	C. Unable to sit comfortably	0
Enter public transport		1

3. Absence of deformity (4 points each if present)
Category
A. Less than 30° fixed flexion contracture
B. Less than 10° fixed adduction
C. Less than 10° fixed internal rotation in extension
D. Limb length discrepancy less than 3.2 cm

2. Function

	Category	Score
Gait (max 33)		
Limp	A. None	11
	B. Slight	8
	C. Moderate	5
	D. Severe	0
Support	A. None	11
	B. Cane for long walks	7
	C. Cane most of the time	5
	D. One crutch	3
	E. Two canes	2
	F. Two crutches	0
	G. Not able to walk	0
Activities (14 possible)		
Stairs	A. Normally	4
	B. Using railing	2
	C. In any manner	1
	D. Unable to do stairs	0
Shoes and socks	A. With ease	4
	B. With difficulty	2
	C. Unable	0

4. Range of motion

	Arc of motion	Index	Max. possible
Flexion	0–45° (45°)	1.0	45
	45–90° (45°)	0.6	27
	90–110° (20°)	0.3	6
	110–130° (20°)	0.0	0
Abduction	0–15° (15°)	0.8	12
	15–20° (5°)	0.3	1.5
	20–45° (25°)	0.0	0
External rotation in extension	0–15° (15°)	0.4	0
	Over 15°	0.0	0
Internal rotation in extension	Any	0.0	0
Adduction	0–15° (15°)	0.2	3
	Over 15°	0.0	0
Extension	Any	0.0	0

Total Motion Point Value = 100.5
Overall range of motion = Total Motion Point Value × 0.05
Record Trendelenburg test as positive, level or neutral

strength and range of active movement. The main objective assessment is geared towards evaluation of the stability of the joint and the general functional ability and balance of the patient. If a lower joint is being replaced it should be remembered that some joint proprioception will be lost as a result of capsule and ligament damage and the excess swelling or bruising in the early stages.

HIP JOINT

The hip joint is the one that is most commonly replaced and has the best success rate of any of the artificial prostheses, with 90% of patients gaining reasonably good clinical outcomes at 10–20 years post-surgery (University of Leeds, National Health Centre for Reviews and Dissemination 1996).

Figure 8.2 A Charnley total hip replacement.
A: The prosthesis.
B: Appearance on X-ray.
(With permission from Dandy & Edwards 2003.)

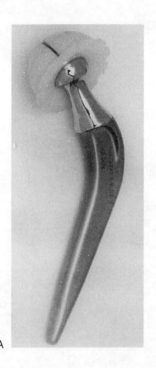

A

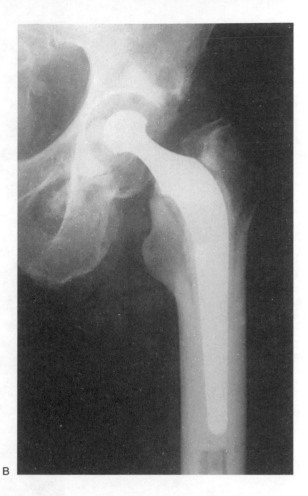

B

Types of hip joint

The commonest type of hip replacement in the UK today is the Charnley low-friction arthroplasty (Hasheminejad et al 1994), which started being used in the 1960s. The femoral component is structured from stainless steel and the acetabular cup from high-density polyethylene (Fig. 8.2).

At the same time, McKee was developing a complete stainless-steel hip joint but the cup's wear capacity was not as good as that of the high-density polyethylene. The modern hip arthroplasties still use a combination of chrome-cobalt molybdenum alloys, or stainless-steel femoral shafts with high-density polyethylene acetabular cup. The acetabular cup may have a metal back in some cases. Fixation of both components can be with or without cement. If no cement is used the femoral component relies on a tight 'press fit',

whereas the acetabular cup relies on either screws or pegs for fixation (Goldie 1992).

Incision sites

There is a huge variety of prosthetic hip replacements available to the surgeon and these are usually of the unconstrained type. Semi-constrained hip joints are available but they are not very common. The normal hip joint has the greatest range of motion of any lower limb joint. Thus an unconstrained joint post-surgery will allow the hip to return to its preoperative motion or greater. The disadvantage of this free movement with no prosthetic constraint is that the joint is prone to dislocation. Dislocation is at greatest risk immediately post-surgery and is common up until 6 weeks post-operation. At this stage the capsule should

Figure 8.3 X-ray showing Charnley total hip replacement with wire fixation of the greater trochanter. (With permission from Rothman & Hozack 1988.)

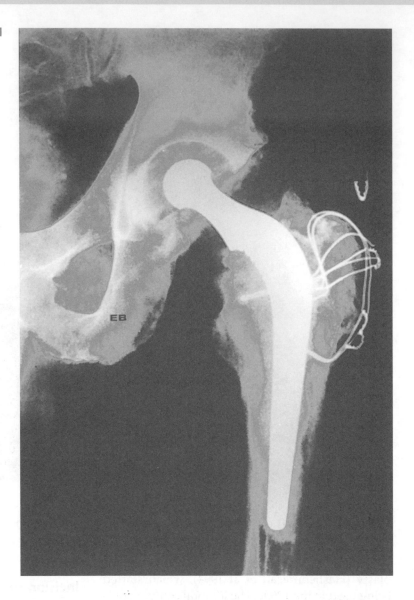

have regrown around the hip joint. It is only when this has occurred that the patient should be advised to aim for full movement of the hip joint. The choices of incision sites for a total hip replacement are:

- *anterolateral*: between the tensor fascia lata and the glutei
- *posterolateral*: through the posterior capsule
- *true lateral*: with the Charnley approach the greater trochanter is excised and reattached with wire fixation (Fig. 8.3). If this occurs, rehabilitation is slower and should be more representative

of an uncemented arthroplasty. The Liverpool approach is an alternative lateral approach that does not remove the greater trochanter.

Each surgeon will have their own preference but it is very important that the therapist knows which incision has been used, and any specific requirements to be undertaken. Irrespective of the type of prosthesis or incision used, a suction drain will be in situ for up to 48 hours postoperatively. The surgeon and/or nursing staff will also dictate management of the wound and this should be made clear to all therapy staff.

Common complications

Dislocation

The position for dislocation depends very much on the incision site used for the operation.

- *Anterolateral and true lateral*: the hip will dislocate if placed in excessive extension, external rotation and adduction, or a combination of all three
- *Posterolateral*: the hip will dislocate in excessive flexion, internal rotation and adduction, or a combination of all three.

Thus for at least 6 weeks and preferably up to 12, the patient's hip should not be placed in these positions.

The patient must be aware of the possibility of dislocation and this should be reinforced, especially immediately following surgery. To assist in the prevention of dislocation the patient should sleep with an abduction pillow between the legs when supine or may lie on their operated side once the drain is out. While in bed it is recommended that the patient's locker be placed on the operated side, so that if the patient leans over, the leg will not roll into internal rotation and adduction (Goldie 1992).

Dislocation of the hip is easily recognizable because it is shorter, externally rotated and in extension if it has dislocated anteriorly, or shorter, flexed and internally rotated if dislocated in the posterior direction and in both cases will be extremely painful. An X-ray of the hip will clearly show the dislocation (Fig. 8.4). Treatment then will be relocation of the hip under general anaesthetic and then a period of bed rest with traction for up to 6 weeks (Dandy & Edwards 2003, Goldie 1992). If the hip is unstable in flexion then a plaster of Paris cast (POP) may be applied to keep the leg in extension.

Wear

Any material will develop signs of wear, e.g. pits and holes in the material or fragments of debris flaking from the material, with repeated loading to its surface. This is true of the high-density polyethylene of the acetabular cup or the tibial plateau. Failure of a total hip joint will occur if the

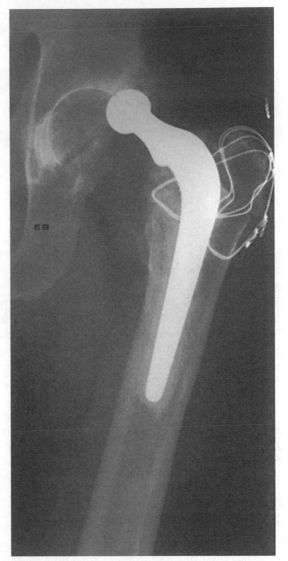

Figure 8.4   X-ray showing dislocation of total hip replacement. (With permission from Rothman & Hozack 1988.)

prosthetic material cannot sustain the forces and starts to flake or crumble. Revision of the cup is essential if signs of debris occur, as the opposing surface will eventually become pitted as well, and the converse will apply should the head of the femur show signs of wear.

Other complications

- Other complications are those common to any surgical procedure. SAQ 5.7 in the fracture chapter highlights the main complications for people on bed rest, and these are very similar to complications following an operative procedure.

Problem–solving exercise 8.1

Which of the common surgical complications from the answer to SAQ 5.7 do you think patients following total hip replacement are most prone to?

(Answer at end of chapter.)

If there is any reason why a patient cannot have a general anaesthetic, e.g. severe respiratory disease, then the procedure could be carried out under an epidural anaesthetic. Brinker et al (1997) reported equally good results when using epidural anaesthesia compared to general for 'length of hospitalization, non-surgical operating room time, intraoperative blood transfusions, intraoperative femur fractures, deep venous thrombosis, deep infections, death or the prevalence of postoperative urinary tract infections'.

Significant differences were found for estimated intraoperative blood loss, surgical time and the drain output, with the epidural group having the 'best' results in unilateral hip replacement surgery.

Venous thrombi

Prophylactic drug therapy against deep vein thrombosis and pulmonary embolism both before and after total hip replacement is routine in most surgical units, although the need for its use has been questioned (McGrath et al 1996). In most cases a programme of prophylactic warfarin or aspirin will be given to reduce the risk of a venous clot (Hull et al 1997). An alternative to this would be intermittent pneumatic compression (IPC) of the lower limbs both during and after surgery (Woolson & Watt 1991). These authors have shown that there is no significant difference between treatment with warfarin, aspirin and IPC, with the mean occurrence of thrombosis being 10%.

It is also common practice, irrespective of which type of prophylactic treatment is used, for patients to wear an elasticated antiembolus stocking on the operated limb, or possibly on both limbs (Woolson & Watt 1991).

Fracture

Femoral fractures, particularly around the stem of the femoral component of the hip, can occur either at the time of surgery or at a later date. The femur can either fracture just distal to the tip of the stem of the prosthesis or the lower tip of the stem can protrude through the lateral wall of the femur (Fig. 8.5). It is common to see bone erosion at the site of the fracture, which may indicate excessive loading at that point (McRae & Esser 2002). It may be possible to fix these fractures without revision of the femoral stem but this is highly unlikely.

Longitudinal fractures around the stem can be repaired successfully with internal fixation using either wires or a screw and plate.

The femoral prosthesis can fracture transversally mid-stem and this may cause an associated fracture of the femur at this point. If the fracture occurs at a late stage postoperatively, signs of loosening often accompany it. It would be normal practice to revise the stem of the prosthesis when this fracture occurs (Dandy & Edwards 2003; Fig. 8.5).

Postoperative thigh pain

Pain can arise in both cemented and uncemented hip procedures but for very different reasons.

Thigh pain immediately following an uncemented hip replacement is quite usual and will diminish once new bone growth has occurred and the implant becomes secure, at any time up to 6 months (Engh et al 1987). Occasionally, patients complain of pain after activity at a point equivalent to the end of the femoral stem. The repetitive compressive loading on the bone distal to the femoral stem may cause the end pain but this has not been confirmed (Maihafer 1990). If a patient has thigh pain following a cemented prosthesis, this is not normal, and signifies loosening of the femoral component. Any signs of unresolving thigh pain should be reported to the consultant surgeon for review. The patient should be reminded of this on discharge, as the loosening pain may not arise until many months or years after the operation.

Figure 8.5 Fractures around the femoral stem. (A: With permission from Dandy & Edwards 2003; B: adapted with permission from McRae 1997.)

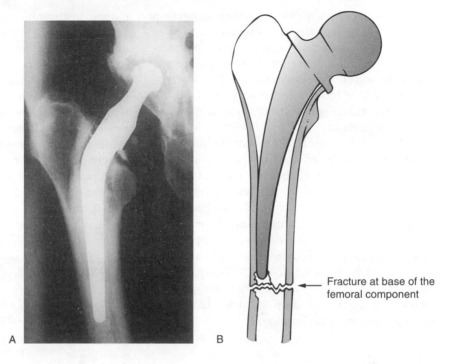

A   B

Fracture at base of the femoral component

Failure

Approximately 0.5–1% of total hip arthroplasties undertaken each year fail (Dandy & Edwards 2003). If failure occurs, revision arthroplasty may be a possibility and it is estimated that approximately 5–7% of all hip replacements will need revision through time (Fitzpatrick et al 1998). The main reason for this is either loosening or deep infection.

As discussed previously, biomechanical loosening between the bone and the cement is inevitable at some stage but the aim is to delay this for as long as possible. Loosening is particularly prevalent around the stem of the femoral component and the patient will complain of pain and discomfort down the thigh and loss of function. On X-ray a dark line is seen at the cement–prosthesis interface, indicating a gap between the surfaces (Fig. 8.6). Loosening of the acetabular component can also occur but the patient now complains of pain in the groin and loss of function (Dandy & Edwards 2003).

Infection

Infection can occur at any time post-surgery although the surgeon takes great care to prevent

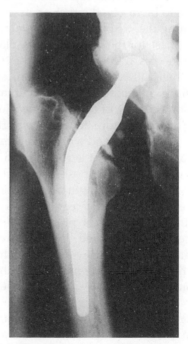

Figure 8.6 X-ray showing loosening of the femoral stem. (With permission from Dandy & Edwards 2003.)

this happening. As with any infection, the patient will have a raised temperature and complain of pain around the groin or thigh. Infections arising after the initial operation period may be secondary to infections elsewhere in the body, e.g. urinary tract or tooth infections. There is also a direct relationship between mouth infections that are present preoperatively and late-onset infection of total hip replacements (Bartzokas et al 1994).

Patients must be advised of the possibility of infection and the need to seek medical help if these should arise. Following management with antibiotics the only option for the surgeon is to undertake a revision arthroplasty. Prior to the revision arthroplasty the infected arthroplasty is removed (excision arthroplasty) and the resulting hole is filled with antibiotic beads. The patient is then kept on bed rest and traction for up to 6 weeks or until the infection subsides. Only then will the revision be undertaken.

Rehabilitation

The hip joint once altered by disease pathology or trauma will develop fixed contractures in flexion, adduction and external rotation. These contractures have to be resolved either preoperatively, in the operating theatre or in the postoperative rehabilitation phase for the operation to be classed as a complete success. If the hip is left in the contracted position then full range of extension, abduction and rotation will remain lost, thus maintaining the altered biomechanics of the presurgical joint.

A flexion contracture tends to emphasize an adduction contracture and will severely exaggerate a discrepancy in apparent leg length and may add to any true discrepancy post-surgery. Therefore, following surgery, the length of the patient's legs should be measured on a regular basis. If a true leg length discrepancy is present, a temporary shoe raise can be supplied. If the discrepancy is over 25 mm then only provide half of this height until the hip and lumbar spine adapt to the change of alignment. If there is an apparent leg length discrepancy only, do not give a shoe raise until the contracture or muscle weakness has been resolved. This is particularly important for an adduction contracture with abductor weakness. As strength and range increase, the apparent discrepancy will

reduce. If it resolves to less than 12 mm, no action should be taken, but wait at least 4 months before reassessment to maximize possible recovery.

The type of prosthesis and the incision site are the main dictators of the rehabilitation regime to be used. Both cemented and uncemented replacements follow a similar regime, except for times of weight bearing. The patient with an uncemented prosthesis will remain partially or non-weight-bearing for between 6 and 12 weeks postoperatively, or on some occasions up to 9 months (Engh & Bobyn 1985). Weight bearing with a cemented prosthesis usually begins on the first day postoperatively (Maihafer 1990).

Problem-solving exercise 8.2

What would you do for a preoperative assessment to a patient awaiting a total hip replacement?

(If you have trouble with this question, look back at the case study of Mrs Jones in Chapter 5 and Problem-solving exercise 5.11 for help.) After you have worked out your answer, read the next section.

- Assess:
  - joint movement and muscle tone around the joint, particularly the range of hip flexion and abduction, extension, rotation and abd/adduction; strength of the glutei group (extension and abduction) and the quadriceps group
  - general functional ability: walking, stairs, sitting to standing and bed mobility. Note the use of walking aids, handholds and how well the function is achieved
  - respiratory function prior to surgery
  - venous return in the lower limbs
- What does the patient know about their surgery?
- Advise the patient of the postoperative regime.

All these points are important but it is particularly important to gain knowledge of the preoperative range of motion, strength and functional ability. There are many studies showing that the successful outcome of a hip replacement is closely related to the preoperative motion available (Rowe et al 1989). These authors studied the function of patients before and following hip replacement and found that the range of active flexion and fixed flexion deformity correlated highly with the Health Assessment Questionnaire, and that a fixed flexion deformity in the presence of limited flexion correlated with the Specific Disability Scale.

Stanic et al (1993) developed a successful and comprehensive evaluation of function for pre- and postoperative use with patients undergoing total hip replacement. The evaluation comprised of passive hip movement, observational gait analysis and kinemetric gait parameters (stride length, time, gait velocity, stance time and joint kinematics). This team showed that all parameters showed significant changes between preoperative and postoperative values, the most notable being an increase in hip extension, reduction of a Trendelenburg gait, and loss of the adduction contracture.

It is particularly important, therefore, to measure these aspects accurately. Advice on how to undertake a full clinical hip assessment can be revised in McRae (1997), Kendall et al (1993) and Norkin & White (2003). As mentioned before, it is important to remember that a full clinical examination is not necessary for a preoperative assessment of a total hip replacement because the joint stability, range of motion, muscle power and proprioception will all change postoperatively. For the lower limb, the weight-bearing functions are obviously the most important to assess.

> ### Problem-solving exercise 8.3
>
> Go back and review Chapters 3 and 5 before answering this question.
>   How can the therapist measure the functions of: walking, stair climbing, sit to stand or forward flexion (e.g. to put on shoes or socks)?
>
> (Answer at end of chapter.)

Following surgery the postoperative assessment will be exactly the same as for a fracture around the hip joint. The greater risk of dislocation means that full range hip, knee, or lumbar spine motion or combined movements should be avoided.

> ### Self-assessment question
>
> ● SAQ 8.2 In what position does a total hip joint replacement dislocate?
>
> (Answer at end of chapter.)

Active postoperative therapy starts from day 1, remembering that the abduction pillow or wedge should remain in situ while the patient is lying supine or on the non-operated side. Also, the patient should be discouraged from performing a straight leg raise on the operated side until full quadriceps and iliopsoas control has returned.

The treatment goals at this time do not differ greatly from those of a patient following a fracture around the hip. These are:

● Restoration of:
  – *joint motion*: hip extension, abduction and rotation are all lost preoperatively therefore these are the most important to start re-educating
  – *muscle strength*: hip abductors, extensors and rotators in particular, but hip flexors must also be strengthened for climbing a stair or step or for putting on a shoe. Quadriceps and hamstrings activity should also be encouraged
● Maintenance of:
  – *vascular function*: foot and ankle pumps, quadriceps activity and deep breathing will all help
  – *respiratory function*
● Education about:
  – *joint preservation techniques* to prevent dislocation, loosening and fracture
  – *bed mobility*
  – *weight bearing*: gait and sitting to standing.

Bed mobility

The patient will need assistance to move up and down the bed and to go into the 'bridging position' for toilet purposes. If the patient has had a posterolateral incision then care must be taken to avoid too much hip extension in the early stages and it may be easier to get the patient out of bed for toileting. Getting the patient in and out of bed should have been taught in the preoperative stage, but if not then this should be done on the first day of mobilizing. Ideally the patient should be assisted out of bed on the operated side with the leg held in abduction. If a posterior surgical approach has been used then the hip should also remain in extension as much as possible.

Muscle re-education

From day 1 postoperatively, isometric exercises for the muscle groups highlighted above should be undertaken at least three or four times a day in the 'neutral' hip position in supine. The therapist will have to be present to help the patient and to ensure that correct muscle activity is taking place. Because of misuse or complete lack of use of these muscles preoperatively, endurance will be limited and an appropriately low-level programme should be initiated. Similarly, active assisted or passive movements should be started at this time but only under the therapist's supervision.

Once grade II muscle activity has been achieved in the neutral hip supine position, isometric activity of the rotators, extensors and abductors can begin in hip flexion. Again, the therapist must be

present to control the hip position and check muscle function. In most cases 'good' muscle function returns quickly and most patients will have active grade III muscle power by one week postoperatively, but this will only be through the limited range of motion allowed during the early postoperative period. Often the quadratus lumborum and the lateral trunk muscles will assist hip abduction activity by 'hitching' the pelvis on the side of abduction. This occurs as a compensatory activity to weak abductors and will appear in both supine and standing positions (Fig. 8.7). The therapist must encourage the patient to maintain a level pelvis while doing hip abduction; if 'hitching' occurs then more assistance should be given to reduce the weight of the limb and make abduction easier. Further explanation of this phenomenon can be gained by reading Kendall et al (1993).

It is very easy for the therapist to miss this compensatory action as the patient may have been doing this for many months preoperatively. Another favourite compensatory action is the use of the abdominal muscles to help flex the hip in the supine and standing positions. Thus the pelvis is tilted in the posterior direction to gain more hip flexion.

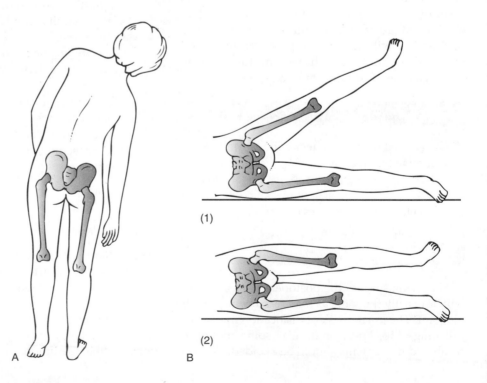

Figure 8.7 Hip abduction with weak gluteus medius. A: Weak gluteus medius in standing. B: Weak gluteus medius in side lying: (1) correct abduction; (2) use of quadratus lumborum to compensate. (With permission from Kendall et al 1993.)

A

B

(1)

(2)

Weight bearing

The start date for weight bearing depends on the incision used, any complications of surgery and gaining a good postoperative check X-ray at approximately 24 hours. Patients with lateral or posterolateral incisions can start weight bearing from day 1, but patients with anterolateral incisions may be delayed until 2 days postoperatively, as extension is the dislocation position. Alternatively the start of sitting can be delayed for patients with a posterolateral incision to prevent dislocation. Patients will be required to sit in a raised chair so that the hip is held at less than 90° of flexion.

Sitting and walking will become easier and more comfortable with the suction drain removed and any intravenous drips disconnected (usually 24–48 hours postoperatively).

During the preoperative phase it is common for the patient to walk with limited hip extension range and weak hip extensors during the final stages of the stance phase of gait. This is compensated for by a backwards rotation of the pelvis, with forward flexion of the trunk and a shorter step length. This action allows the opposite side of the pelvis to rotate forward so that the opposing leg can gain the correct position for weight bearing and achieve a reasonable step length (Perry 1992). This becomes a 'learned' response but once the patient starts walking postoperatively this compensation must be corrected as quickly as possible. Likewise weak hip abductors preoperatively will be compensated by leaning to the weight-bearing side or dropping the pelvis on the opposite side (Trendelenburg sign). A shortened leg on the osteoarthritic side will also mean that the patient may lean to the same side on weight bearing. Adequate strength in the hip extensors, flexors and abductors is required before any of these can be remedied.

When the patient starts to weight bear, a frame or crutches should be used to increase stability, reduce the weight taken across the 'new' hip joint and reduce the load on the hip musculature. It is very common for the patient to flex forward at the hip and lumbar spine because of weak hip extensors and previous loss of hip extension range (Kendall et al 1993). This must be discouraged from the start, to help re-educate unused muscles and reinforce 'correct' walking pattern (Perry 1992).

In cemented joints weight bearing is increased until minimal assistance is required from a walking aid. In the 1990 survey of the 'normal' rehabilitation practice for a cemented hip arthroplasty most patients were discharged from hospital at 10–12 days postoperatively, walking with one or two sticks and able to climb a step or steps (Association of Orthopaedic Chartered Physiotherapists 1991). The admission time for patients with total hip replacement since then has changed radically and the mean NHS hospital stay for primary hip replacements has decreased from 11 to 8 days and for revision surgery from 16 to 11.5 days (National Audit Office 2003). These are now similar to the times in the private sector, where the recommended average length of stay for a primary replacement is 6 days and 9 days for a revision.

It is also now commonplace to have an early discharge programme or hospital at home scheme, where patients who are medically fit with no surgical complications are discharged at 4–5 days post-operation to be looked after by the community team. A nominated lead person will co-ordinate the necessary services, which will include nursing, occupational therapy, home help, etc. as well as physiotherapy. From the literature, patients on these schemes do not regain functional return as quickly as those on a hospital-based rehabilitation programme but it is as yet not possible to know if there are other longer-term issues (Ganz et al 2003).

Patients with an uncemented prosthesis will also follow this pattern but will remain on crutches or a frame for much longer (6–12 weeks). It is even more important for these patients to be encouraged to walk with good hip extension during the stance phase of gait and to prevent forward flexion of the trunk, as walking aids will reinforce this posture.

Discharge

On discharge from hospital it is very unusual for patients with total hip replacements to be referred for outpatient physiotherapy. Therefore it is important that fact sheets on exercise, joint preservation and limitations should be given to the patient. It has been predicted that, if patient information and advice was more readily available, the length of hospital stay could be reduced further (National Audit Office 2003). The Arthritis and Rheumatism Council provide excellent leaflets on all these subjects but most orthopaedic departments have developed their own advice sheets to accommodate their particular requirements.

> **Problem–solving exercise 8.4**
>
> What actions should the patient avoid until 6 weeks postoperatively? After you have worked out your answer, read the next section.

Patients should avoid the following:

Anterolateral and true lateral incision: Excessive extension, external rotation and adduction, or a combination of all three

Posterolateral incision: Excessive flexion, internal rotation and adduction, or a combination of all three.

Functions:

- Sitting in low chairs (less than 53 cm in height)
- Bending forward to put on shoes, socks, cut toenails, etc.
- Crossing the legs in sitting or lying
- Twisting the legs in sitting or lying
- Driving
- Jumping or running
- Contact sports.

These actions are self-explanatory but as patients regain strength and motion and enjoy the freedom from pain, they may carry out these actions subconsciously. The surgeon will decide when the patient should return to driving and sport, but this very much depends on the activity and the person involved.

In the last few years there has been an increase in patients wishing to participate in sport following joint replacement. In a survey of orthopaedic practitioners at the Mayo Clinic, McGrory et al (1995) listed the sports recommended after joint replacement as sailing, swimming, scuba diving, cycling, golfing, and bowling after hip and knee replacement procedures and also cross-country

skiing after knee arthroplasty – i.e. low-impact non-contact sports. High-impact or contact sports – e.g. running, water-skiing, football, baseball, basketball, hockey, martial arts, soccer – should be prohibited.

Mallon et al (1996) also suggested that golf could be resumed following hip or knee replacement surgery without increasing the risk of dislocation, loosening and hence revision, but not until after 6–12 weeks following surgery.

Outcome

A patient with an uncomplicated cemented hip replacement should be able to achieve functional independence as defined by Zavadak et al (1995):

- Get in and out of bed with minimal assistance including raising from lying to sitting
- Easily move from sitting to standing and vice versa
- Walk approximately 100 m with the assistance of one or two sticks
- Be able to climb two or three steps with the help of a banister.

These goals may not be achieved by discharge, as it takes a variable time to reach them (Zavadak et al 1995), stair climbing being the most difficult procedure. Those with hip replacements find it difficult to achieve getting in and out of bed or rising from lying to sitting. It may take up to 6 months before the patient has confidence to return to full function and by this time the musculature should be strong enough to support normal activity.

Borstlap et al (1994) reported that a single total hip replacement solved the problems of most people with a primary diagnosis of osteoarthrosis, but was only partially helpful to those with rheumatoid arthritis because of their multiple joint problems. There is no evidence, as yet, to show that the lack of a rehabilitation programme reduces the longevity of a total hip replacement, but only time and the number of revision arthroplasties being undertaken will answer this question completely.

Wykman and Olsson (1992) studied the outcome of single hip replacements versus bilateral. The patients with bilateral surgery did not gain full functional independence until the second hip had been replaced. Even on reaching a good post-operative outcome after the second replacement this was significantly different to the achievements of patients with a single joint replacement.

Treatment of surgical complications

External hip protectors

In some orthopaedic clinics hip protectors are used to prevent hip damage from falls and to offer stability to a 'new' hip replacement (Cameron & Quine 1994). For the patient with ongoing hip complications following replacement or a history of falling, these devices do offer reassurance but they are cumbersome and it is not surprising that patients do not like wearing them (Cameron & Quine 1994).

Revision arthroplasty

If repeated complications arise (e.g. dislocation, infection) or the prosthesis reaches the end of its natural life and begins to loosen, a revision arthroplasty will have to be undertaken.

Mallory (1992) voiced the concern that the age-range of the hip-replacement population is broadening with an average age of 69 years in 1979 and now 57 years. As a result, a greater number of hip replacements will need to be undertaken because of failure. The total number of people getting hip replacements is also increasing – 43 000 total hip replacements are carried out each year on the NHS in England and Wales (National Audit Office 2003) with a further 3304 hip replacements being undertaken in Scotland in 2001(Health Technology Board Scotland 2002). Even with the advances in design and surgical technique, the number of hip replacements needing revision through reaching the end of their natural life is immense (Mallory 1992).

Following a revision arthroplasty a period of bed rest may ensue. If this is the case then the role of the physiotherapist is to maintain the motion and muscle strength of the lower limbs, maintain circulation and respiratory function and prevent the complications of bed rest. Specific treatment for the affected joint will depend on whether an excision arthroplasty has taken place; then the therapist must maintain isometric muscle power around the joint and some active joint motion.

The joints above and below the excised joints should be exercised as much as possible, allowing for the fact that the patient has very little control of the excised joint in the early stages.

Once the revision joint has been inserted, the hip can be treated exactly as for a primary replacement, but greater care must be taken, particularly if the joint had been revised because of repeated dislocation. The muscles around the revised joint will take longer to regain their strength because of repeated surgical trauma. Therefore it will also take a greater time to regain functional independence.

Excision arthrodesis (Girdlestone's procedure) is now less common because of advances in revision surgery. Postoperative management of an excision arthroplasty requires the patient to have good muscle control around the hip. A considerable shoe raise (>7.5 cm) is necessary to accommodate the leg length discrepancy, which will increase as the end of the femur telescopes into the acetabulum on weight bearing. It is possible for the patient to mobilize with a frame or crutches but the outcome is not wonderful.

Hip replacements are one of the most successful orthopaedic surgical procedures today (National Audit Office 2003, National Institute for Clinical Excellence 2000) but the role of the physiotherapist is not totally clear. The reduction in hospital stay requires that physiotherapy input into patient care is multiple; before they enter hospital, in hospital and after they are discharged. The mode of delivery of physiotherapy has changed to be less hands-on and more involved with patient information and education. There is no research, as yet, to show whether the change in physiotherapy input will have an effect on prosthetic outcome or the quality of functional return.

KNEE JOINT

The development of knee replacements was slower than that of the hip, because of the complexity of the joint structure and biomechanics. The knee (tibiofemoral and patellofemoral joints) is the middle joint of the lower limb and therefore acts as the link for all the forces on the lower limb. The knee joint relies strongly on its ligaments, joint surface congruity and muscle control for stability (Nordin & Frankel 1989). In knee pathology

Figure 8.8
Unicompartmental knee replacement. X-rays of an osteoarthritic knee A: before and B: after knee replacement. C: Anteroposterior and D: lateral views of a different type of prosthesis. (With permission from Dandy & Edwards 2003.)

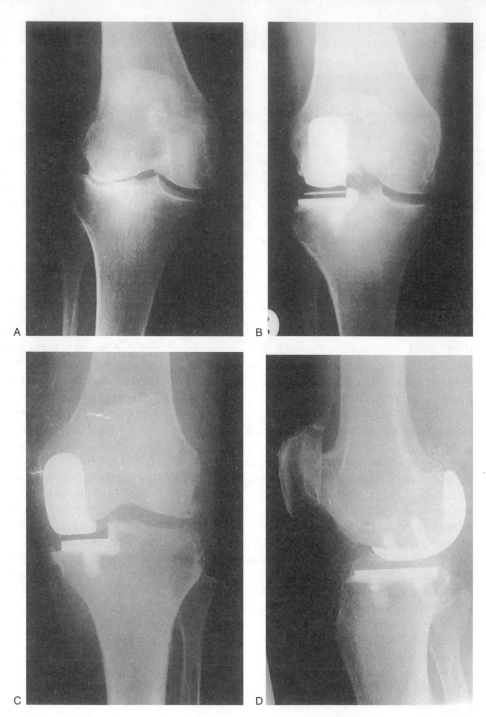

these three factors are altered, so the design of the knee replacement has to enhance the normal knee joint congruity to compensate for lost antero-posterior stability. This is particularly important as the anterior cruciate ligament is sacrificed in the operative procedure and in some cases the posterior cruciate will also be removed. The design of the prosthetic tibial replacement varies depending on the presence of the posterior cruciate ligament. The medial and lateral collateral ligaments are not

Figure 8.9 Types of total knee replacement. A: Unicompartmental arthroplasty. B: Unconstrained total knee replacement. C: Constrained hinge total knee replacement. (With permission from Dandy & Edwards 2003.)

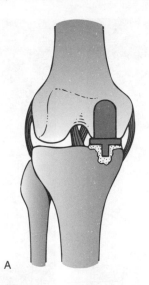

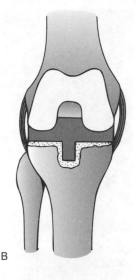

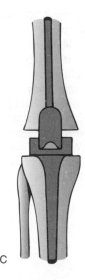

A   B   C

removed during surgery but may be stretched or damaged from previous pathology, if this is so, then operative repair may be necessary. There is controversy about the replacement or resurfacing of the patella when the tibiofemoral joint is replaced. Surgeons hold differing beliefs depending on their experience and the type of tibiofemoral replacement to be undertaken.

As a result of these issues the prosthetic knee will never totally replace the normal knee. The aim of the orthopaedic surgeon therefore is to prolong the life of the natural knee joint as much as possible before undertaking a knee arthroplasty because of the known short life-span of the replacement joint (Dandy & Edwards 2003). A number of other surgical procedures can be undertaken prior to a total knee replacement:

- Intra-articular lavage via an arthroscope
- Debridement (trimming of soft tissue and wash-out of joint)
- Capsular and soft tissue repair
- Meniscectomy or meniscal repair
- Tibial osteotomy
- Hemiarthroplasty or unicompartmental replacement (Perrot & Menkes 1996).

If only one joint surface was affected, a MacIntosh surface replacement made from metal used to be inserted over the tibial plateau (Crawford Adams & Stossel 1992). It is now more common for a tibial osteotomy (realignment of the tibial joint surface; Perrot & Menkes 1996) or unicompartmental arthroplasty to be performed (Figs 8.8, 8.9). An unconstrained unicompartmental arthroplasty is inserted if both joint surfaces of one compartment of the knee joint are affected by disease pathology, usually osteoarthrosis. Goodfellow and O'Connor, in Oxford, were predominantly responsible for designing and developing the unicompartmental joint, using the concept of the Oxford meniscal knee replacement (Goodfellow et al 1988).

Non-surgical management is also encouraged, including patient education, psychological support, reassuring patients that such pain is a reversible state, use of splints, weight reduction and unconventional therapies such as homeopathy, acupuncture and transcutaneous electrical nerve stimulation (Perrot & Menkes 1996).

Types of knee joint

The first prosthetic knee designs were predominantly of the constrained type using a metal hinge with a purely uniaxial motion (e.g. Shiers or Wallidus) (Crawford Adams & Stossel 1992). Metal and plastic unconstrained total knee replacements such as the Polycentric, Freeman–Swanson and Geomedic were first introduced in the late 1960s (Walker 1987; Fig. 8.9). The evolution of the current designs of semi-constrained (Fig. 8.10) and unconstrained prostheses has mainly occurred

Figure 8.10   A, B:
X-ray of
Insall–Burstein total
knee replacement.
(With permission
from Dandy &
Edwards 2003.)
C: Insall–Burstein
knee replacement.
(With permission
from Niwa et al
1987.)

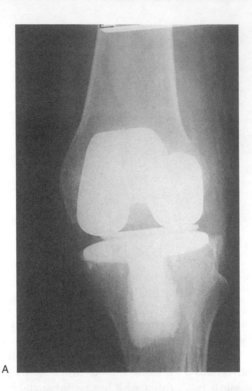

A

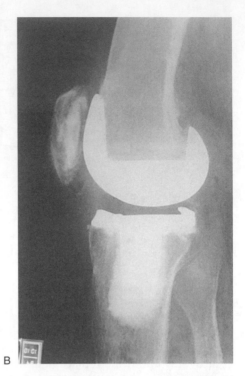

B

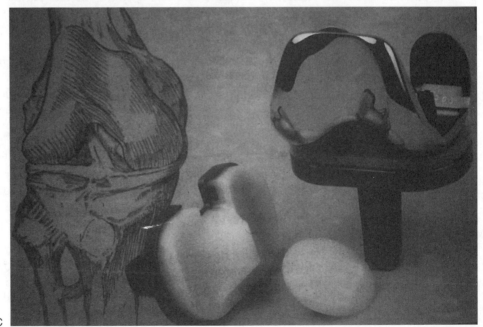

C

because of advances in computer-aided technology. The precision and accuracy of these designs offer a greater chance of survival but this is still dependent on the surgical procedure, where errors in alignment of as little as 3° can lead to failure (Dandy & Edwards 2003).

Once again, fixation of the prosthesis to the bone can be with or without cement. Semi- and unconstrained prostheses have short stem or 'lug' attachments to the underlying bone, while the constrained 'hinge' joints tend to have far longer stems into both the tibia and femur. Greater forces are taken across the knee joint surfaces than the hip, so the risk of loosening is far higher (Sahlstrom et al 1994). This is particularly so in the constrained joints, where there is only one axis of motion; therefore the rotatory and shear forces occur between the bone and the cement. In semi- and unconstrained joints the tibial component is often cemented in place but the femoral component is not, while both components of a hinge joint are usually held by cement (Fig. 8.10(A, B)). Uncemented components are held by bone ingrowth around the roughened surface of the prosthesis.

Criteria for knee replacement

An un- or semi-constrained prosthetic joint is used if the patient complains of:

- severe tibiofemoral pain, which may be accompanied by patellofemoral pain
- loss of general function and/or knee joint mobility
- severe deformity of the knee joint.

If severe loss of knee stability were present in combination with any of the above, a constrained joint would have to be used as it offers much greater internal control. A constrained or hinge joint would also be used as a revision arthroplasty following removal of an un- or semi-constrained joint. If a hemiarthroplasty were removed then a semi-constrained joint would act as the revision prosthesis.

Complications

> ### Problem–solving exercise 8.5
>
> Re-read the complications of total hip replacement and the complications outlined in the introduction and identify the common complications specific to a knee joint replacement.
>
> (Answer at end of chapter.)

These are not dissimilar to the complications following a hip replacement, except that the risk of dislocation is far less in the tibiofemoral joint, although not uncommon at the patellofemoral joint. However, because the knee has to endure far greater forces than the hip, the risk of loosening is much higher at the knee joint. The forces are much greater on the medial compartment compared to the lateral, and this can lead to specific loosening of the prosthesis (Sahlstrom et al 1994). Loosening of the tibial prosthesis can be noticed on X-ray or the patient may complain of continuing pain in the lower knee joint radiating down the tibia, usually on the anterior aspect. This pain differs from deep infection pain, which is usually contained to the joint and is not as specific as the tibial pain.

Signs of 'wear' on the tibial plateau are also seen, particularly on the medial aspect. It is usual to have forces of up to four times body weight across the tibial plateau during normal walking (Nordin & Frankel 1989) and, because of the normal adduction moment on weight bearing, the medial component has to endure more stresses (Sahlstrom et al 1994). Although the design of the prosthetic tibial component tries to limit the effects of wear by distributing the load more evenly, there will still be a greater stress on the medial side of the knee, particularly on weight bearing. If wear of the prosthetic surface does occur, debris may be found within the knee joint and this may stir up an inflammatory reaction. Arthroscopy and joint wash-out can remove debris but this greatly increases the risk of infection, which is a far greater enemy to a knee joint replacement.

The risk of a deep vein thrombosis (DVT) or pulmonary embolus is also equally high for all total joint replacements. Swelling and pain in the centre of the calf, which increases with passive dorsiflexion in knee extension, must give concern that a DVT is present.

Lastly, the risk of either a wound infection or a deep joint infection is equally as high as for the hip, but the consequences are far worse. If the joint becomes loosened or infected, removal and revision is the obvious choice, but it is far more difficult to undertake than in the hip (Dandy & Edwards 2003). Revision surgery requires that the prosthesis and all the cement be removed before a new, larger prosthesis is inserted (Goldie 1992). Thus bone stock is always sacrificed with a revision replacement, particularly in cases where a custom-made constrained joint is inserted (Dandy & Edwards 2003). Infection in a knee prosthesis is difficult to resolve and an excision arthroplasty does not have the same successful results as in the hip. Once the knee joint has been excised, the gap is filled with antibiotic beads or antibiotic-impregnated cement for 6 weeks and a new knee is then inserted.

Following excision arthroplasty of the hip, the joint can gain some stability through good muscle control, but this is not so for the knee, where an external splint is always needed to give support. After this surgery either a compression or nail and graft arthrodesis can be undertaken to permit a stronger limb to bear weight. The vast loss of bone stock from the excision of the total knee replacement is not replaced when the arthrodesis is undertaken, so the leg ends up considerably shorter than the other side (Crawford Adams & Stossel 1992). Cosmetically, this is not pleasing, particularly as a large shoe raise will have to be worn to provide compensation during weight bearing. Also the forces across the arthrodesed knee joint make success difficult to achieve and loosening of the internal metalwork or failure may occur. An external rigid splint may have to be worn even after surgery.

The only option left if the infection is not treated successfully or if an excision arthroplasty fails is an above-knee amputation. Even after amputation the patient does not necessarily return to a good level of function (Pring et al 1988).

Surgery and postoperative management

The knee is normally approached through a midline incision, curved slightly medially to avoid the patella (Crawford Adams & Stossel 1992). Suction drains will be inserted for at least 24 hours (Goldie 1992). During the operation care is taken to align the joint correctly in all planes and make sure that the soft tissue tension is balanced (Crawford Adams & Stossel 1992). Resurfacing of the patella may also take place. The posterior aspect of the patella is shaved until the entire roughened surface is removed and then a small, high-density polyethylene button is inserted. The button has to be of the correct dimensions, particularly width, so that it will run smoothly in the patellar groove of the femoral component.

Following surgery there are two main forms of management that can be chosen – the use, or not, of a continuous passive motion (CPM) machine. If a CPM machine is not used, the knee will be maintained in the extended position by a pressure bandage alone or with either a splint or a plaster of Paris. The knee is kept straight for up to 7 days postoperatively, limiting the start of an active exercise regime.

If a CPM machine is used, passive knee mobilizing begins at some time from immediately post-surgery up to 4 days post-operation. The recommendation for an immediate postoperative start of CPM comes from many good researchers (Coutts 1983, Harms & Engstrom 1991, Johnson 1990, McInnes et al 1992, Wasilewski et al 1990). A few authors have advised delaying application until the second or third day postoperatively to allow the knee to 'settle' in extension prior to flexing (Gose 1987, Maloney et al 1990, Ritter et al 1989). The variation in length of time on the CPM machine during a 24 hour period ranges from 20 hours (Ritter et al 1989, Romness & Rand 1988) to 3 hours (Gose 1987). Basso & Knapp (1987) compared the results of treatment between two groups receiving either 20 hours or 5 hours of CPM immediately following knee replacement. No significant differences were found in range of motion, knee joint effusion, pain or length of stay in hospital, so they recommended the shorter application time. It is now common practice to limit CPM use to approximately 6 hours per day (Harms & Engstrom 1991).

Johnson (1990) indicates that, if the range of flexion is controlled to a maximum of 40° over the first 72 hours, wound integrity will not be jeopardized. Flexion range should be increased by 10° per day until 80–90° of passive and ideally active flexion is gained (Coutts 1983, Harms & Engstrom 1991, Johnson 1990).

The repeated motion on the CPM machine will cause an increase in the volume of blood exuded via the suction drain and wound (Coutts 1983). The increased pumping action has a general effect on the vascular flow in the lower limb and this helps to reduce the tendency for postoperative DVT (Vince et al 1987) and will also reduce joint effusion (Harms & Engstrom 1991, McInnes et al 1992, O'Driscoll et al 1983).

There are many obvious differences between these two regimes but the greatest is that the non-CPM regime promotes extension before flexion and the CPM regime flexion before extension. The therapist must take this into account when preparing the rehabilitation programme, and discuss the issues with the patient.

Rehabilitation

Preoperative

Prior to surgery the postoperative regimen must be discussed with the patient and the range of knee motion, and quadriceps strength including lag, must be recorded. It is likely that a preoperative fixed flexion deformity of the knee will still be present after the operation. The patient should be shown any form of immobilization – splint, POP back slab, etc. – prior to surgery and advised on how, when and why it is to be worn. If a CPM machine is to be used, the patient should try this before surgery and initial measurements can be made for ease post-surgery. It is important that the CPM machine is set up correctly and that the patient understands how it works and any problems that may occur – pressure under the ischial tuberosity, correct positioning of the knee, emergency release switch, etc. (Coutts et al 1989). If possible, isometric quadriceps exercises should be encouraged preoperatively but these may be very difficult because of pain, effusion and deformity. If no walking aids have been used before then the patient should practise using them.

Early postoperation stage

Irrespective of use of the CPM or not, isometric quadriceps, glutei and isotonic foot pumps should be started from day 1 post-operation.

Self-assessment question

- SAQ 8.3 Why is it particularly important for a patient following a total knee replacement to carry out isometric quadriceps exercises immediately postoperatively?

(Answer at end of chapter.)

No continuous passive motion

If the knee is immobilized, then no active exercise to the knee can begin until this is removed. During this period, active motion of the ankle, toes and hip on the operated side should be encouraged, remembering that a straight leg raise will not be possible at this early stage. Indeed straight leg raises should only be used as an isometric quadriceps exercise and not as a test of quadriceps function.

The immobilization device can stay in situ for any time between 3 and 7 days (Harms & Engstrom 1991, Johnson 1990) but as soon as this is removed active assisted knee flexion should begin. A friction-free board, therapist assistance or a pulley system have all been used to promote assisted flexion but the patient should try to undertake the action actively where possible.

Problem–solving exercise 8.6

What state would you expect the knee to be in on release from immobilization?
What should you be concerned about?

(Answer at end of chapter.)

At this stage the patient may be very apprehensive about moving the limb and encouragement should be given as well as physical assistance. There is a great difference between initial movement of a hip and knee post-replacement. Patients with hip replacements do not have the same anxieties about moving the joint, bursting the stitches, etc. This is partly because they cannot easily see the hip wound, but also because there is less inhibition to the surrounding musculature.

Once movement has started, there will be an increase in pain and the patient may feel aching in the quadriceps/hamstrings muscles or around the patella. Passive mobilization of the patella and the scar may help to reduce pain in this area and make it easier to gain flexion. Care must be taken if a patellar resurfacing has taken place and consultation with the surgeon may be necessary before doing mobilization techniques to the patella.

A progressive exercise regime should be undertaken at least twice per day for at least 20 minutes but will vary depending on general strength, endurance and postoperative complications. By the seventh postoperative day the patient will normally have 50–70° of active knee flexion and fixed flexion deformity of 4–8° (Harms & Engstrom 1991, Johnson 1990).

Assisted weight bearing begins from day 2 post-operation and is usually undertaken with an immobilization device until good quadriceps control has been achieved (Harms & Engstrom 1991).

As with the total hip replacement patients, an early discharge scheme may be in operation. Patients with no surgical complications will be discharged home at 5–6 days so long as they have assistance at home. When this type of scheme is in operation, CPM is not normally used so that the patient has good knee extension with limited knee flexion prior to discharge. Return of knee flexion will be undertaken at home along with isometric and isotonic extension work.

Continuous passive motion

As mentioned above, CPM may be applied in the surgical recovery room or ward during the first 24 hours after surgery (Fig. 8.11). If this is the case then the therapist may be responsible for the application and care of the machine. The patient should keep a record of the time on and off the machine and any problems experienced.

The CPM will only move the knee passively through the desired range, so from day 1 on the machine there must be definite exercise times. The rehabilitation emphasis must be towards gaining static and controlled inner-range quadriceps contraction. Therefore, active knee flexion should not be encouraged until quadriceps function is achieved (Coutts et al 1989). Passive mobilization techniques to the patella may be necessary at this stage to ensure the return of flexion, but this is not as essential as for the non-CPM group. Active assisted knee flexion will always return much more quickly than with the non-CPM group (Coutts 1983, Harms & Engstrom 1991, Johnson 1990, McInnes et al 1992).

Figure 8.11 Continuous passive motion machine. (Kinetic CPM, courtesy of Smith & Nephew, Richards Ltd. 2003.)

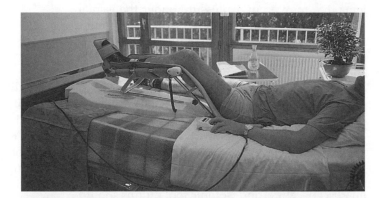

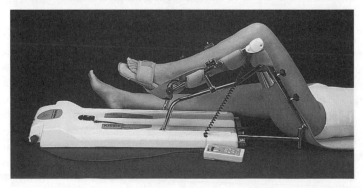

By day 7 post-operation the patient should easily have 70–90° of flexion but will have a similar degree of fixed flexion deformity to the non-CPM group (Gose 1987, Ritter et al 1989, Romness & Rand 1988). There is evidence that the longer the patient spends on the CPM the smaller the fixed flexion deformity (Basso & Knapp 1987). Maloney et al (1990) advocate the use of a bolster under the heel while the leg is on the CPM to ensure that the knee goes into full extension.

Patients on CPM have a greater quadriceps lag (Ritter et al 1989) and should be advised to wear a splint at night, or when off the CPM, to reduce the possibility of holding the knee in flexion, encouraging a quadriceps lag (Harms & Engstrom 1991, Ritter et al 1989).

Once again, weight bearing with a splint can start on postoperative day 2 and without the splint only when quadriceps control has been established. Unsupported weight bearing is often a day or two later in the CPM group because of the presence of a greater quadriceps lag.

Harms & Engstrom (1990) indicate that, following knee replacement, patients who achieve 60–70° of flexion by day 7 and 70–80° at day 14 postoperatively have 'the optimal rate of return of knee movement'. These guidelines should be used for patients, whether on CPM or not.

Comparison between regimes with and without CPM indicate that the CPM group will:

- always gain a greater degree of knee flexion (Coutts 1983) at an earlier stage (Vince et al 1987)
- have an easier return of knee flexion (Harms & Engstrom 1991)
- have less effusion (McInnes et al 1992)
- have smaller risk of manipulation (Coutts 1983, McInnes et al 1992)
- have a shorter stay in hospital (Coutts 1983, Johnson 1990)
- have less risk of DVT (Vince et al 1987).

There will be a greater financial outlay to purchase CPM machines but this expense has been costed to be less than that incurred by the additional treatment (i.e. manipulation) and length of hospital stay necessary because of not using CPM (McInnes et al 1992).

By 1 year following operation there is very little difference in the performance of the knee joint

(Wasilewski et al 1990). An average of 101° of knee flexion is to be expected, with a minimal fixed flexion deformity of 4° and no extensor lag (Johnson 1990). Disadvantages of CPM in the early stage relate to increased time in bed, loss of independence if on CPM for long periods, discomfort, incidence of common peroneal nerve palsy, time taken to maintain the machine and non-compliance from the patient (McInnes et al 1992).

There have been no longitudinal studies of a CPM group to see if there are disadvantages, either biomechanical or physical, at a later stage.

Problem–solving exercise 8.7

A patient with a 3-day-old new knee joint is complaining of a hot painful knee joint following inner-range quadriceps exercise. On inspection, the knee is slightly more swollen than prior to treatment. Why do you think this has occurred and what would you do about it?

Answer

Possible causes are: infection, DVT, too much exercise too soon.

The patient's body temperature needs to be checked to see if there are any signs of infection.

Also check to see if there are any signs of a DVT in the calf (swelling, pain and discomfort). The knee also swells and becomes hot and painful if there is inflammation present. This could be part of the normal healing process but it is also possible that the patient was doing too much exercise too quickly. All these signs should be reported to the nursing staff and recorded in appropriate medical/nursing or paramedical notes. Ice may be applied to the knee, if sensation is intact, and the leg elevated to help reduce the signs.

It is very difficult to know when and how hard to 'push' the patient, so start slowly and progress from exercise session to exercise session: every patient is different.

The symptoms above can occur at any stage of the rehabilitation process and the three thoughts of infection, DVT or too much too soon, should be kept in mind. At the later stages, loosening or joint wear should be added to this list.

The knee can also become hot and painful if flexion is 'pushed' too much. This may happen in the non-CPM group because they are not moving into flexion as regularly as the CPM group. If knee joint flexion has not reached 60–70° by day 7 then it may be prudent to start the patient on CPM, taking knee flexion up to its maximum and keeping the machine on for a minimum of 6 hours a day to complement normal exercise sessions. Flexion range should be increased by at least 10° per day as for the CPM regime but this should be pushed as much as possible. On this 'added' passive flexion regime, the knee should reach 80–90° by day 14.

If a CPM machine is not available then manipulation under anaesthetic (MUA) may be indicated. Under general anaesthetic the patient's knee is forced into flexion, stretching any intra-articular adhesions that have developed. Following an MUA, CPM could be used to augment therapy but if not then the therapist must work hard with the patient to maintain the passive flexion range before gaining active flexion and extension. Either post-MUA or with the 'added' CPM regime, some degree of active knee extension will be lost, but this will return in time.

The alternative problem is when an extensor lag or fixed flexion deformity will not resolve. This can be a particular problem for the CPM group and occurs if there is an imbalance between the gain of flexion and of extension (Harms & Engstrom 1991). Progression of passive flexion should be stopped until there is an increased range of flexion or reduction of the extensor lag. To reduce the fixed flexion deformity the posterior aspect of the knee must be stretched and isometric quadriceps exercises encouraged in this new position.

Problem–solving exercise 8.8

How would you stretch the posterior aspect of a prosthetic knee replacement?

(Answer at end of chapter.)

Whatever the technique used to gain extension the therapist should not force the knee into extension by applying a large anteroposterior force down through the extended knee. Apart from causing excessive pain, this will increase hamstring spasm, and therefore more flexion, the force may also affect the fixation of the joint. Gentle manual mobilization techniques (Gd I or II Maitland mobilizations) can be used to help increase extension, but only with caution.

An extensor lag will only decrease if the inner range quadriceps strength increases and any joint effusion is kept to a minimum. Therefore it is essential that the patient carry out specific inner-range extension exercises on an hourly basis. This becomes imperative when weight bearing is commenced, as often the patient is more anxious to get up walking than to undertake specific extension exercises.

Functional rehabilitation

In either group (CPM or non-CPM) functional retraining will take place once weight bearing without a splint commences. Wearing a splint will not encourage a normal walking pattern and therefore walking should be limited where possible. Weight bearing without the splint will encourage quadriceps control so long as there is no large extensor lag (>15°). Closed chain exercises in the parallel bars, e.g. foot placement, low-level step-ups (5–8 cm) or small-arc cycling in extension, will all encourage extension without putting the joint under excessive strain. Practising sitting to standing from various heights and stair climbing will also promote muscle strengthening, joint mobility and proprioception.

All functional activities must be undertaken under supervision in the early stages and correction of compensatory patterns must be encouraged. If there are ongoing difficulties with function gains, loss of proprioception may be the main problem. The suggestion that the use of a CPM machine enhances the return of this sensation has not been supported by research evidence (Coutts 1983). Barrett et al (1991) assessed the proprioception of patients following knee replacement and found that initially this was particularly poor; some degree of progression was made over time but preoperative levels were not reached.

Problem–solving exercise 8.9

What compensatory patterns might occur when a patient with a knee replacement walks?

(Answer at end of chapter.)

An overall leg length discrepancy may be present post-surgery but this is far less common than in the hip joint. The discrepancy is usually less than 1 cm and can be accommodated, unless the patient has limited movement in the hip and lumbar spine. Only then should a temporary heel raise be applied.

Outcome

Dandy & Edwards (2003) consider that a knee replacement is successful if:

- the knee straightens
- the knee gains flexion to 100°
- the leg takes the patient's weight
- the joint is stable.

These outcomes are far lower than those expected following a hip joint replacement and indicate the limited expectations of the joint. These indicators must be made clear to the patient, indicating that it is considered to be a good outcome if 80% of patients are still able to achieve these goals at 5 years post-surgery (Dandy & Edwards 2003).

There are other beneficial outcomes from undertaking a knee joint replacement. Ries et al (1996) showed that in 13 patients there was 'a trend toward improvement in cardiovascular fitness 1 year after total knee arthroplasty and a significant improvement 2 years postoperatively for patients who had been able to resume routine functional activities because of the arthroplasty'. If full knee motion is not regained following surgery, the patient should gain an increase in general function and fitness after a period of time.

A walking aid may be used by a number of patients but this is usually one stick; exceptions to this may be patients with rheumatoid arthritis whose general pathology may limit return to full mobility. Often assistance is needed for stair climbing or descending and the patient may not feel confident doing this and will use a banister.

Avoidance of twisting and turning, high-impact forces, such as are sustained during jumping and running, and sudden jarring movements is essential for at least 3 months postoperation; some surgeons extend this to 6 months. Driving can be very difficult because of the repeated small arc motion needed to use the accelerator and clutch, not to mention the jarring movement of the brake pedal.

Loss of proprioception is normal with any joint replacement but removal of the anterior cruciate and joint capsule, with joint effusion, exaggerates this loss following a knee replacement. Knee joint proprioception is definitely needed for driving and return of this may be used, along with inner-range quadriceps strength and range of motion, as a guide to when to recommence driving.

As mentioned earlier, return to sporting activity may be possible following knee arthroplasty but consultation with the surgeon is essential before any sport is recommenced, or recommended to the patient.

Case study 8.1: Mr Nicholls

Mr Nicholls is a 70-year-old gentleman with a 20-year history of osteoarthrosis. He is a retired carpenter (retired at 60 due to problems with his knees, hips and right shoulder). He had a right hip replacement 4 years ago but over the last year the pain in the right knee has increased markedly and his mobility is severely limited. He has been admitted to the orthopaedic ward for a right knee replacement.

He lives with his wife in a terraced house with steep stairs. His bed was moved downstairs 6 months ago and there is a downstairs toilet.

On observation, Mr Nicholls is rather overweight and moves with difficulty, complaining of pain both at rest and on movement. Right knee is swollen with decreased muscle bulk, fixed flexion deformity (15°) with marked osteophyte formation and joint thickening felt on palpation. (These findings are mirrored on the left side but with no flexion defor-mity). Range of movement is decreased and there is marked tenderness medially and posteriorly.

Mr Nicholls's cervical spine is stiff with some discomfort on movement, the right shoulder, left knee and left hip have reduced range, and he has pain in them.

Functionally, Mr Nicholls can get up from a chair if the seat is high and there are arms. He needs help getting in and out of bed and it is difficult to turn over. He sleeps with a pillow under his right knee and reports that he has not had an unbroken night's sleep in the last 3 months because of the pain.

He can walk a short distance with two sticks. He is now unable to drive (his wife cannot drive).

He cannot get into the bath. There is a separate shower at home but it is upstairs and so difficult to get to. There is a high seat for the toilet and grab rails already fitted.

Problem-solving exercise 8.10

Try to work out a realistic set of goals of treatment for this gentleman and suggest possible interventions you think may be of use in this case.

Which other members of the healthcare team might be involved?

After you have worked out your answers, read the next section.

Physiotherapy goals for Mr Nicholls

Mr Nicholls has a lot more problems to deal with than the previous case study, Mrs Stamford (Chapter 7), however your approach with regard to physiotherapy input may be very similar. It is also important to keep in mind which other members of the healthcare team may be involved and how and when you need to communicate with them as appropriate. Another essential point to remember is the patient's viewpoint – what needs does he perceive that he has?

This patient has been admitted for a total knee replacement – your intervention is likely to be affected by a number of factors:

- Orthopaedic surgeons often have specific post-operative regimens for their patients. In the ideal situation the physiotherapist will have been involved in the initial design of this regimen.
- In some hospitals there are systems whereby the physiotherapist is involved throughout the management of the patients, i.e. seeing them in orthopaedic clinic before admission, then while in hospital and finally through to the home vis-its and occasionally post-discharge. In other sit-uations you will only see patients while they are on the ward.

Hopefully you can see how these factors would affect both the amount and type of your intervention.

Mr Nicholls has a long history of osteoarthrosis and is quite disabled. He will probably have had physiotherapy before. Your goals of treatment may involve the following:

1. Reduction of pain
2. To maintain or increase range of movement in the joints not involved in the operation
3. To work on range of movement in the new right knee joint – hopefully to reach 90° for good function
4. To maintain and increase muscle strength if possible, particularly quadriceps and gluteal muscles
5. To maximize function within the limits of the patient's abilities
6. Education/advice/support as necessary for both patient and carer, encouraging self-care and management.

These goals would need to be tailored specifically for Mr Nicholls and related to his environment and abilities.

Possible interventions

1. Much of the pain will be relieved by the knee replacement itself (once the soreness of the

wound has gone). Mr Nicholls is used to using two sticks; you might change his walking aid if you and the patient feel it would be helpful. For example, elbow crutches or a walking frame may be useful, at least initially, to relieve weight and in turn reduce pain. This can then be changed as Mr Nicholls improves. It is unlikely that you would carry out any local pain-relieving techniques.

2. For increase of range in the operated knee there is often use of CPM, plus a set of exercises as appropriate, depending on the postoperative regimen used. Active knee flexion in half lying with a friction-free board and a 'donut' under the heel should be encouraged whenever possible. Sitting over the side of the bed, when grade 2+ quadriceps control has been regained, doing flexion and extension will help restore movement.

3. Increase in range, muscle power and function are usually addressed by some sort of exercise regimen, starting with bed exercises and then becoming more active as the patient mobilizes. Exercise sheets are sometimes used – these can be standardized or if appropriate computer software is available. A scheme could be designed specifically for Mr Nicholls. Quadriceps strength in particular must be emphasized; return of this will give more knee stability, proprioception and therefore greater balance control and safety in walking. If Mr Nicholls has a quadriceps lag then it is better to provide a knee extension splint of some kind so that no uncontrolled force can be exerted inadvertently, especially on walking.

4. Hydrotherapy may be indicated if a pool is available on site. This type of treatment can reduce pain through warmth and weight reduction. It is useful for general exercise, which would be important for a patient such as this who has widespread problems. It is also useful for increasing exercise tolerance.

5. Education, advice and support resources will vary from place to place. This could be on a one-to-one basis, with the therapist talking to Mr Nicholls and his wife, or might be in a group. Some hospitals have information available in written and/or audiovisual forms. Occasionally this support is continued at home by community services, especially if there is a 'fast track' early-discharge system in operation. Possible advice for Mr Nicholls might include:

- 'do's and 'don't's following joint replacement
- information on joint protection
- advice on home exercise and amounts of general activity
- dietary information (as he is overweight)
- available aids and appliances
- services available in the local area and how to access them
- benefits he may be entitled to
- useful addresses.

It is also important to encourage the patient and his wife to ask questions, particularly if anything is worrying them.

The other members of the healthcare team who might be involved include:

- Mr Nicholls and his wife (plus any other family or friends who may help out)
- Orthopaedic surgeon
- Nursing staff
- Occupational therapist
- Social worker/social services
- Dietitian
- Community staff, e.g. physiotherapist, occupational therapist, nurse, home help
- General practitioner
- Self-help groups (if available in the locality)
- Volunteer helpers.

This list may be longer or shorter for each patient you come into contact with.

SUMMARY OF HIP AND KNEE REPLACEMENT

Hip and knee replacement surgery has excellent outcomes for the majority of patients (80% at 5 years). Unfortunately when complications arise they can be major. Realistic expectations must be encouraged and the patient should be made aware of all possibilities – good and bad.

This is particularly true for the younger patient (under 65 years) for whom joint survival is especially important. The therapist must place emphasis on knowing the surgical regime to be used and the normal postoperative management. Understanding the complications and how they present, and informing the consultant or GP if you are anxious about the new joint or patient progression, are all important.

Return of full joint function will only be gained if the soft tissue length and strength is returned and this takes time, good physical therapy and compliance from the patient.

UPPER LIMB JOINT REPLACEMENT

The shoulder, elbow, wrist, metacarpophalangeal (MCP) and interphalangeal (IP) joints can all be replaced with artificial arthroplasties, although their survival is limited. These surgeries are very specialized and are not routinely seen in most orthopaedic wards, except where surgical management of rheumatoid arthritis is undertaken or if a consultant has a particular interest. Many physiotherapists will not encounter these types of replacement and advice should be sought from either the senior physiotherapy staff or the consultant involved. In some cases it may be prudent to contact a local therapy 'expert' if there is only limited expertise available in house.

Unlike the lower limbs, the upper limbs only bear minimal weight, unless the person uses a walking aid. Therefore the artificial joints do not have to cope with the same biomechanical demands as the lower limb joints but do require good range of motion and stability. Rheumatoid arthritis is the main pathology associated with upper limb replacements and the achievable main outcome is pain relief with return of movement and function being an added benefit.

Shoulder joint

The shoulder is the upper limb joint most commonly replaced, constrained or semi-constrained joints being the type of choice. The arthroplasties emulate the modified ball and socket joint of the shoulder and can provide almost full range of shoulder movement and full pain relief (Kessel & Bayley 1986). The results of surgery show that the patient's postoperative movement depends on the state of the joint prior to the surgery and the surrounding muscle strength. Pain relief is usually good but joint movement may be only marginally greater than the preoperative range. The stability

of the normal shoulder joint is dependent on the strength of the capsule and the surrounding ligaments and muscles (Kessel & Bayley 1986).

Unfortunately, the underlying pathology, usually rheumatoid arthritis, disrupts both the capsule and adjoining ligaments and this is compounded by the surgical procedure. As rotator cuff problems are often associated with rheumatoid arthritis or secondary osteoarthritis, the shoulder is often weak and unstable prior to surgery. The constrained shoulder replacements (e.g. Bayely-Walker prosthesis) have good inherent stability but the unconstrained joints (e.g. Neer prosthesis) rely on the muscles around the shoulder joint to provide this. In many cases these muscles are weak and thus in the early stages post-surgery the joint must be protected from adverse movement. Some postoperative treatment regimes will include stabilization in the scapular plane to allow fibrous repair of the shoulder capsule and ligaments before active shoulder movement is allowed.

Treatment regimes vary considerably depending on the type of joint and the surgical procedure and it is advisable that the regimen is discussed with the consultant or senior staff before active or passive shoulder movement is attempted.

Rehabilitation of both range of movement and the adjoining muscle strength will provide return of both stability and function. Shoulder movement may start from 7 days postoperatively but some surgeons will delay active movement until 4–6 weeks post-surgery.

It is important to aid return of stability so therapists should concentrate on isometric muscle contraction in the stabilized position initially, with the rotator cuff muscles being most important. Gradually the other muscles, especially deltoid, biceps and triceps will be included, but emphasis must still be placed on the external rotators as these will be considerably weaker than the other muscles. Once movement is allowed, isometric contractions through range will encourage more control of shoulder joint movement, before isotonic muscle work is introduced.

When exercise or function is not being undertaken then the shoulder must be supported in the position of safety, which will be dictated by the surgical procedure used and may be either in a sling or collar and cuff by the side or in the scapular plane position of 80° flexion, neutral rotation and 45° cross adduction, with a 'wedge' supporting the arm.

Although shoulder replacements have been available for a number of years there is limited published research on their outcome. It is estimated that the complication rate is less than 5% and loosening occurs in 3% (Johns Hopkins Department of Orthopaedic Surgery 2000).

The take-home message for shoulder replacements is stability first and then movement, liaise with medical and senior physiotherapy staff to find out the postsurgical routine, and return of muscle strength in a controlled range of motion is the major treatment objective. The patient may be disappointed with the lack of return of movement but many functions can be rehabilitated, with the help of gadgets or adapted movement, and relief of pain is usually certain.

Elbow joint

The elbow joint requires strength and stability as it is often the end of the movement arc for lifting. It has complex biomechanics and it is very difficult to emulate these in a prosthetic joint. Stability is a major issue and constrained hinge joints were therefore designed to supply this. This type of elbow joint unfortunately does not allow rotation and the fixation around the stem–bone interface can loosen more easily because of this. The Strathclyde elbow arthroplasty is a semi-constrained (snap-fit) joint that offers good return of movement and stability.

Once again pain relief post-surgery is good and a functional range of motion is usually achieved. The majority of elbow replacements are inserted in patients with rheumatoid arthritis and their symptoms will have been severe for them to have been considered for this type of surgery. The range of movement may be restricted, so the replacements have good longevity. Potential problems with wound healing, infection, nerve damage or dislocation can occur in approximately 1–5% of cases but about 90% of patients with rheumatoid arthritis will have a good functioning elbow at 5 years. But only 50–70% of patients with other pathologies, e.g. osteoarthrosis or fracture, will have a good result at 5 years (OxMed.com 2002).

As with any elbow injury, forced passive movement should not be undertaken at any time during rehabilitation as this may predispose the tissue to myositis ossificans.

Wrist/hand joints

The wrist does not have a good replacement history and replacement is undertaken very rarely, mainly for the relief of pain. The MCPs and IPs, however, can be replaced and offer both relief of pain and return of some movement. As the function of the hand requires dexterity and strength, return of function following MCP or IP arthroplasty is again limited but is often far better than the preoperative state. Such replacements with silicone elastomer implants are only done by a few specialist hand surgeons and are not seen routinely in the orthopaedic ward. Therefore specialist hand therapists will also be involved in the rehabilitation of these patients and advice should be sought from them should the need arise.

CONCLUSIONS

The role of the physiotherapist in joint replacement rehabilitation is changing and the emphasis on getting the patient out of hospital quickly has resulted in the shorter-term objectives being addressed in hospital while longer-term issues are left to information sheets or follow-up clinics. Thus we must be clear in the message we give to patients and indicate the precautions that might give their prosthetic joints greater longevity. Remember the dos and don'ts; muscle strength will take many months to return and may not do so fully; and exercises will have to be undertaken regularly for some time. Even when the patient feels better, exercises should be continued to ensure real benefit.

It will not be until longer follow-up review of the patients has been undertaken, comparing the results of hospital rehabilitation with early discharge, that the true advantages of these schemes will be known. Until then we must concentrate on giving good advice, with achievable short-term goals, and if possible become involved in postoperative follow-up clinics. The government has proposed that specialist joint replacement units should be established throughout the country (National Audit Office 2003) to manage patients more appropriately. This may assist in understanding and researching the rehabilitation process.

ANSWERS TO QUESTIONS AND EXERCISES

Self-assessment question 8.1 (page 237)

- **SAQ 8.1** How would you measure apparent and true leg length discrepancies?

  Answer:

  Apparent: with the patient in supine, lying with the head, shoulders, pelvis and lower limbs aligned. Place the end of the tape measure on the xiphisternum, extend it down to the medial malleolus and record the length on this side before measuring the other. If there is an adduction contracture then the 'good' leg should be adducted to the same degree as the contracture for comparison. Apparent shortening will demonstrate whether there is a pelvic obliquity and may be accompanied by true shortening.

  True: with the patient in supine and the pelvis level the heels will not be level if a true discrepancy is present. To identify where the discrepancy is, three measurements need to be taken:

  - from the anterior superior iliac spines on each side of the pelvis to the medial malleolus on the same side (complete limb length)
  - from the greater trochanter to lateral joint line (femoral length)
  - from the medial knee joint line in flexion to the medial malleolus that side (tibial length).

  Measurements from each side and between apparent and true can then be compared.

  Leg length discrepancy may be present in the femoral neck but this is very difficult to measure and may present as an apparent deformity. If the pelvis is mobile and can be levelled, and there is no true leg length discrepancy in the presence of an apparent difference, then there will be a shortening of the femoral neck. (McRae 1997, Chapter 10, page 151–153).

Problem-solving exercise 8.1 (page 242)

- Which of the common surgical complications from the answer to SAQ 5.7 do you think

patients following total hip replacement are most prone to?

Answer: Infection, deep vein thrombus or pulmonary embolus, or respiratory problems.

Problem-solving exercise 8.2 (page 244)

See information in text.

Problem-solving exercise 8.3 (page 245)

- How can the therapist measure the functions of: walking, stair climbing, sit to stand or forward flexion (e.g. to put on shoes or socks)?

  Answer:

  Walking: Measure distance walked, time taken to achieve this (McNicol et al 1980). Observe and note any gait abnormalities (Perry 1992).

  Stair climbing: Record the time taken, pattern used and use of aids (e.g. banister or walking aid) to perform the function.

  Sit to stand: Again the time taken and the pattern used should be noted. Here the position of the feet, use of the hands and the trunk motion are particularly important (Ada & Westwood 1992).

  A video of the performance of any of these activities will be particularly useful and will help the patient to recognize improved performance of these activities.

  Forward flexion: **Remember that this can be measured preoperatively but not postoperatively until at least 3 months.** Measuring the distance from fingertip to floor represents both lumbar and hip movement but if hip movement alone is to be recorded then a goniometer or electrogoniometer should be used. If this is not possible, again a video of the activity will be helpful. Markers to the anterior and posterior superior iliac spines, greater trochanter, lateral femoral condyle and lateral malleolus will assist observation of the video.

Self-assessment question 8.2 (page 245)

- **SAQ 8.2** In what position does a total hip joint replacement dislocate?

  Answer: You would be correct if you answered:

- *anterolateral and true lateral incision*: the hip will dislocate if placed in excessive extension, external rotation and adduction, or a combination of all three

- *posterolateral incision*: the hip will dislocate in excessive flexion, internal rotation and adduction, or a combination of all three.

Problem-solving exercise 8.4 (page 248)

See information in text.

Problem-solving exercise 8.5 (page 253)

- Identify the common complications specific to a knee joint replacement.

Answer: Dislocation, loosening, wound infection, deep joint infection, deep vein thrombus or pulmonary embolus, wear of the prosthetic surface.

Self-assessment question 8.3 (page 255)

- **SAQ 8.3** Why is it particularly important for a patient following a total knee replacement to carry out isometric quadriceps exercises immediately postoperatively?

   Answer:
- To reduce joint effusion: contraction of the four components of the group compresses the suprapatellar pouch and so helps to remove excess fluid from the knee joint
- Pain acts as an inhibitor to muscle activity, so early contraction of the quadriceps is important to overcome this
- The patient is more than likely to have had a fixed flexion deformity preoperatively and the quadriceps function will be non-existent in the inner range. Encouragement of early activity will help to achieve the return of inner-range strength.

Problem-solving exercise 8.6 (page 255)

a. What state would you expect the knee to be in on release from immobilization?
b. What should you be concerned about?

   Answer:
a. The knee will appear bruised, swollen and may be covered with antiseptic dye. A single or double suction drain will be protruding from the joint and there will be an obvious surgical scar (as described earlier). The knee should lie in more extension than preoperatively but this may not be apparent because of swelling. The muscles around the knee will appear flaccid and the patient may feel the leg to be extremely heavy.
b. Wound healing – are any open parts of the wound infected or necrosed? This information can be gleaned from the nursing staff or doctors but it is not uncommon for the therapist to be present when the immobilization is removed. Also you will need to inspect the wound when flexion starts so that any leaking, bleeding or gaping can be observed and recorded. A premobilizing look at the wound is essential.

Problem-solving exercise 8.7 (page 257)

See information in text.

Problem-solving exercise 8.8 (page 258)

- How would you stretch the posterior aspect of a prosthetic knee replacement?

   Answer:
- Immobilization in POP, knee extension splint, serial casting or reversed dynamic traction are all possible techniques
- Encourage passive knee extension stretch at all times, e.g. keep the feet elevated with knees straight when in bed or sitting
- Encourage isometric quadriceps exercises in as much extension as is possible and inner-range quadriceps exercises to maximum extension.

Problem-solving exercise 8.9 (page 259)

- What compensatory patterns might occur when a patient with a knee replacement walks?

   Answer:
- Dependent use of walking aids – limited balance, anxiety
- Keep the knee straight during stance – compensation for weak quadriceps

- Reduced hip extension and push off during stance on the operated side – compensation for a generally stiff knee and not wanting to move it
- Excessive flexion of the hip and ankle on operated side during swing phase – compensation for limited knee flexion

- Shortened step length – compensation for lack of extension

Problem-solving exercise 8.10 (page 260)

See information in text.

References

Ada L, Westwood P 1992 A kinematic analysis of recovery of the ability to stand up following stroke. Australian Journal of Physiotherapy 38: 135–142

Andriacchi TP, Hurwitz DE 1997 Gait biomechanics and the evolution of total joint replacement. Gait and Posture 5: 256–264

Association of Orthopaedic Chartered Physiotherapists 1991 Survey of uncomplicated, cemented total hip replacements. AOCP, London

Barrett DS, Cobb AG, Bentley G 1991 Joint proprioception in normal osteoarthritic and replaced knees. Journal of Bone and Joint Surgery 73B: 53–56

Bartzokas C, Johnson R, Jane M et al 1994 Relation between mouth and hematogenous infection in total joint replacements. British Medical Journal 309: 506–508

Basso D, Knapp L 1987 Comparison of two continuous passive motion protocols for patients with total knee implants. Physical Therapy 67: 360–363

Borstlap M, Zant J, Vansoesbergen M, Vanderkorst J 1994 Effects of total hip replacement on quality of life in patients with osteoarthritis and in patients with rheumatoid arthritis. Clinical Rheumatology 13: 45–50

Brinker M, Reuben J, Mull J et al 1997 Comparison of general and epidural anaesthesia in patients undergoing primary unilateral THR. Orthopedics 20: 109–115

Cameron I, Quine S 1994 External hip protectors – likely noncompliance among high-risk elderly people living in the community. Archives of Gerontology and Geriatrics 19: 273–281

Coutts F, Hewetson D, Matthew J 1989 Continuous passive motion of the knee joint: use at the Royal National Orthopaedic Hospital, Stanmore. Physiotherapy 75: 427–430

Coutts R 1983 The effect of continuous passive motion on total knee rehabilitation. Orthopaedic Transactions 7: 355–356

Crawford Adams J, Stossel C 1992 Standard orthopaedic operations, 4th edn. Churchill Livingstone, Edinburgh

Dandy D, Edwards D 2003 Essential orthopaedics and trauma, 4th edn. Churchill Livingstone, Oxford

Echternach J 1990 Clinics in physical therapy: physical therapy of the hip. Churchill Livingstone, New York

Engh C, Bobyn J 1985 Biological fixation in total hip arthroplasty. Slack, Thorofare, NJ

Engh C, Bobyn J, Glassman A 1987 Porous-coated hip replacement: the factors governing bone in-growth,
stress shielding and clinical results. Journal of Bone and Joint Surgery 69: 145

Fender D, Harper WM, Gregg PJ 1999 Outcome of Charnley total hip replacement across a single health region in England. Journal of Bone and Joint Surgery 81B: 577–581

Fernandez Galinski D, Puig M, Rue M et al 1996 Pain evaluation in elderly patients after orthopaedic surgery under regional anaesthesia. Pain Clinics 9: 303–309

Fitzpatrick R, Shortall E, Sculpher M 1998 Primary total hip replacement surgery: a systematic review of outcomes and modelling of cost effectiveness associated with different prostheses. Health Technology Assessment 2: 1–64

Franzen H, Johnsson R, Nilsson LT 1997 Impaired quality of life 10 to 20 years after primary arthroplasty. Journal of Arthroplasty 12: 21–24

Ganz SB, Wilson PD, Cioppa-Mosca J, Peterson MG 2003 The day of discharge after total hip arthroplasty and the achievement of rehabilitation functional milestones: 11-year trends. Journal of Arthroplasty 18: 453–457

Garellick G, Malchau H, Herberts P 1998 Specific or general health outcomes measures in the evaluation of total hip replacement. A comparison between the Harris Hip Score and the Nottingham Health Profile. Journal of Bone and Joint Surgery 80: 600–606

Goldie B 1992 Orthopaedic diagnosis and management. Blackwell Scientific, Oxford

Goodfellow J, Kershaw C, Benson M, O'Connor J 1988 The Oxford knee for unicompartmental osteoarthritis. Journal of Bone and Joint Surgery 70B: 692–701

Gose J 1987 Continuous passive motion in the postoperative treatment of patients with total knee replacements. Physical Therapy 67: 39–42

Hajat S, Fitzpatrick R, Morris R et al 2002 Does waiting for total hip replacement matter? Prospective cohort study. Journal of Health Services and Health Policy 7: 19–25

Harms M, Engstrom B 1991 Continuous passive motion as an adjunct to treatment of the total knee arthroplasty patient. Physiotherapy 77: 301–307

Harris WH 1969 Traumatic arthritis of the hip after dislocation and acetabular fractures: treatment by mold arthroplasty. Journal of Bone and Joint Surgery 51A: 737–755

Hasheminejad A, Birch N, Goddard N 1994 Current attitudes to cementing techniques in British hip surgery.

Annals of the Royal College of Surgeons of England 76: 396–400

Health Technology Board Scotland 2002 Press release – 14 August: Comment on the use of metal on metal hip resurfacing. Available online at: www.htbs.co.uk/news/pressrel.asp?did = 786

Hull R, Raskob G, Pineo G et al 1997 Subcutaneous low-molecular-weight heparin vs warfarin for prophylaxis of deep vein thrombosis after hip or knee implantation – an economic perspective. Archives of Internal Medicine 157: 298–303

Johns Hopkins Department of Orthopaedic Surgery 2000 Patient guide to shoulder replacements. Johns Hopkins University and Health System, Baltimore, MD. Available online at: www.hopkinsmedicine.org/orthopedicsurgery/ sports/shoulder/replacement/index.html

Johnson D 1990 The effect of continuous passive motion on wound healing and joint mobility after knee arthroplasty. Journal of Bone and Joint Surgery 72A: 421–426

Joshi AB, Markovic L, Hardinge K, Murphy JCM 2002 Conversion of a fused hip to total hip arthroplasty. Journal of Bone and Joint Surgery 84A: 1335–1341

Kendall F, McCready E, Provance P 1993 Muscle testing and function. Williams & Wilkins, Baltimore, MD

Kessel L, Bayley I 1986 Clinical Disorders of the Shoulder. Churchill Livingstone, Edinburgh

Kilgus DJ, Amstutz HC, Wolgin MA, Dorey FJ 1990 Joint replacement for ankylosed hips. Journal of Bone and Joint Surgery 72A: 45–54

Kili S, Wright I, Jones RS 2003 Change in Harris hip score in patients on the waiting list for total hip replacement. Annals of the Royal College of Surgeons of England 85: 269–271

Kirwan JR, Currey HL, Freeman MA et al 1994 Overall long-term impact of total hip and knee replacement surgery on patients with osteoarthritis and rheumatoid arthritis. British Journal of Rheumatology 33: 357–360

Maihafer G 1990 Rehabilitation of total hip replacements and fracture management considerations. In: Echternach J (ed) Clinics in physical therapy: physical therapy of the hip. Churchill Livingstone, New York, ch 6

Mallon W, Liebelt R, Mason J 1996 Total joint replacement and golf. Clinics in Sports Medicine 15: 179

Mallory T 1992 Total hip replacement in the 1990s: the procedure, the patient, the surgeon. Orthopaedics 115: 427–430

Maloney W, Schurman D, Hangen D et al 1990 The influence of continuous passive motion on outcome in total knee arthroplasty. Clinical Orthopaedics and Related Research 256: 162–168

McGrath D, Dennyson W, Rolland M 1996 Death rate from pulmonary-embolism following joint replacement surgery. Journal of the Royal College of Surgeons of Edinburgh 41: 265–266

McGrory B, Stuart M, Sim F 1995 Participation in sports after hip and knee arthroplasty – review of literature and survey of surgeon preferences. Mayo Clinic Proceedings 70: 342–348

McInnes J, Larson M, Daltroy L et al 1992 A controlled evaluation of continuous passive motion in patients undergoing total knee arthroplasty. Journal of the American Medical Association 268: 1423–1428

McNicol MF, McHardy R, Chalmers J 1980 Exercise testing before and after hip arthroplasty. Journal of Bone and Joint Surgery 62B: 326–331

McRae R 1997 Clinical orthopaedic examination, 4th edn. Churchill Livingstone, Edinburgh

McRae R, Esser M 2002 Practical fracture treatment, 4th edn. Churchill Livingstone, Oxford

Murray MP, Gore DR, Brewer BJ, Zuegge RC 1976 Comparison of functional performance after McKee–Farrar, Charnley and Muller total hip replacement. Clinical Orthopaedics and Related Research 121: 33–43

National Audit Office 2000 Hip replacements: getting it right first time. Report by the Comptroller and Auditor General, HC417, April. Stationery Office, London

National Audit Office 2003 Hip replacements: an update. Report by the Comptroller and Auditor General, HC956, July. Stationery Office, London

National Institute for Clinical Excellence (NICE) 2000 Guidance on the selection of prostheses for primary total hip replacement. Stationery Office, London

Nilsdottir AK, Lohmander LS 2002 Age and waiting time as predictor of outcome after total hip replacement for osteoarthritis. Rheumatology 41: 1261–1267

Niwa S, Paul JP, Yamamoto S 1987 Total knee replacement. Springer, Tokyo

Nordin M, Frankel V 1989 Biomechanics of the musculoskeletal system. Lea & Febiger, Philadelphia, PA

Norkin CC, White DJ 2003 Measurement of joint motion: a guideline for goniometry, 3rd edn. FA Davis, Philadelphia, PA

O'Driscoll S, Kumar A, Salter B 1983 The effect of the volume of effusion, joint position and continuous passive motion on intra-articular pressure in the rabbit knee. Journal of Rheumatology 10: 360–363

OxMed.com 2002. Total elbow replacement. Available online at: www.Oxmed.com/docs/datafiles/ elbow%20replacement.html

Perrot S, Menkes C 1996 Nonpharmacological approaches to pain in osteoarthritis – available options. Drugs 52: 21–26

Perry J 1992 Gait analysis: normal and pathological function. Slack, Thorofare, NJ

Pettine K, Amlid B, Cabanela M 1991 Elective total hip arthroplasty in patients older than 80 years of age. Clinical Orthopaedics and Related Research 266: 127–132

Pring D, Marks L, Angel J 1988 Mobility after amputation for failed total knee replacements. Journal of Bone and Joint Surgery 70B: 770–771

Ries M, Philbin E, Groff G et al 1996 Improvement in cardiovascular fitness after total knee arthroplasty. Journal of Bone and Joint Surgery 78A: 1696–1701

Ritter M, Gandolf V, Holston K 1989 Continuous passive motion versus physical therapy in total knee arthroplasty. Clinical Orthopaedics and Related Research 244: 239–243

Romness D, Rand J 1988 The role of continuous passive motion following total knee arthroplasty. Clinical Orthopaedics and Related Research 226: 34–37

Rothman R, Hozack W 1988 Complications of total hip replacements. WB Saunders, Philadelphia, PA

Rowe PJ, Nicol AC, Kelly IG 1989 Flexible goniometer computer system for the assessment of hip function. Clinical Biomechanics 4: 68–72

Sahlstrom A, Lanshammer H, Wigren A 1994 Ground reaction force and its moment with respect to the knee joint centre in a total condylar arthroplasty series. Clinical Biomechanics 9: 125–129

Söderman P, Malchau H, Herberts P 2001a Outcome of total hip replacement: a comparison of different measurement methods. Clinical Orthopaedics and Related Research 390: 163–173

Söderman P, Malchau H 2001b Is the Harris Hip Score system useful to study the outcome of total hip replacements? Clinical Orthopaedics and Related Research 384: 189–197

Söderman P, Malchau H, Herberts P et al 2001c Outcome after total hip arthroplasty: part II. Disease specific follow-up and the Swedish National Total Hip Arthroplasty Register. Acta Orthopaedica Scandinavia 72: 113–119

Stanic U, Herman S, Merhar J 1993 Evaluation of rehabilitation of patients with total hip replacements. IEEE Transactions on Rehabilitation Engineering 1: 86–93

University of Leeds, National Health Centre for Reviews and Dissemination 1996 Total hip replacement. (University of Leeds, Nuffield Institute for Health, University of York, NHS Centre for Review and Dissemination.) Effective Health Care 2: 1–12

Vince K, Kelly M, Beck J, Insall J 1987 Continuous passive motion after total knee arthroplasty. Journal of Arthroplasty 2: 281–284

Walker 1987 Cited in Niwa et al 1987

Wasilewski S, Woods L, Torgerson W, Healy W 1990 Value of continuous passive motion in total knee arthroplasty. Orthopaedics 13: 291–295

Woolson S, Watt J 1991 Intermittent pneumatic compression to prevent proximal deep vein thrombosis during and after total hip replacement. Journal of Bone and Joint Surgery 73A: 507–511

Wykman A, Olsson E 1992 Walking ability after total knee replacement. Journal of Bone and Joint Surgery 74B: 53–56

Zavadak K, Gibson K, Whitley D et al 1995 Variability in the attainment of functional milestones during the acute-care admission after total joint replacement. Journal of Rheumatology 22: 482–487

Chapter 9

Bone diseases

Anne-Marie Hassenkamp

CHAPTER CONTENTS

OBJECTIVES

By the end of this chapter you should:

- Have gained insight into the various classifications of different bone diseases
- Have gained an understanding of the different ways in which the physiotherapist can contribute to this area of orthopaedics
- Have gained some confidence in how you can draw on your previously acquired knowledge and experiences by using problem-solving approaches.

KEY WORDS

Orthopaedics, bone disease, tumours, infections, nutrition, metabolic disorders, degenerative conditions, physiotherapy management, assessment.

Prerequisties

In order to get the most from this chapter you need to refresh your knowledge of the problem-solving approach (you may want to refer to the earlier chapters). Browsing through the available orthopaedic journals will help you to develop an insight into the current debates in this area with regard to medical and surgical management. This will allow you to develop an appreciation of the differing roles the physiotherapist can play in the varying arenas of bone disease rehabilitation.

INTRODUCTION

Bone diseases cover an enormous area in the field of orthopaedics, as will become clearer when you look at the classification of these. While a lot of our patients have a frank diagnosis of a specific bone disease (e.g. Paget's disease), others will present with often more hidden signs of this problem, which need careful eliciting in a masterful assessment (e.g. osteoporosis). This aspect of our practice – yet again – is the most important one when dealing with patients complaining of bone problems. If in doubt, go back to Chapter 3 to refresh your own ideas and convictions in this area. Without good assessment skills it is very difficult to plan a reasonable and cohesive management strategy for and with patients who are in need of problem solving that covers not only their immediate musculoskeletal problem but also their future outlook on life and its management.

Having said this, we have already indicated that this is not a one-off difficulty but a long-term one.

In contrast to people with soft tissue injuries, who often refer themselves to a physiotherapist or are referred by their general practitioner, this group of patients will most probably be referred by a specialist (e.g. an orthopaedic surgeon, paediatrician or physician). Communication with the referrer about assessment findings, treatment goals and outcomes, and long-term management is absolutely vital. In this case the physiotherapist is not a single practitioner but a member of a multidisciplinary team, which should of course include patients and/or their carers. Physiotherapy management therefore has to take team issues into account.

Worthington (1994) explored the different aspects of the multidisciplinary team. Uniprofessional models of working have identified a lot of repetition (Jones et al 1995) and variability (Hands & Wilson 1997) putting the patient's outcome of rehabilitation at risk (Ovretveit 1997). The idea of multidisciplinary teams is not new. As far back as 1979 the Royal Commission on the NHS (Bruce 1980) stated that 'we are in no doubt that it is in the patients' interests for multidisciplinary teams to be encouraged'. The difficulties of moving into multidisciplinary working from single professional practice is demanding and difficult and a challenge for all involved in rehabilitation (Hassenkamp 2003, Lowe & O'Hara 2000).

Self-assessment question

- SAQ 9.1 What is your own experience of working in a multidisciplinary team? Try to be specific about who was part of it and in which area of practice it occurred. What do you think was special about this setting for a multidisciplinary team to become involved? Who was perceived to be the leader of the team, and did that balance up with his/her contribution to the overall management of the patient (or did it seem to follow a more established hierarchical set-up)? How were decisions arrived at? Did your initial undergraduate education prepare you for this aspect of practice? How did you get into this aspect of practice if your training did not include it?

It is important to remember that people with a diagnosis of one of the many different bone diseases can literally belong to any age group. We see babies and young children who might be diagnosed with, for example, neurofibromatosis (von Recklinghausen's disease); we might see adults with metabolic problems (e.g. osteoporosis) or tumours, and we often see older patients with, for example, Paget's disease. While these problems often occur in the age groups mentioned they are also well known in other client groups.

Thinking about these different client groups will make you recognize that we as physiotherapists could be meeting them in all sorts of different settings. We might see them in our own hospital departments or wards, in the GP's practice, in their own homes in a domiciliary capacity, in private practice settings. All of these naturally require quite different approaches from the physiotherapists. Good communication skills are therefore absolutely vital. It is good to remember at this point that these skills, like any others, need practising and supervision if they are meant to be of a high order (Thomson et al 1997). The 'common-sense' approach to communication is not really acceptable when we are dealing with patients or their relatives in distress.

Self-assessment question

- **SAQ 9.2** How will you be able to detect whether your communication skills are effective and appropriate? How do you view your patients? You might find Linda Finlay's paper (Finlay 1997) helpful in your reflections.

Earlier on I mentioned that people with bone diseases might have to live with a long-term, at times irreversible problem. In contrast to working with patients with soft tissue injuries or other short-term problems, you will have to change your approach in order to incorporate this aspect. Many of these skills are, of course, exactly the same as in other physiotherapy encounters but obviously the goal setting and treatment planning with the patient must be different in light of the life-long nature of this scenario. Lifestyle questions must therefore be addressed, work positions must be explored and the changing nature of the problem with regard to the future (e.g. ageing) has to be attended to. We need to allow the patient's problem-solving skills to become enhanced and focused.

This life-long aspect of real pathology in contrast to more transient injury makes it particularly important to view the patient as a participator in goal setting and assessment of outcome. Who sets the patient's goals? It is much easier for the physiotherapist to set disease-specific goals than to involve patients in the details of their very personal list of functional priorities. Does patient-focused goal setting really happen and what are the patient's experiences of this? Payton & Nelson (1996) interviewed a group of patients about their views on whether they had an important input in goal setting and treatment planning. Most of their sample felt that their participation in this was not great but they believed that they gave important feedback that influenced the outcome of the actual therapy. When asked if they valued physiotherapy input they were very positive and felt that they had confidence and trust in their physiotherapist. Payton & Nelson's interesting study seems to indicate that the goal setting and treatment planning aspects with patients is the weakest aspect of our interaction with them while the patient's participation in treatment evaluation is the strongest.

The goal attainment scale (GAS; Kiresuk et al 1994) is a widely used outcome measure in rehabilitation. It is a measurement approach that accommodates multiple individual patient goals and has a scoring system that allows for comparisons between patients. Rockwood et al (1997) compared the GAS with several standardized outcome measures in the area of rehabilitation and were able to demonstrate that the GAS was more responsive to change than the other chosen measures. Fisher & Hardie (2002) came to a similar conclusion when looking at its use as an outcome measure in a multidisciplinary pain management programme. They also commented on the therapeutic tool aspect of the GAS as well as on the fact that it was a reliable outcome measure. Reid & Chesson (1998) used the GAS to look at patient-set goals versus physiotherapy-set goals in a group of patients with stroke. Their study identified that patients rarely reached their expected levels of their own goals but scored much higher on the ones set by their physiotherapists. This is an interesting verdict on our model of practice vis-à-vis the patient. The literature on the use of GAS within rehabilitation settings is growing steadily. In an ideal setting the GAS can be used as an outcome measure for the input of the whole multidisciplinary team and could be evaluated by any member of the team.

CLASSIFICATION OF BONE DISEASES

Many different classifications appear in the literature but the one still mostly referred to was established by Wynne-Davies & Fairbank (1976; Box 9.1).

Another way of classifying these abnormalities has been recommended by Dandy (1998; Box 9.2). He suggests an order that looks at the probable cause of the disease.

As you can see, the field of bone diseases is enormous and not easily classified.

Box 9.1   Classification of bone diseases (Wynne–Davies & Fairbank 1976)

1. **Bone dysplasias and malformations**
   - Achondroplasia
   - Osteogenesis imperfecta
   - Diaphyseal aclasis
   - Ollier's disease
   - Paget's disease
   - Polyostotic fibrous dysplasia
   - Neurofibromatosis
   - Fibrodysplasia ossificans progressiva
2. **Inborn errors of metabolism**
   - Gaucher's disease
   - Histiocytosis X
3. **Metabolic bone disease**
   - Hyperparathyroidism
   - Nutritional rickets
   - Other forms of rickets
   - Nutritional osteomalacia
   - Other forms of osteomalacia
   - Vitamin C deficiency
4. **Endocrine disorders**
   - Senile osteoporosis
   - Hypopituitarism
   - Gigantism
   - Acromegaly
   - Hypothyroidism
   - Glucocorticoid excess

Self-assessment question

- **SAQ 9.3** Which of these diseases have you come across? Try to remember as much as possible about them with regard to:
  - the age and sex of the patient
  - the part of the body affected – or did it involve the entire body?
  - the general physical condition of the patient
  - where you met this patient – in hospital? as an outpatient? in the community?

Reading through the lists in Boxes 9.1 and 9.2 you will immediately recognize some conditions and not others. While any of these might come the physiotherapist's way, some will do so with more regularity than others.

Box 9.2   Classification of bone diseases (Dandy 1998)

1. **Abnormalities of bone structure altered by hormones**
   - Growth hormones
   - Sex hormones
   - Thyroid hormones
   - Parathyroid hormones
   - Vitamin C
   - Vitamin D plus calcium
   - Calcitonin
   Collagen forms part of bone and abnormalities here can lead to:
   - Scurvy
   - Osteogenesis imperfecta
   The bone structure can further be influenced by abnormalities of mineralization, which in turn leads to bone loss:
   - Osteomalacia – decreased mineralization
   - Osteolysis – increased removal of osteoclasts
   - Osteopenia – decrease in osteoid tissue
   Often these three occur together and are referred to as osteoporosis.

   Abnormalities of the osteon structure
   - Paget's disease
   - Fibrous dysplasia
   - Other dysplasias

   Abnormalities of cartilage
   - Mucopolysaccharidosis
   - Achondroplasia
   - Diaphyseal aclasis

2. **Osteochondritis**

   Due to vascular abnormalities
   - Perthes disease
   - Kienböck's disease
   - Köhler's disease

   Due to damage to the apophyses
   - Osgood–Schlatter disease
   - Sever's disease
   - Sinding-Larsen's disease
   - Scheuermann's disease

   Others
   - Osteochondritis dissecans
   - Calvé's disease

3. **Bone infections**
   - Osteomyelitis
   - Septic arthritis

Once you have reflected on your encounters with patients with bone diseases you might have already formed an opinion as to the frequency of some of these conditions, as well as their preferred sites and behaviours.

In this chapter I will concentrate on manifestations of bone disease in adults that we as physiotherapists come across and hence will deal with the special happenings and demands of and in that age group.

A shorter list of the main bone diseases, which we as physiotherapists come across more frequently than others, follows. You will immediately realize that this is not a complete list compared with the classifications in Boxes 9.1 and 9.2.

- Dysplasia
  - Paget's disease
- Degenerative
  - Osteoarthrosis
  - Osteochondritis
- Nutritional/metabolic
  - Rickets
  - Osteoporosis
  - Osteomalacia
  - Vitamin C deficiency
- Infections
  - Tuberculosis
  - Osteomyelitis
  - Periostitis
- Tumours
  - Benign
    - Osteoma
    - Chondroma
    - Osteochondroma
    - Giant cell tumour
  - Malignant
    - Osteosarcoma
    - Chondrosarcoma of bone
    - Fibrosarcoma of bone
    - Ewing's tumour
    - Multiple myeloma
    - Secondary (metastatic).

ANATOMY AND PHYSIOLOGY OF BONE

The lists in Boxes 9.1 and 9.2 of different classifications of bone disease and their possible causes necessitate a short review of the anatomy and physiology of bone itself. Any good anatomy/physiology text will help you with this.

Long bones consist mainly of articular cartilage at the top covering the bone of the epiphysis below which the epiphyseal plate is located (in growing bone). The bone of the diaphysis protects the marrow cavity of the bone, which of course is the site of blood cell production. Sherwood (1995) gives a good and concise overview of the physiology of bone:

Growth of long bones is a result of growth hormones.

Bones are made up of a kind of connective tissue, which consists of cells on the one hand and an extracellular matrix on the other that is produced by these cells, which are known as osteoblasts. The matrix is made up of collagen and hence is responsible for the tensile strength of bone. Clearly, though, bone is not really rubbery, as this description might imply. Bone is made hard by the calcium phosphate crystals within this matrix. However, if bones were made up mostly of these crystals they would be hard, brittle and easily breakable. Bones are incredibly strong, light and not brittle because of the structural interweaving of organic scaffolding hardened by inorganic crystals.

The important elements of bone therefore are calcium carbonate, calcium phosphate, collagen and water. Their relative compositions vary with age and health. Calcium carbonate and calcium phosphate make up nearly 60–79% of bone weight. Water makes up about 25–30% of the total bone weight (Hall 1991) and is directly related to its strength. Not all bones are made up in the same way. The smaller the proportion of calcium phosphate and calcium carbonate and the greater the proportion of non-mineralized bone tissue the more porous the bone is. If 5–30% of bone tissue is occupied by non-mineralized tissue (i.e. the less porous a bone is) it is referred to as cortical bone. If 30–90% of bone volume is occupied by non-mineralized tissue the bone is called cancellous bone and is rubbery and spongy. Most bones have an outer layer of cortical bone and an internal layer of cancellous bone. Cortical bone is stronger and hence more able to sustain stress, while cancellous bone is more flexible and hence more able to deal with deformation (Hall 1991).

How does bone grow in thickness?

Sherwood (1995) explains how new bone is added to the outer surface of the bone as a result of osteoblast activity inside the sheath of connective tissue that covers the outer side of the bone. The osteoblasts all come from the bone marrow and are related to structural cells. They come from one nucleus and work together to build bone. This new bone is called osteoid and is made up of bone collagen and other proteins. They control calcium and mineral deposition. While this is happening on the outside, osteoclasts situated inside the bone are engaged in breaking down the bone tissue nearest the marrow cavity. Osteoclasts are large cells that come from bone marrow and are related to white blood cells. They often fuse together, meaning that they often have more than one nucleus. They lie on the surface of the mineral next to the dissolving bone. As the shaft circumference is enlarged the marrow cavity is enlarged as well to keep pace with these changes.

How does bone grow in length?

This happens via a different mechanism from the one causing increase in thickness. Sherwood (1995) reports that this process is located mainly in the epiphyseal plate, where a proliferation of cartilage cells can be observed. Cell division on the outer edge of the plate right next to the epiphysis causes thickening of the cartilaginous plate and hence a pushing away of the epiphysis from the diaphysis. As this process happens near the epiphyseal border the old cartilage cells close to the diaphyseal border die off and are replaced by osteoblasts, which move upwards towards the epiphysis. These osteoblasts then model new bone around the persistent survivors of the disintegrating cartilage until the inner aspect of the diaphysis, where it meets the epiphyseal plate, is entirely replaced by bone. Once this whole process is completed the diaphysis has increased in length and the epiphyseal plate has resumed its original thickness.

Once the osteoblast has done its bone-creating duty it becomes buried inside the extracellular matrix as this calcifies. Osteoblasts do not really die off, though, but turn into osteocytes and lay down an extensive tunnel system to receive their nutrients and get rid of waste. In the final new bone one therefore sees a multitude of little canals, which the osteoblasts have formed.

All the processes discussed so far are possible because of the activities of growth hormone.

What is the role of growth hormone in bone growth?

Growth hormone – also known as somatotropin – is responsible for the increase in both thickness and length in bone. It is a protein produced by the pituitary gland and works directly on the proliferation of epiphyseal cartilage. As described above, this allows for more bone formation and osteoblast activity. Growth hormone works on the epiphyseal plate, hence allowing for increased bone length. For this to happen, however, it relies on the epiphyseal plate remaining open (i.e. cartilaginous). The plate closes or ossifies under the influence of sex hormones once adolescence is over. This is the reason why people do not grow in height after this period.

Growth hormone is important not only during childhood growth but also during adulthood (Lifshitz 2003) after bone growth stops. It continues to help regulate metabolism in a number of different ways. It also is vital to maintaining healthy body composition, proper bone density, heart muscle function and cholesterol levels.

Bone formation and removal normally happen all the time. This is important for:

- keeping the skeleton in a state of maximum efficiency for its mechanical uses and the demands made on it
- maintaining the free plasma calcium level.

This leads to the conclusion that mechanical factors are the most important factors in adjusting the strength of bone. The greater the mechanical or physical stress on it the greater the rate of bone formation. Athletes' bones are more massive than those of sedentary people (Sherwood 1995). The other side to this is that loss of mechanical stress (e.g. during prolonged bed rest) results in loss of bone mass.

The actual rate of bone formation and removal is again controlled by hormones. The growth and sex hormones actions have already been discussed. The other important hormone to mention with regards to bone is parathyroid hormone. It withdraws calcium from the bone fluid, which is found in the multitude of little canals between the buried osteoblasts (now called osteocytes). In contrast to plasma, bone has calcium in abundance. In this way the actual integrity of the bone is not interfered with at all and all the necessary plasma calcium comes from this bone fluid.

If by any chance there is an acute lack of calcium (e.g. from dietary problems), the parathyroid hormone stimulates the local dissolution of bone and promotes the transfer of calcium (and other ingredients) from the bone itself into the plasma. On the whole, this process does not leave any discernible effects on the bones. It is clearly a life-saving strategy for the body. Once the calcium levels have risen again the superfluous calcium is re-deposited in the bone. However, if this process were to be maintained over many months there would be a widening of the canals filled with body fluid, which would eventually cluster together to form cavities.

COMMON REASONS FOR REFERRALS TO PHYSIOTHERAPY OF PATIENTS WITH BONE DISEASES

The diagnosis of bone disease in itself is not usually a reason for referral. In fact, as stated previously, the actual diagnosis is often secondary with regard to rehabilitation. What is important are the actual findings in terms of loss of function, pain and what these mean to the patient.

We meet this group of patients after surgery, which might have been aimed at, for example, correcting a deformity, replacing a 'worn out' joint, salvaging a limb (e.g. removing a tumour) or after a fracture. All of these happen more often in a ward situation within a hospital.

On the other hand, we might come across this group of patients when they complain of pain or an inability to live life in the way they have been used to. These patients might be met in our outpatient departments as well as in GP practices or community settings.

As medication and surgical approaches change so does the role of the physiotherapist. Where there were once regimens involving lengthy stays in hospital that required the physiotherapist to combat the effects of prolonged bed rest, our role now is mostly much more proactive, taking advantage of a more active general treatment management.

Strong bones are needed to provide a lever for muscles and ligaments. When they are weakened, for whatever reason, postural problems automatically follow. This will result in functional losses due to muscle weakness and perhaps gait abnormalities. The analysis of gait patterns and their rehabilitation is an area physiotherapists are involved in all the time. We therefore see such patients in our gyms and departments for (for example) general strengthening, muscle imbalance work and gait re-education.

Prevention of future problems is of course a major aspect of our work in habilitation (a more holistic approach than purely rehabilitation). Prevention is mostly much easier than the treatment that is necessary once a problem has occurred. It therefore makes a lot of sense to spend time and expertise to home in on this. Clearly for someone with a lifelong locomotor problem this is vital and no management approach is acceptable that does not focus on this point.

GENERAL DISORDERS OF THE SKELETON IN CHILDREN

These fall into two main areas: those characterized by loss of bone mass (osteoporosis) and those where mineralization is defective (osteomalacia). The WHO definition of osteoporosis is 'A systemic skeletal disease characterized by micro-architectural deterioration and low bone mass giving rise to an increased susceptibility to fracture'. In adults, classification of osteoporosis is achieved through the use of bone mineral density T scores in which the specific value obtained using a DXA measurement of the lumbar spine or hip is related to the population mean for young healthy adults. DXA measures bone mass, not density. For children this classification is less clear and hence one assumes the presence of osteoporosis if a child has had fragility-type fractures in association with low bone density.

Most of these conditions are very rare and hence are not often seen by physiotherapists. A lot of them are congenital. It seems that most are caused in the fetal stage of development by a dominant mutant gene (Crawford Adams & Hamblen 1998). It is important to remember that not all of these conditions manifest themselves at birth but may only reveal themselves later on.

Self-assessment questions

- **SAQ 9.4** What are the mechanisms involved in bone growth? If in doubt, re-read the physiology review above.
- **SAQ 9.5** How would you expect the presence of bone disease to influence the healing time of a hip fracture in an elderly woman?

World-wide the most common disorder of the skeleton remains rickets, which is caused by a deficiency of vitamin D and sunlight leading to a defective calcification of growing bone (Crawford Adams & Hamblen 1998). The sight of thin children with weak and very bendy bones is very rare now in Western societies, where diet and exposure to sunlight have improved.

Osteogenesis imperfecta is a hereditary genetic disorder characterized by bone fragility with an increased tendency to fracture. The defective gene affects collagen, causing defective type 1 collagen synthesis that results in either abnormal collagen fibres or too few fibres. This affects bone formation and turnover (Clark 2001, Rauch et al 2000).

Osteomalacia – another vitamin D deficiency problem – is another condition frequently encountered by physiotherapists. It is often seen as a side effect of Crohn's disease, which involves a resorption problem that leads to bone mineral loss. Vogelsang et al (1995) tried to determine whether long-term dietary supplementation with low doses of vitamin D helped to prevent bone loss and the development of osteomalacia in patients with Crohn's disease. They concluded from their positive results that long-term oral vitamin D supplementation seemed to be an efficient means of preventing bone loss in these patients and hence a method of preventing osteomalacia.

OSTEOPOROSIS

Patients with osteoporosis form the biggest subgroup of people with endocrine bone problems. It is caused amongst other factors by a general decrease in calcium in bone (see earlier mention under children's heading). Osteoporosis in adults can occur without any symptoms and may therefore be difficult to detect. Young women with eating disorders (e.g. anorexia nervosa) can lose bone with dramatic speed and sustain stress fractures. The same can happen to young women involved in high-level endurance sports (marathon running, gymnastics, etc.). It seems that alcohol and smoking can be risk factors for osteoporosis (Eisman 1998, Ilich et al 2002, Lane & Nydick 1999).

Osteoporosis is a metabolic disease of bone characterized by reduced bone mass that results in an increased risk of fractures. It is by far the commonest bone disease (Ritson & Scott 1996). Women, particularly postmenopausal women, are at a greater risk than men, as low oestrogen levels contribute to brittle bones (Miller et al 1998). Dinan & Rutherford (1994) reported that, in the UK, one in 12 men over the age of 70 years and one in four women over 60 have osteoporosis. A recent study even identified that nearly half of postmenopausal women have undetected low bone mineral density (Siris et al 2001).

Bone mass increases throughout childhood and early adult life, arriving at its peak in the third decade. It is dependent on hormones, exercise, diet, genes, lifestyle and illness (Adami 1994). For the assessment of the level of bone turnover in women with vertebral osteoporosis, serum osteocalcin and urinary pyridinoline appear to be the most sensitive markers to date (Delmas 1993, Delmas et al 1997). On the other hand, the measurement of general bone resorption and formation seems to lack a particular specific and reliable test so far and hence patients are usually asked to undergo a whole battery of tests in order to investigate these two general indicators.

Osteoporosis is characterized in the spine by a thinning of the cortices of the vertebrae and a thinning of the individual trabeculae, with resultant widening of the vertebral canal.

Turner (1991) reminds us that fractures of the proximal femur and distal radius are regarded as typical osteoporotic fractures. These mostly seem to occur in elderly women. On the other hand as Spector (1990) claims, vertebral fractures occur three times as often as hip fractures but remain undetected more frequently. These can occur almost spontaneously after a cough or sneeze and can lead to chronic pain, a crushing down of vertebrae on top of each other and hence an increased thoracic kyphosis and loss of height. A wedge-shaped vertebra is a classical radiological finding in osteoporosis (Fig. 9.1). While these studies are old, the numbers cited have not really changed.

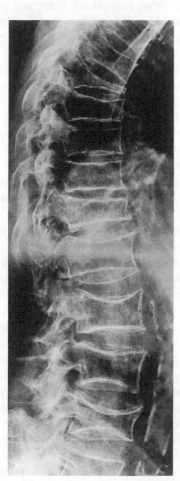

Figure 9.1 X-ray of an osteoporotic spine. (With permission from Crawford Adams & Hamblen, 1998.)

Turner (1991) reviews the possible causes of accelerating bone loss and finds that it occurs in:

- post-gastrectomy patients who have poor calcium absorption
- people who diet excessively or who have diets deficient in calcium or vitamin D
- post-hysterectomy patients
- people who suffer from anorexia nervosa and related diseases
- females who exercise excessively – affecting normal menstruation
- people with a history of osteoporosis
- people receiving long-term steroids
- people with metabolic or glandular disorders (e.g. hyperparathyroidism)
- people who have to submit to immobilization (e.g. patients with spinal cord injuries)
- postmenopausal women.

Management of osteoporosis

Primary prevention

This is aimed at young women and usually takes the form of specifically targeted advertising. It covers the known precursors, e.g. diet and exercise.

Secondary prevention

This is aimed at the high-risk group, i.e. women in their forties. In this pre- or perimenopausal period it is important that women are informed about hormone replacement therapy and correct diets, especially concentrating on vitamin D and calcium. Weight-bearing exercise or activities are essential but the high-impact jarring of some sports might be counterproductive. Postural exercises and general fitness should be encouraged to promote good posture. Fall prevention training is another important ingredient for this group of patients as the fear of falls is often a seemingly insurmountable problem (Li et al 2003, Nitz & Choy 2004).

Tertiary management

Here symptoms have occurred and actual treatment is necessary. This could happen at any stage in life. Intervention is mainly concerned with the relief of pain, the possible loss of mobility and deformity. The initial spinal deformity can make it difficult to treat patients in our usual treatment position – supine or prone lying. Clearly, other positions need to be explored. Any change in spinal shape will obviously cause a change in respiration, which needs to be checked and if necessary included into a treatment plan. Walking is a good self-treatment avenue, as is any kind of fitness and strength training (Feskanich et al 2002). See also the international clinical guidelines for osteoporosis (Meunier et al 1999).

Exercises have already been mentioned. The aim of these is to maximize the bone mass by loading the skeleton and contracting muscles.

Ritson & Scott (1996) investigated the treatment techniques commonly used by Scottish and Swedish physiotherapists. These two groups also included electrotherapy (especially transcutaneous nerve stimulation) for pain relief and hydrotherapy for general mobility.

These authors drew up a list of 10 exercises obtained from the literature, ranked in order of benefit to those at risk of osteoporosis:

1. Running/jumping
2. Walking
3. Strength training
4. Extension
5. Postural exercise
6. Flexibility
7. Swimming
8. Cycling
9. Flexion
10. Bed rest.

None of these avenues, however, really addresses the disability experienced by women with osteoporotic spinal fractures. Helmes et al (1995) reported their initial results in trying to validate the Osteoporotic Functional Disability Questionnaire (OFDQ). The domains of the OFDQ include: quantitative indices of pain, a standard 20-item scale, 26 items relating to functional disability, a scale of social activities, and confidence in the ability of prescribed osteoporosis treatment to reverse disability. The authors reported the test–retest reliability to vary between 0.76 and 0.93, with internal consistency between 0.57 and 0.96.

They also showed that the OFDQ correlated significantly with relevant spinal pathology and showed significant improvements in activities of daily living and socialization when active exercisers were compared to inactive patients with osteoporosis. Helmes et al (1995) therefore concluded that the OFDQ was a reliable instrument that correlated well with objective measures of osteoporotic spinal damage. It is also sensitive to changes in disability brought about by participation in an aerobic exercise programme. As physiotherapists, we are in need of a more bio-psychosocial measuring tool and might investigate this further.

LOCAL AFFECTIONS OF BONE

These might not all be caused by genetic problems. The most important ones are infections, tumours, osteochondritis and cystic changes.

Osteomyelitis can manifest itself in childhood when organisms reach the bloodstream, or on the other hand at any stage in life as a consequence of an open fracture or surgical intervention.

Tuberculosis, which used to account for a large number of local bone infections, is much rarer in the Western patient population now, although still a major problem in some countries. Its infection is chronic, develops slowly and is much more hidden than a lot of conditions that develop faster (e.g. osteomyelitis). Tuberculosis is often confined to one particular joint (e.g. hip) but can spread to other parts of the body, where all sorts of complications can arise, e.g. compression of the spinal cord by an abscess of the spinal column. In contrast to a lot of other patients with bone diseases, this group of patients will have general malaise with high temperatures, a raised erythrocyte sedimentation rate (ESR) and a positive Mantoux test (Crawford Adams & Hamblen 1998).

Tumours are either benign or malignant. As physiotherapists we come across them as either the primary tumour or, when malignant, as a metastatic occurrence. Both of these settings are regular pictures in any orthopaedic practice. Make sure you refer to the National Service Framework for Cancer (Department of Health 1995).

Osteochondritis occurs usually in young people or children and seems to be caused by the development of bony nuclei inside the bone, which leads to a softening of the bone structure.

SPECIAL TESTS

- *X-rays* are of course the primary special tool for the doctor. Of particular interest are the length and width of bones, the state of the epiphyses, the size of the spinal canal, the symmetry of the vertebrae, any outgrowths of bones and translucency of bones.
- *Magnetic resonance imaging (MRI)* is a routinely used, modern, non-invasive, reliable screening tool that has the advantage of giving a good view of the soft tissues.
- In suspected tumours *biopsies* may be necessary.
- *Blood tests* show if the plasma calcium levels are normal or low, if alkaline phosphates are increased (e.g. osteomalacia) and if the calcium balance is normal or negative.
- *Bone (radio-isotope) scans* are invaluable in the detection of, for example, Paget's disease.
- *DXA scans* are the investigation of choice for osteoporosis and osteopenia. Bone mineral density (BMD) within 1 SD of the young adult reference mean (YARM) is the normal baseline; BMD between −1 and −2.5 SD below YARM identifies osteopenia while anything higher than −2.5 SD below YARM confirms the diagnosis of osteoporosis.

It is important for the physiotherapist to be able to interpret these results as possible clues to the background diagnosis. Our forte, however, is the physical assessment rather than the tests avenue.

It is important that you have a good idea about your assessment priorities as a physiotherapist before you start assessing someone with a bone disease problem. You might want to quickly reflect on some of the issues raised in Chapter 3. This area is often led by highly specialized technological tests and screening that focuses on a particular area of the skeleton. In the presence of all this technological information it can be easy to forget that some of these problems will be entirely hidden and it may only be through a skilful assessment that suspicion of a problem connected to bone disease is aroused.

ASSESSMENT OF THE PATIENT WITH BONE DISEASE

Subjective assessment

The aim of this aspect is to gain an insight into the patient's problem. Remember that some of these underlying problems can be completely hidden. However, pain is nearly always the reason for referral. One needs to ascertain the mechanical, social and psychological elements that might contribute to the whole picture. Remember that metabolic pain is non-mechanical in nature with a propensity to be worse at night (reduced metabolic rate). The patient's lifestyle and the way he uses his body have to be established by carefully interviewing him. The patient must have the opportunity to express his own thoughts and feelings about the problem and what he is hoping to gain from physiotherapy. It is all too easy to jump to certain conclusions after having read the diagnosis of the referrer. As physiotherapists we should attempt to build up a relationship with the patient, enabling him to focus on a particular aspect of the wide variety of possibilities. We do not really treat a condition but a person, with a specific problem caused by that condition. The patient is likely to experience problems that will have to be tackled in terms of the rest of his life rather than a few weeks of treatment. This might necessitate that his partner is involved in this aspect of the assessment.

Remember to introduce questions focusing on possible mineralization loss, e.g. hysterectomy, gastrectomy or long-term use of steroids or any blood thinning agent. The resultant loss of bone mineralization might only become visible on X-ray once more than 30% has been lost. This is to say that the clinical interview might raise suspicions long before radiographic findings can confirm them. Mostly, our assessments try to identify a mechanical pattern and hence a cause for the patient's problem. With this patient group, however – dealing with permanent changes rather than an injury – you want to make absolutely sure that you understand any non-mechanical hints the patient might give you. Considering the life-long aspect of these conditions, it is important that a measure of disability with subjective as well as objective markers can be introduced. Disability is experienced in very different ways by different patients and according to their diagnosis. Clearly, someone with osteoporosis will feel himself to be differently affected from someone with cancer. There are therefore very different disability measures to be employed for each of these client groups.

Objective assessment

The aims of this do not really differ very much from any other orthopaedic assessment in as much as the assessment attempts to elicit and isolate the patient's main problem through focused tests and examinations. Special physical tests are dictated by the physical findings rather than the diagnosis. They are altered to suit the different client groups, e.g. children, adults or the elderly, and to take account of possible contraindications.

Bone structure and alignment are a very important area to concentrate on with these patients. Don't forget to look at the shape and size of long bones with regard to Paget's disease.

Posture

As mentioned earlier in this chapter, a change in bone strength, length or shape is bound to have an effect on muscles and ligaments and hence on posture. Posture is probably one of the most difficult areas of any physical assessment. In order to assess abnormalities of posture you must re-familiarize yourself with the hallmarks of normal posture.

Roaf (1978) defined posture as the position the body assumes in preparation for the next movement. Mere uprightness, he continued, is not true posture since it involves balance, muscular control, co-ordination and adaptation. With this definition in mind it becomes clear that postural defects are very common. Barlow (1952) assumed that about 70–80% of adolescents presented with postural problems and he considered this number to rise with increasing age. Grieve (1989) comments on the monumental task involved in classifying and meaningfully assessing the rich variety of emotional, hormonal, mechanical, neurophysiological and social factors that might all influence posture.

On the whole, one assumes that postural problems can be abolished. If, however, permanent soft tissue shortening, bone and joint changes have manifested themselves, postural problems may have clearly led to a deformity. Congenital and acquired deformities tend to produce asymmetrical changes and thus predispose to degenerative changes. On the other hand, though, degenerative changes can produce changes in body contour and attitude. These can manifest themselves at every level and therefore need careful attention in an assessment.

Grieve (1989) reminds us that the interpretation of our objective findings is very important. Things are not always what they seem and a deformity might not result in pathology.

Bad posture can have a markedly negative effect and augment the patient's problems as well as causing them. It can:

- limit range of movement
- increase discomfort and pain (back pain, headaches, arm and shoulder pain etc.)
- create pain in the temporomandibular joint
- decrease lung capacity
- affect bowel function
- change normal muscle patterning
- change the length and flexibility of soft tissue structures
- generally interfere with musculoskeletal potential.

Self-assessment question

- **SAQ 9.6** What pointers might you have come across in your assessment that will alert the physiotherapist to the fact that disability is a bigger problem than the measured impairment?

(Answer at end of chapter.)

Case study 9.1: Mrs Bell

Mrs Bell is a 58-year-old mother of three grown-up children who has started to notice pain in her lumbar spine over the past year or so. She particularly finds any static posture or position extremely uncomfortable. On the whole, short rests help her but she now feels severely curtailed in her activities.

PAGET'S DISEASE

Paget's disease is a common disease also called osteitis deformans. About 3% of the population over 40 years of age (Apley 2001) can show signs of it. It is a slowly progressive problem affecting one or several bones but never crossing joint spaces. It got its name from Sir James Paget, who first described it in 1879. In spite of a lot of research into its cause this is as yet unknown, although it is interesting to note that it is virtually unknown in some areas (e.g. Norway, Japan).

The affected bones increase in width and become thicker. They lose their normal consistency, increase their blood supply and hence become spongy and weakened, leading to an increase in fractures (Crawford Adams & Hamblen 1998, Dandy 1998).

The disease can remain localized to one bone for years before affecting others (skull, femur, pelvis, clavicle and spine). The patient complains of often quite severe pain (often worse at night) but is able to continue with life as before. The diagnosis can be confirmed by

- a raised alkaline phosphatase level in the plasma
- raised hydroxyproline in the urine
- 'hot spots' on the isotope (bone) scan.

On examination, the painful bone is characteristically bent, thickened and hot to touch. As bone formation and resorption is increased, spaces are being created by this absorption that are slowly going to be filled by vascular tissues (Apley 2001). The body reacts to this by forming new osteoid tissue on either side of the cortex that does not get converted into mature bone tissue. The bone is therefore much thicker on the one hand but also much weaker on the other, easily giving way under load and fracturing. Nerves can easily be compromised because of the decrease in available space caused by the increase in bone circumference.

The X-ray is characteristic and is a vital part of confirming the diagnosis (Figs 9.2–9.4).

Management

Mr Johnson's physician has already prescribed some painkillers and bisphosphonates (Siris 1998). These latter drugs are a class of synthetic compounds used in the treatment of various metabolic bone diseases as well as Paget's disease. Rosen &

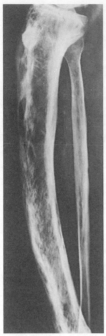

Figure 9.2 X-ray showing Paget's disease of the tibia. (With permission from Crawford Adams & Hamblen, 1998.)

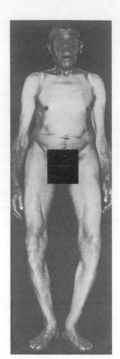

Figure 9.3 Typical appearance of a patient with widespread Paget's disease. (With permission from Crawford Adams & Hamblen, 1998.)

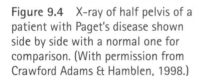

Figure 9.4 X-ray of half pelvis of a patient with Paget's disease shown side by side with a normal one for comparison. (With permission from Crawford Adams & Hamblen, 1998.)

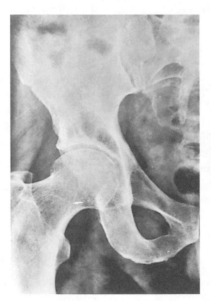
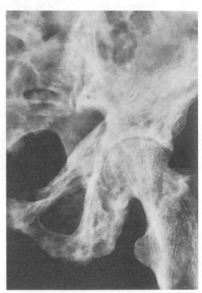

Kessenich (1996) published an interesting review of the effect of these bisphosphonates. They identified several studies that had compared these drugs with placebo but found a paucity of comparative research comparing the effects of these drugs with other pharmacological agents. They were nevertheless convinced that the effects documented so far for bisphosphonates made them the treatment of choice for Paget's disease (and some other metabolic diseases).

OSTEOSARCOMA

Osteosarcoma is a malignant tumour also known as osteogenic sarcoma. It occurs predominantly in younger people or even children but can also appear as a complication of Paget's disease in older adults. Osteosarcoma occurs more often in males than females, with a ratio of roughly 2:1 (Maxwell 1995). It arises from the bone-forming cells and most often appears at the lower end of the femur, the upper end of the tibia and the upper end of the humerus. Crawford Adams & Hamblen (1998) describe how osteosarcomas classically destroy the bone structure before bursting into the surrounding soft tissues. Any type of connective tissue may be represented, giving the tumour a widely varying histological appearance. Always present, however, are areas of neoplastic new bone or osteoid tissue.

Metastasis of this tumour occurs early via the blood stream, particularly to the lungs. Dandy (1998) reports an average survival rate of about 30%, although this is improving all the time.

Clinically there is pain and a local increasing swelling. On examination, this swelling is usually found at the end of bones near to the joint (Figs 9.5, 9.6; Crawford Adams & Hamblen 1998).

The patient often implicates a minor injury disproportionate to the extent of the pain and the change seen in the affected region.

The X-rays show the proliferation of bone and the destruction of the metaphysis. Often one can identify the Codman's triangle, which is the appearance of new bone formation under the corners of the raised periosteum.

Magnetic resonance imaging is the best way of identifying spread into the surrounding soft tissues.

Management

The rest of the body (especially the lungs and the rest of the skeleton) needs to be scanned to

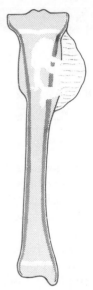

Figure 9.5 Osteosarcoma. (With permission from Crawford Adams & Hamblen, 1998.)

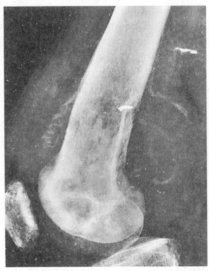

Figure 9.6 X-ray of osteosarcoma at the lower end of the femur. (With permission from Crawford Adams & Hamblen, 1998.)

identify possible metastases. Chemotherapy, in conjunction with amputation, has increased the survival rate greatly from the original 25–30% (Crawford Adams & Hamblen 1998). Chemotherapy is usually started before surgery and then continues for about a year afterwards. As drug

therapy has increased, radical resection has often replaced amputation. Simon (1988) reported in excess of 70% disease-free survival after 5 years with this mixed approach.

Fulton (1994) discusses the different rehabilitation strategies as follows. First of all the care has to be comprehensive, which means that the needs of the whole person have to be addressed, i.e. the psychological, social, vocational, economic and physical factors shaping someone's life. Fulton continues by quoting Habeck et al (1984). It is necessary to use an interdisciplinary approach, which should include both the patient and his or her family. The members of this team also include the physician or surgeon, nurses, therapists and ancillary personnel. The remaining elements of the framework of the rehabilitation of cancer patients will be as follows (Habeck et al 1984).

- Goals for rehabilitation should be derived from the effects of medical problems in accordance with prognostic expectations. Dietz (1974, 1985) argues that these goals can be:
  - preventive (when disability can be predicted)
  - restorative (when patients can be expected to have only minimal or residual handicap)
  - supportive (when patients have to cope with ongoing disease or permanent disability)
  - palliative (when patients are managing advanced disease and basic disability cannot be corrected but where training can enhance performance).

  Dietz (1985) considers that these goals will be determined by an aggregate of factors relevant to the individual – age, type and stage of neoplastic disease, other concomitant disease, inherent physical ability, social background, basic education and job or work experience.

- Intervention should occur as soon as the likelihood of disability is anticipated. Fulton (1994) and Dietz (1985) argue that any rehabilitation programme for a cancer patient should be instituted as soon as possible. They comment further that preventative goals (e.g. breathing control, general muscle and joint range maintenance and fitness exercises) are crucial and the role of the physiotherapist is firmly established within this framework. Fulton (1994), citing the work of Folkman & Lazarus (1980), states that as patients with a cancer diagnosis often initially feel out of control the exercises might help them to regain some control of their bodies and hence give them a general psychological advantage.

- Rehabilitation needs must be reassessed on a continuing basis and addressed throughout. Fulton (1994) reiterates the point that rehabilitation needs must be met throughout all phases of the disease: diagnosis, primary treatment, adjuvant therapy, secondary recurrence and palliation. She draws attention to the fact that goals must be realistic for the current stage of the patient's disease process and abilities.

- Education must be regarded as a major component of the rehabilitation process. By focusing on the rehabilitation process the multidisciplinary team is able to focus on the patient's abilities rather than the disease. The aim of rehabilitation at this stage is therefore to concentrate on reducing the degree to which disabilities become permanent or interfere with everyday life, irrespective of how long that life might be.

Fulton (1994) continues her review by stating that the main problems for effective rehabilitation of the cancer patient seem to involve attitudinal problems and a poor level of knowledge about the disease and the rehabilitation process. It is important to remember that part of the role of the physiotherapist is to identify problems with the rehabilitation process that are not purely physical (e.g. anxiety and depression), as the physiotherapist often spends more time with the patient than other team members do. This might then result in a helpful referral to the psychologist on the team.

Fulton (1994) suggests that it is essential for the physiotherapist to address more specific issues in order to plan the most effective rehabilitation. S/he therefore must make it his/her business to fully understand all aspects of the different stages of the disease, to be familiar with the medical tests and their implication and to have a realistic view of the disease process. This realistic outlook will have a direct influence on the physiotherapist's goal. If the therapist is unrealistic or unknowledgeable about the disease process the short-term goals can result in inappropriate programmes and

hence can lead to trauma, both physical and psychological, for the patient and a feeling of helplessness for the physiotherapist. In the long term, Fulton reminds us, the patient can lose out in rehabilitation achievement and the physiotherapist might feel deskilled and impotent.

A physiotherapist's checklist of medical tests and their implication so far prior to starting an assessment might look something like this (Fulton 1994):

1. What sort of cancer is it? Which organ and cell type are involved?
2. What is the stage of the patient's cancer? Is the patient dealing with an isolated growth or has metastasis taken place already? If so, have the metastases spread to the lung, other organs or another bony site?
3. What kind of treatment has been adopted? Is it surgery, chemotherapy and radiotherapy? Is it only one of these? Remember that some side effects of cancer treatment may only start many years after the diagnosis.
4. What is the patient's prognosis? (This is changing all the time, mostly for the better.)
5. Which members of the multidisciplinary team are involved in the rehabilitation process?
6. Are there any obvious contraindications to certain modalities of physiotherapy?

With regard to the last point, Maxwell (1995) reviews the contradictory evidence regarding ultrasound therapy and tumour metastases. It has certainly always been thought that ultrasound therapy was contraindicated, as it was felt that it could disrupt tumours and hence increase the risk of metastasis. This, Maxwell argues, is due to the micromassage effect, which could cause the separation of weakly bound tumour cells and the disruption of the very delicate tumour vessels. Once a tumour cell has been dislodged it can be disseminated by three different routes (Maxwell 1995):

- Tumours growing in cavities may show a transcoelomic spread, in which shed fragments attach themselves to and become implanted into the apposing serosal or mucosal surfaces to form secondary tumours

- The more prevalent route for carcinomas is via the lymphatic system; hence the assessment of local lymph nodes is vital
- Tumours can also spread via the blood stream; it seems that the amount of tumour material escaping into the blood stream is directly related to the size of the vessels in the tumour.

Maxwell (1995) reminds us that physiotherapists must be aware of the differential diagnosis of musculoskeletal tumours and the possibility that some musculoskeletal tumours might mimic conditions for which some physiotherapeutic modalities (e.g. electrotherapy) might be helpful. A good and thorough assessment based upon constant vigilance is required if such malignant tumours are not to be mismanaged.

Fallowfield (1990) noted that the mere knowledge that one has a life-threatening disease is enough to seriously impair one's quality of life. The psychosocial problems cancer patients might have to battle are provoked by the actual knowledge of their diagnosis (Fallowfield 1990). They are concerned about lack of information, the uncertainty of the prognosis, possible guilt about the causality and the fear of a painful and undignified death. In addition, these patients have to cope with radical treatments, such as surgery that may be mutilating and/or lead to loss of body image and/or rejection by their partner. Radiotherapy is linked to anxiety and depression and can cause nausea and vomiting, lethargy and skin problems. Chemotherapy is linked to nausea and vomiting, hair loss, mouth ulcers, hot flushes and other side effects. All these lead to a disruption in economic, social and sexual terms resulting in depression and anxiety and hence a loss of quality of life (Fallowfield 1990). Some work has been done with the profile of mood states (POMS) with cancer patients (Silberfarb et al 1983).

Problem-solving exercise 9.3

Alan is facing rigorous chemotherapy, perhaps radiotherapy, and either an above-knee amputation or a radical resection of his tumour involving the upper end of his tibia, his knee and the lower end of his femur and resulting in a massive total knee replacement.

What are the general strategies going to be? Irrespective of Alan's prognosis, what are realistic goals for him?

What members of the multidisciplinary team will the physiotherapist have to work with?

Refer to Chapters 3 and 8 if you are stuck.

SUMMARY

This chapter has attempted to give you a framework to assess and then manage patients with bone diseases. In contrast to e.g. soft tissue injuries or fractures you need to be able to form an assessment strategy that will include not just the search for a mechanical cause but that will help you to identify not-mechanical disease states. It is not necessary to 'know the medical diagnosis' but to come to a reasoned and well-thought-out treatment plan.

ANSWERS TO QUESTIONS AND EXERCISES

Self-assessment question 9.2 (page 271)

- **SAQ 9.2** How will you be able to detect whether your communication skills are effective and appropriate?

  Answer: The patient will be relaxed and co-operative. S/he will be able to be specific and precise during the subjective and objective assessments, and will be able to adhere to advice or to treatment approaches that have been planned collaboratively.

Self-assessment questions 9.4, 9.5 (page 276)

See information in text.

Self-assessment question 9.6 (page 280)

- **SAQ 9.6** What pointers might you have come across in your assessment that will alert the physiotherapist to the fact that disability is a bigger problem than the measured impairment?

  Answer: For example, the patient may be off work, may be avoiding daily tasks such as domestic chores and may be withdrawing from social interactions.

Problem-solving exercise 9.1 (page 281)

See information in text.

Self-assessment question 9.7 (page 281)

- **SAQ 9.7** Listening to Mr Johnson's story, what have you identified so far that would suggest Paget's disease?

Answer:

- His age
- The main site of his problem (his (R) thigh) and the fact that pain and deformity seem to appear together
- The possibility of associated symptoms (headaches, increased kyphosis).

Problem-solving exercise 9.2 (page 283)

See information in this chapter and in Chapter 3.

Self-assessment question 9.8 (page 283)

- **SAQ 9.8** What are the important aspects of this patient's history with regard to his diagnosis?

Answer:

- The problem began with a seemingly insignificant injury
- The patient noticed a non-mechanical behaviour of his pain
- The patient noticed swelling.

Problem-solving exercise 9.3 (page 286)

See information in Chapters 3 and 8.

References

Adami M 1994 Optimising peak bone mass – what are the therapeutic possibilities? Osteoporosis International Supplement 1, S27–S30

Apley AG 2001 System of orthopaedics and fractures, 7th edn. Butterworths: London

Barlow W 1952 Postural homeostasis. Annals of Physical Medicine 1: 77

Bruce N 1980 Teamwork for preventive care. Research Studies Press, Chichester

Clark C 2001 Osteogenesis imperfecta: an overview. Nursing Standard 16(5): 47–54

Crawford Adams J, Hamblen DL 1998 Outline of orthopaedics, 11th edn. Churchill Livingstone, Edinburgh

Dandy D 1998 Essential orthopaedics and trauma, 3rd edn. Churchill Livingstone, Edinburgh

Delmas PD 1993 Biochemical markers of bone turnover. Journal of Bone and Mineral Research 8(suppl 2): S549–S555

Delmas PD, Bjarnason NH, Mitlak BH et al 1997 Effects of raloxifene on bone mineral density, serum cholesterol concentrations, and uterine endometrium in postmenopausal women. New England Journal of Medicine 337: 1641–1647

Department of Health 1995 National service framework for cancer. HMSO, London

Dietz JH Jr 1974 Rehabilitation of the cancer patient. Its role in the scheme of comprehensive care. Clinical Bulletin 4: 104–107

Dietz JH Jr 1985 Rehabilitation of the patient with cancer. In: Cabresi P, Schein PS, Rosenberg SA (eds) Medical oncology: basic principles and clinical management of cancer. Macmillan, New York

Dinan S, Rutherford O 1994 Osteoporosis. Asset 2: 14–21

Eisman JA 1998 Genetics, calcium intake and osteoporosis. Proceedings of the Nutritional Society 57: 187–193

Fallowfield L 1990 The quality of life. The missing measurement in health care. Human Horizons Series. Souvenir Press, London

Feskanich D, Willett W, Colditz G 2002 Walking and leisure-time activity and risk of hip fracture in postmenopausal women. Journal of the American Medical Association 288: 2300–2306

Finlay L 1997 Good patients and bad patients. How occupational therapists view their patients/clients. British Journal of Occupational Therapy 60: 440–446

Fisher K, Hardie RJ 2002 Goal attainment scaling in evaluating a multidisciplinary pain management programme. Clinical Rehabilitation 16: 871–877

Folkman S, Lazarus RS 1980 An analysis of coping in a middle aged community sample. Journal of Health and Social Behaviour 2: 219–239

Fulton C 1994 Physiotherapists in cancer care. A framework for rehabilitation of patients. Physiotherapy 80: 830–834

Grieve GP 1989 Common vertebral joint problems, 2nd edn. Churchill Livingstone, Edinburgh

Habeck RV, Romsaas EP, Olson SJ 1984 Cancer rehabilitation and continuing care: a case study. Cancer Nursing 7: 315–319

Hall SJ 1991 Basic biomechanics. Mosby/Yearbook, St Louis, MO

Hands D, Wilson J 1997 Integrated care management. Healthcare Risk Resources International, Melbourne

Hassenkamp A 2003 Shifting the goalposts. Proceedings of WCPT, Barcelona

Helmes E, Hodsman A, Lazowski D et al 1995 A questionnaire to evaluate disability in osteoporotic patients with vertebral compression fractures. Journals of Gerontology Series A – Biological Sciences and Medical Sciences 50: M91–M98

Ilich JZ, Brownbill RA, Tamborini L, Crnevic-Orlic Z 2002 To drink or not to drink: how are alcohol, caffeine and past smoking related to bone mineral density in elderly women? Journal of the American College of Nutrition 21: 536–544

Jones J, Tidwell B, Travis H et al 1995 Nutritional support of the hospitalized patient: a team approach. Journal of Mississippi Health Care State Medical Association 36: 91–99

Kiresuk TJ, Smith A, Cardillo JE (eds) 1994 Goal attainment scaling: applications, theory and measurement. Laurence Erlbaum, Hillsdale, NJ

Lane JM, Nydick M 1999 Osteoporosis: current modes of prevention and treatment. Journal of the American Academy of Orthopaedic Surgeons 7: 19–31

Li F, Fisher KJ, Harmer P et al 2003 Fear of falling in elderly persons: association with falls, functional ability, and quality of life. Journals of Gerontology Series B – Psychological Sciences and Social Sciences 58: 283–290

Lifshitz F (ed) 2003 Pediatric endocrinology, 4th edn. Marcel Dekker, New York

Lowe F, O'Hara S 2000 Multidisciplinary team working in practice: managing the transition. Journal of Interprofessional Care 14: 269–279

Maxwell L 1995 Therapeutic ultrasound and tumour metastasis. Physiotherapy 81: 272–275

Meunier PJ, Delmas PD, Eastell R et al 1999 Diagnosis and management of osteoporosis in postmenopausal women: clinical guidelines. International Committee for Osteoporosis Clinical Guidelines. Clinical Therapy 21: 1025–1044

Miller P, Lukert B, Broy S 1998 Management of postmenopausal osteoporosis for primary care. Menopause 5: 123–131

Nitz JC, Choy NL 2004 The efficacy of a specific balance-strategy training programme for preventing falls among older people: a pilot randomised controlled trial. Age and Ageing 33: 52–58

Ovretveit J, Matthias P, Thompson T 1997 Interprofessional working for health and social care. Macmillan, London

Payton O, Nelson C 1996 A preliminary study of patients' perceptions of certain aspects of their physical therapy experience. Physiotherapy Theory and Practice 12: 27–38

Rauch F, Travers R, Parfitt AM et al 2000 Static and dynamic bone histomorphometry in children with osteogenesis imperfecta. Bone 26: 581–589

Reid A, Chesson R 1998 Goal attainment scaling: is it appropriate for stroke patients and their physiotherapists? Physiotherapy 84: 136–144

Ritson F, Scott S 1996 Physiotherapy for osteoporosis. A pilot study comparing practice and knowledge in Scotland and Sweden. Physiotherapy 82: 390–394

Roaf L 1978 Posture. Academic Press, London

Rockwood K, Joyce B, Stolee P 1997 Use of goal attainment scaling in measuring clinically important changes in cognitive rehabilitation patients. Journal of Epidemiology 50: 581–588

Rosen CJ, Kessenich CR 1996 Comparative clinical pharmacology and therapeutic use of bisphosphonates in metabolic bone diseases. Drugs 51: 537–551

Sherwood L 1995 Fundamentals of physiology. A human perspective, 2nd edn. West Publishing, Minneapolis, MN

Silberfarb PM, Holland J, Anbar D et al 1983 Psychological response of patients receiving two drug regimens for lung carcinoma. American Journal of Psychiatry 140: 110–111

Simon MA 1988 Limb salvage for osteosarcoma. Journal of Bone and Joint Surgery 70A: 307

Siris ES 1998 Paget's disease of bone. Journal of Bone and Mineral Research 13: 1061–1065

Siris ES, Miller PD, Barrett-Connor E et al 2001 Identification and fracture outcomes of undiagnosed low bone mineral density in postmenopausal women. Journal of the American Medical Association 286: 2815–2822

Spector TD 1990 Trends for admissions of hip fractures in England and Wales 1968–1985. British Medical Journal 300: 1173–1174

Thomson DJ, Hassenkamp AM, Mansbridge C 1997 The measurement of empathy in a clinical and a non-clinical setting. Does empathy increase with clinical experience? Physiotherapy 83: 173–180

Turner P 1991 Osteoporotic back pain – its prevention and treatment. Physiotherapy 77: 642–646

Vogelsang H, Ferenci P, Resch H et al 1995 Prevention of bone mineral loss in patients with Crohn's disease by long-term oral vitamin D supplementation. European Journal of Gastroenterology–Hepatology 7: 609–614

Worthington J 1994 Team approach to multidisciplinary care. British Journal of Therapy and Rehabilitation 1: 119–120

Wynne-Davies R, Fairbank TJ 1976 Fairbank's atlas of general afflictions of the skeleton. Churchill Livingstone, Edinburgh

Chapter 10

Gait assessment in the clinical situation

Fiona Coutts

CHAPTER CONTENTS

OBJECTIVES

By end of this chapter you should:

- Have reviewed the terminology and phases of normal gait and how this changes with age
- Have an overview of gait assessment to be used in the clinical situation
- Recognize gait deviations using observational analysis
- Understand the assessment implications and treatment of gait problems.

KEY WORDS

Gait analysis, gait assessment, observational analysis, kinematics, walkway, key component analysis.

Prerequisites

Re-read the chapter on assessment (Ch. 3) and the case studies in Chapters 3 and 4.

   Review normal gait and its terminology in any of the following:

- Trew M, Everett T 2001 Human movement: an introductory text, 4th edn. Churchill Livingstone, Edinburgh, ch 10, p 173–184
- Whittle M 2003 Gait analysis, an introduction, 3rd edn. Butterworth Heinemann, Oxford, ch 2, p 42–88.

- McRae R 1997 Clinical orthopaedic examination, 4th edn. Churchill Livingstone, Edinburgh.

The biomechanics of 'normal' gait is presented in many texts, from a brief overview (Craik & Oatis 1985) to the more detailed (Winter 1987 or Perry 1992). The excellent book by Michael Whittle listed above is thorough but less complex than the previous two.

INTRODUCTION

The ability to move for functional reasons is a basic necessity of life, and normally takes the form of walking (gait). Gait is a function that we tend to take for granted unless there is an abnormality or discomfort that alters the pattern of our gait and renders it more difficult. A gait problem is often a symptom that the patient will introduce in an initial assessment and that the therapist can use as a marker of effective treatment, e.g. 'pain after I walked to the shops...', 'My leg feels heavy when I am walking...', etc.

Rose (1983) suggests that 'gait assessment' is a problem-solving exercise that involves the complete process of subjective and objective evaluation of gait, physical examination of the patient and a review of the treatment decisions undertaken in the clinical situation. The physiotherapist is the main person to undertake this evaluation and the consequent treatment, so a good understanding of gait is essential.

This chapter will explore the basic requirements of normal gait and then take you through the process of observing and measuring gait, examples from two case studies will be used to understand the main gait problems and recording of findings.

INDIVIDUAL GAIT PATTERN

Gait has been defined by many authors but Perry (1992) notably describes it: 'Walking uses a repetitious sequence of limb motion to move the body forward while simultaneously maintaining stance stability' (Perry 1992, p 3) and 'Walking is the simple act of falling forward and catching oneself' (Perry 1992, ch 14, p 673). These definitions clearly describe the need for balance and dynamic control

of movement, where the body is required to control its progress over the base of support to allow stepping to take place. Everyone does this slightly differently and there is no 'absolutely correct' pattern.

Each person has his/her own individual gait pattern, which s/he is used to and can adapt to suit different weather and environmental conditions. Throughout a lifespan the gait pattern alters as the body systems adjust to neurological and musculoskeletal development (up to 7 years of age), and then decline (50+ years). The child develops initial control of moving, starting with the less demanding tasks such as sitting to standing, then standing balance and progressing to walking, until s/he masters, by the age of 7 years, the basic adult gait pattern (Sutherland et al 1980). From the age of around 1 to 7 years the child gait pattern is modified as growth and developmental maturity continue. Once established the basic adult gait pattern remains the same throughout life. Decline in strength and motor control in the older years (see Chapter 2) slows down the gait and adjustments in the pattern have to be made accordingly (Winter et al 1990).

As gait is individual there is a wide range of what is normal and a more detailed account of these ranges can be found in many textbooks; in particular, Whittle (2003) gives an excellent review of these. I would advise that at this point you consult one of the textbooks mentioned above to review the normal gait parameters before progressing with this chapter.

TERMINOLOGY AND DEFINITIONS OF NORMAL ADULT GAIT

The gait terminology used in this chapter is taken from that outlined by Jacqueline Perry (1992) from Rancho Los Amigos and is widely acknowledged and recognized.

The two main periods of the adult gait cycle (GC) are the stance phase (~60% of GC) and the swing phase (~40% of GC; Fig. 10.1). The stance phase has two tasks that must be undertaken: weight acceptance and single limb support. Swing limb advancement (SLA) is the only task in the swing phase of the gait cycle. Each of the periods is divided into phases, four in the stance phase, three in the swing phase and one phase that links both (Fig. 10.1).

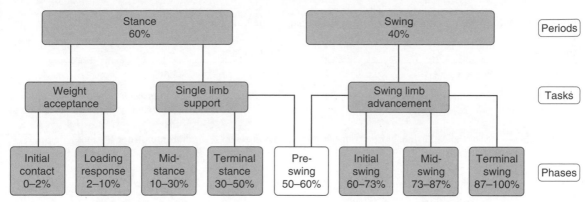

Figure 10.1   The gait cycle.

Table 10.1   Phases of the gait cycle

	Phase	Definition
STANCE	Initial contact	The moment when the foot hits the ground
STANCE	Loading response	The body weight is transferred on to the lead limb
STANCE	Mid stance	The body progresses over a single stable limb
STANCE	Terminal stance	Progression over the stance limb continues and the body moves ahead of the limb and weight is transferred on to the forefoot
TRANSITION	Pre-swing	A rapid unloading occurs as weight is transferred to the other limb
SWING	Initial swing	The thigh advances as the foot is lifted clear of the floor
SWING	Mid-swing	The thigh continues to advances and the knee, having reached maximum flexion, now extends, keeping the foot clear of the floor
SWING	Terminal swing	The knee extends and the limb prepares to take the load at initial contact

From Rancho Los Amigos Medical Centre 1989 Observational gait analysis handbook. Los Amigos Research and Education Institute, Downey, CA

In each of the phase boxes (Fig. 10.1), there is an approximate percentage of the adult gait cycle for that phase. The two tasks in the stance period have very different time elements, with the time for single limb support being much greater than that for weight acceptance. Therefore, control of the trunk on a single limb and moving the body over the foot takes up the majority of the task in the stance phase. In contrast, the three phases of the swing period are all relatively equal in length, indicating a smooth movement with no alteration to the velocity of the lower limb.

Table 10.1 outlines the names of the periods, the basic tasks and phases of the gait cycle. The definitions of the phases are denoted with the main action(s) for that task, and are provided to help

you understand what happens specifically during each of the phases.

The phases of the adult gait cycle can also be recognized by specific joint or muscle action taking place. Table 10.2 therefore describes the main muscle action or joint movement of the lower limbs occurring at each phase. You should note that the task 'Pre-swing' is a transition task between the stance and the swing phase but I have included it under the swing phase in this table for convenience.

The initial contact of the foot with the ground is usually made by the posterolateral aspect of the calcaneus, with the ankle and knee held in neutral and the hip in the maximum flexion (25°) required for the gait cycle. The body weight is then transferred on to the lead leg during loading response

Table 10.2   Main muscle and joint action for each phase of the gait cycle

Stance phase		Swing phase	
Task	Action	Task	Action
Initial contact	Maximum hip flexion	Pre-swing	Maximum ankle plantar flexion, start of knee flexion, greatest plantar flexion torque
Loading response	Slight knee flexion, ankle plantar flexion	Initial swing	Maximum knee flexion
Mid-stance	Vertical alignment of the hip, knee and ankle	Mid-swing	Hip returns to maximum flexion
Terminal stance	Maximum hip extension, greatest hip extensor torque, maximum ankle dorsiflexion	Terminal swing	Knee, ankle in neutral

and the knee flexes marginally (up to 15°) to act as a shock absorber. The ankle plantar flexes to 10° so that the whole of the foot touches the floor for the start of weight bearing and the hip remains in the same degree of flexion.

At the start of single limb stance the body progresses over the foot in 'mid-stance' with both the hip and knee moving into extension and the ankle from plantar flexion to neutral and then into dorsiflexion. At the midpoint of 'mid-stance' the ankle is in neutral and the body is aligned vertically over the hip and knee. In the second part of single limb support, terminal stance, the body progresses forward so that the weight is transferred from the middle of the foot to the forefoot, via the lateral aspect. During this time the hip extends to its maximum during the gait cycle (20°) and the ankle moves from neutral to maximal dorsiflexion (10°). The knee continues to move into extension but this is a passive action subsequent to the active movement at the hip and ankle.

Pre-swing marks the full transference of weight on to the other limb, which is in initial contact. The ankle on the reference limb moves into maximal plantar flexion (20°) and the concentric contraction of gastrocnemius and soleus produces the greatest moment during the gait cycle. The simultaneous action of ankle plantar flexion and knee flexion to approximately 40° results in the hip flexing to neutral.

At the start of the swing phase the knee continues to flex (60°), as does the hip (15°), and the ankle starts its return to neutral by dorsiflexing to 10° of plantar flexion. With these combined actions the foot is lifted clear from the floor and the thigh accelerates forward to progress the free-moving limb. Through mid-swing the hip continues to flex (to 25°) and the ankle gets to neutral. The knee starts to extend, being eccentrically controlled by the hamstrings. The last phase of the gait cycle prepares the foot for initial contact by the knee actively extending to neutral, the hip remaining in 25° flexion and the ankle remaining in neutral.

In Table 10.2 the action describes the main requirements of each of the tasks of the gait cycle and the demands made at that time. If the body cannot undertake the required action at the appropriate time, the person will have an abnormal gait pattern. Small alterations can be accommodated by the body and will not be noticed by the individual. If the alterations are numerous or large, the consequences can have a great effect on the overall walking pattern as well as on individual joint movement.

TIME AND DISTANCE DATA

Temporal spatial data are those which represent movement (e.g. length, time, distance, velocity) and in walking this constitutes the mainstay of the objective assessment. Michael Whittle, in his text on gait analysis (Whittle 2003), provides a detailed summary table of the main time and distance data over the ages. This is complemented by the work of Öberg et al (1993), who reported similar data taken in the clinical environment.

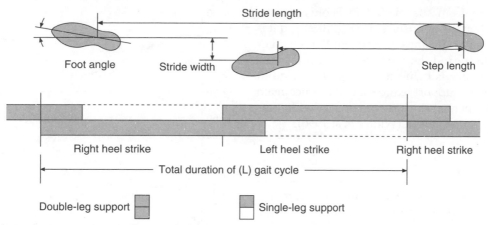

Figure 10.2   Measurement of step and stride lengths.

Self-assessment question

• **SAQ 10.1** What are the walking speeds, cadence and stride lengths for males and females ages 18–40 years and over 65 years?

(Answer at end of chapter.)

The large degree of variance across each of the age groups for both males and females should be noted. There is no one numerical value for velocity, cadence or stride length or any of the many gait variables that can be collected. The variables are all collected at the natural free walking speed but with injury or disease this can be altered so it is important to ask patients if they are walking more slowly or quickly than previously. Footwear can also alter the pattern of the normal gait cycle. For assessment the patients' normal footwear should be used if they cannot walk without their shoes on.

Despite such a wide range of 'normal', overall our individual gait characteristics remain the same throughout life, so that a fast walker will always be a fast walker, and someone who takes long steps will always do so, despite the advancement of age, unless injury or disease intervenes.

There are, however, some overall changes to the gait pattern that normally occur with advancing years and these include reduction in walking speed, increase in the width of the base of support and reduction in step length (Winter et al 1990). So it is important to refresh the more specific changes that occur with advancing years.

Alterations in the gait pattern with age

In fact the gait parameters seem to adapt a bimodal layout, with the childhood years up to 7 and the elderly years after 70 having very similar characteristics:

• a wide base of support
• a short step length
• a more waddling gait
• an alteration in gait speed compared to the adult pattern.

In small children the gait is often faster than the adult gait (Whittle 2003) as the feet try to maintain the centre of gravity over the centre of balance, but the reverse is so for the elderly gait pattern, when there is a significant reduction in gait velocity to allow greater control of balance (Winter et al 1990). It is in the intervening years that the gait pattern has the more recognizable 'mature' pattern.

Stride and step differences are the major distance components of gait and, as Winter et al (1990) indicate, these differ in the younger and older gait cycle. Stride length is the distance from the foot contact (usually the heel) on one side to the same foot contact on that side (e.g. right heel to right heel; Fig. 10.2), while step length is the foot contact from one side to the heel contact on the opposite side (e.g. right heel to left heel). Base of support is the distance from the medial malleolus on one side to that on the opposite side (Fig. 10.2) and it is the other major distance component that changes with age. In the toddler the base of support is very wide as balance is being developed. In the adult gait the base of support reduces and then once again in the older person the base of support widens as balance is compromised (Winter et al 1990).

Toe clearance

Toe clearance is the vertical distance from the great toe to the floor during the swing phase of the gait cycle. It is particularly important in the elderly as this distance decreases by at least 50% with age. During the adult gait, toe clearance is 1.5–2 cm and in the elderly gait it is less than 1 cm (Elbe et al 1991, Prince et al 1997). This normal change is easy to assess in the clinical situation by videoing the walk from the sagittal aspect. Increasing toe clearance is something that the patient can try to alter to help reduce the chance or incidence of falls. The patient should be encouraged to increase the degree of hip and/or knee flexion through mid-swing to compensate for reduced toe clearance.

Movement differences through the years

Figure 10.3 gives a graphical representation of the sagittal plane joint movements in the hip, knee and ankle in younger people (adult gait) and those over 70 years of age (elderly gait). The main differences that occur are:

- at the start of the stance phase and the end of the swing phase in the hip joint
- at loading response and slightly throughout swing phase in the knee joint
- predominantly at the end of the stance phase but slightly at the start of the stance phase and throughout swing in the ankle joint. (Constructed with data from Winter 1987, Winter et al 1990 and Perry 1992.)

This graph should help you to see where the main joint movement differences occur with age and to understand the age changes in gait to decide the correct treatment for gait abnormalities.

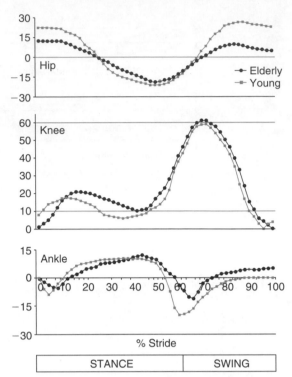

Figure 10.3 Comparison of young and elderly hip, knee and ankle sagittal plane movement.

Self-assessment question

- **SAQ 10.2** Using Figure 10.3 and the three points above, discuss why you think these differences occur.

(Answer at end of chapter.)

By now you should have an understanding of the gait cycle, in particular the movement, distance, and velocity data and how these differ with age. The next stage is to consider how as a physiotherapist you can evaluate the gait cycle and recognize abnormalities.

GAIT ASSESSMENT IN THE THERAPEUTIC ENVIRONMENT

The most accurate and informative biomechanical data on the gait cycle are collected through use of three-dimensional motion analysis systems in gait laboratories. Unfortunately, the laboratories are not available to most patients or physiotherapists because of their high cost and the time taken to complete the task (Krebs et al 1985). Also, interpretation of biomechanical data is complex, time-consuming and not readily understood by most therapists, and this has added to the difficulties of transferring the knowledge gained from the laboratory to the therapy situation. Some physiotherapists, however, do have access to biomechanical data from gait laboratories and may need help to decipher the findings, and there are several papers available to assist this understanding (Bowker & Messenger 1988, Kopf et al 1998, Mendeiros 1984, Rose 1983, Whittle 1996, Yack 1984). Detailed knowledge of biomechanical interpretation is not something that you need to know at this time and should be left until you need to explore specific patient data.

Therefore, for most clinically based physiotherapists, gait assessment will be undertaken in the physiotherapy department, hospital corridor, patient's home, school or workplace, etc. Means of assessing gait variables within these environments must be reliable, valid, user-friendly and cost-effective.

> ### Problem–solving exercise 10.1
>
> List the difficulties that need to be overcome when doing gait assessment outside of a laboratory situation.
>
> (Answer at end of chapter.)

Why do gait assessment?

Before carrying out the assessment it is important to ask the specific question: 'What are the objectives of this gait assessment?' There are many possible answers, including:

- to give an overall impression of the performance
- to allow the patient to become aware of specific gait problems
- to measure the speed and distance of walking
- to measure overall fitness, etc.

In each therapeutic situation the answer will differ and you have a range of skills and tools to measure the effectiveness of treatment. Evaluation of

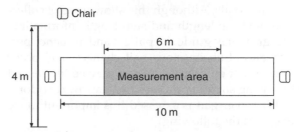

Figure 10.4 A standardized 10 m walkway.

gait will either be subjective (judgement through observation of events) or objective (judgement through numerical measuring/recording of events). Both of these are important to gait evaluation but subjective analysis is the most commonly used in the therapeutic environment.

Subjective assessment of gait

Observation and subjective recording of gait will never be totally superseded as the mainstay of gait assessment in the therapeutic environment because of ease of use, but you should be aware of all the limitations and alternatives available to you.

To accurately assess gait through observation it is important to have a standardization measurement 'walkway', so that the environment for the assessment can be kept the same. Then one of the factors that affects reliability has been controlled.

Environment for the walking test

Ideally the environment for the walking test should be well lit, quiet, and cleared of all equipment. The walking space should ideally be 10 m in length (Robinson & Smidt 1981) with adequate room so that the therapist can move to the front, back and side of the patient (Whittle 2003). Any distractions to the patient (e.g. mirrors, people) should be removed and video cameras, if used, should be kept as far out of the walking field as possible. Chairs should be provided at the ends of the walkway so that the participant can rest (Fig. 10.4) and discreet distance markers on the floor or wall may help if a timed walk is to be undertaken.

Robinson & Smidt (1981) recommend a more structured 10 m walkway with adhesive tape applied to the floor to mark out a grid of 10 m × 0.30 m with numbered transverse strips at

3 cm intervals. Although this allows ease of collection of stride length and step length information, the 'grid' may guide the patient and influence performance. Subconscious gait changes may occur in different environments and may be influenced by cueing such as gridlines or a narrow corridor.

Wherever gait is assessed it is important to try to obtain the following:

- Minimum of 10 m
- 2 m warm-up and warm-down
- Chair at either end
- Skin markers (contrast colour)
- Stop watch
- Quiet area with space on all four sides (if possible)
- Good lighting
- Same footwear.

A 10 m walk is extremely difficult to obtain in the 'home' environment but in the clinic it is essential always to use the same area for gait assessment so that the variables are reduced. In the home situation only a short walk (2–3 m) may be possible and the patient will have to undertake this many more times for you to be able to observe the movement problems. It is also more difficult to 'stand away' from the patient to get a clear view of a specific part of the overall walk.

Worsfold & Simpson (1996) noted that patients who declared a fear of falling and difficulty in walking both indoors and outdoors were more at ease walking in the corridor than in any other environment. This set-up obviously limits how well you can see specific abnormalities and the objective of the gait assessment will have to change to accommodate the limited evaluation possible.

Wherever the gait assessment is taking place, try to standardize the environment so that repeat assessments are more meaningful; this will reduce variability and increase the reliability of your observation.

Observational analysis

There is no agreement as to what should be assessed in observational analysis of gait and many authors have reported issues with poor observational ability, personal bias and experience, poor training of the technique and limitations of visual perception (Krebs et al 1985). Therefore it is not surprising that poor intra- and inter-rater reliability has been found by many researchers (Goodkin & Diller 1973, Krebs et al 1985, Patla et al 1987, Eastlack et al 1991).

While researching observational skills using videotaping, Krebs et al (1985) found a total agreement of 67.5% when three therapists assessed the gait of 15 children. Likewise, Eastlack et al (1991) only found slight to moderate agreement ($\kappa = 0.11$–0.52) when 54 therapists assessed three patients with rheumatoid arthritis. In patients following stroke, Hughes & Bell (1994) ascertained significant agreement between three raters for the swing phase parameters of gait but not for the stance phase or for the overall description of the gait characteristics.

Although observation of specific parameters may be flawed, observation can provide the therapist with a general impression of the quality of movement and help to assess the overall functional walking ability of the patient. Things to look at include:

- How do patients interact with their environment?
- Do they walk near the wall?
- How do they manoeuvre around obstacles?
- How do they use their walking aid?
- Are they easily distracted?
- Can they handle different environments (outdoors, slopes, rough ground, busy streets, etc.)?

Problem-solving exercise 10.2

Take each of the points above and work out what might happen to the person's gait if they are observed to have problems with these issues.

(Answer at end of chapter.)

This material is valuable and gives 'real life' information. Videotaping in the non-clinical environment is difficult so you must have specific objectives of observation, and these will differ depending on the level of ability of the patient.

Video-taping

Video-taping of the gait assessment will enhance the observational skills of the therapists by allowing repeated viewing at slower speeds or freezing specific frames for closer inspection. The advantage to patients of videoing the event is that they should be less fatigued, as the number of repetitions will be reduced, and that they will see a recording of their performance and become aware of any deviations. The disadvantage of any observation, but especially one involving the presence of video cameras, is that the patient can be acutely aware of the 'performance' and gait pattern modification can occur to put on a good show (Rose 1983). Securing privacy within the room, keeping cameras as unobtrusive as possible and ensuring that the patient is at ease will assist in obtaining 'normal' movement. Standardization of the position of the video camera(s) (usually to view the sagittal or frontal plane or both), the 'walkway', the level of light and the general environment will all help to allow comparison of findings from one day to the next and to focus the eye of the reviewer.

If there is no video camera available but you wish to use your observational skills to get an impression of the gait pattern, there are certain issues that you need to consider. To observe the overall walking pattern stand away from the 'walkway' and think of the overall components that can change:

- Timing and speed of limb movement
- Obvious joint problems – increased or decreased
- Obvious joint deformity
- The overall pace of walking
- Are step lengths equal?
- Limb position during stance and swing
- Overall body posture
- Width of base of support
- Heaviness of the footfalls.

For the more detailed assessment of gait, more objective measures have to be taken.

Objective assessment

Objective measures fall into several categories:

- Measurement of time and distance data
- Measurement of joint and limb motion
- Measure of overall walking ability.

Time and distance data

Walking tests are now an accepted part of the measurement of gait (Butland et al 1981, Singh et al 1992, Wade 1992). The walking test can be set by either time or distance, e.g. the 2-, 6- or 12-minute walking test or the 3 m or 10 m walking test. Walking tests have been used to assess general respiratory fitness (Singh 1992), pre- and postoperative performance in patients with orthopaedic problems (McNicol et al 1980, 1981) or overall gait disability in the neurological area. The 10 m timed walk test has been used extensively in the assessment of neurological gait (Wade 1992). Smith (1993) suggests that in laboratory assessment of gait only one walking trial is necessary for intrapatient assessment but the mean of three trials should be used for interpatient assessment.

The test requires that either the time taken to walk a set distance or the total distance walked over a set time is recorded to give an indication of the walking velocity and cadence. Many researchers and clinicians have used gait velocity to reflect change in gait performance as a result of treatment (e.g. McNicol et al 1980, 1981, Robinson & Smidt 1981, Wade 1992). There is a significant correlation between the walking velocity and many other components of gait, e.g. balance ability, quadriceps strength and length of the tendo achillis (Steadman et al 1997a) and velocity is therefore often used as a clinical outcome measure. Wade et al (1987) also showed that walking velocity correlated with the clinical assessment of the gait pattern following stroke.

The number of steps or strides can also be counted to measure cadence and there are recognized normal values for these measures (Whittle 2003).

The longer walking tests (either time or distances) should be used to assess the gait of more able patients (Butland et al 1981, Gulmans et al 1996). The 3-minute test has been used in elderly people (Wolfson et al 1990) and was found to have low variability within one session and was repeatable over 24 hours in elderly patients (mean age 83.6 years, SD 5.8; Worsfold & Simpson 1996). The greatest advantage of this test is that it can be used in both the clinical and the home environment without adaptation.

Stride and step measurement

Stride and step length can only be measured if there is a representation of foot contact; usually heel strike is taken. Recording on to a Dictaphone whenever the patient's foot makes contact with a measured point on the floor grid can provide the number of steps/strides taken and step/stride length, and record the distance from the starting point. Other measures can also be used to measure steps/strides length.

Simple methods of gait analysis
- Footprint analysis (Clarkson 1983, Kippen 1993, Shores 1980, Volpon 1994), the use of ink or paint on the soles of the feet
- Event markers, e.g. pens attached to the heels, talcum powder on floor, sand, etc.
- Ticker tape analysis (Law & Minns 1989)
- Calculation – overall length walked divided by the number of strides will give the mean overall stride length, or the number of steps will give the mean overall step length (McNicol et al 1980, 1981). This technique is not as accurate as direct measurement of the step and stride length.

Complex and more expensive methods
- Instrumented shoes, foot switches (Rowe et al 1989, Whittle 2003, Yack 1984)
- Pressure mats or walkways systems (Silvino et al 1980, SMS Health Care Ltd. 1998, Wall et al 1981)
- Personal-computer-based systems (Wall 1991, Wall & Crosbie 1996, 1997).

The ultimate measurement tools are the Optoelectric Motion Analysis systems (infra red or visible light; Davis 1997, Whittle 1996) but these are confined to gait analysis laboratories in most cases.

The other distance parameter that can be measured is the dynamic width of support or walking base (normal 50–100 mm; Whittle 2003), i.e. the horizontal distance between the centre of the feet during double support time. The static base of support measured from the standing posture just prior to walking (87.5 mm; Perry 1992) is only a true representation of base of support during the mid-stance phase of gait. As the width of the base of support increases dynamic balance ability increases (Winter et al 1990). The wider the dynamic base of support the less the subject has to use muscle control at the hips and ankles and vice versa (Perry 1992). Alternatively, the patient may not widen the base of support but lower the centre of mass by flexing the knees on walking. The base of support will look normal but comparison of knee flexion in the static and dynamic standing posture will indicate the problem.

Joint and limb motion

Joint and limb motion can only be a subjective observational guess unless electrogoniometers (Rowe et al 1989) or an Optoelectric Motion Analysis system are available in the therapeutic situation.

When observing limb segment motion several parameters can be estimated:

- Range and timing of motion
- Starting position of the joint and limb segments (including deformities)
- Acceleration of the limb segments.

Measuring joint angles directly from the television screen (from freeze frame on videotape) is prone to error and therefore cannot give true objective data, only a guestimation of joint angle. The advent of video-based computer systems using an ordinary personal computer means that cheaper and easier objective measures are starting to be available for use in the therapeutic environment (Wall & Crosbie 1996, 1997).

The observation of joint motion or limb segment position is particularly difficult and unreliable without the use of videotape. A video recorder with a freeze frame and jog per frame facility is also preferable, allowing you time to study the position of the body or limb segments. A systematic approach to joint and limb motion is required for enhancing observational techniques and for consistency of results. Patla et al (1987) report that the 22 therapists they studied predominantly used a variety of starting points when studying specific body segments, i.e. foot to head, hip to foot, etc. Once the therapists had established a systematic approach, they kept to it. There is no evidence in the literature to indicate whether the observer should start at the foot and work up to the head or vice versa, or concentrate on the lower limb before the trunk. Whichever approach is used a routine should be established, practised and used for all patients. Ideally all planes of motion should be observed but realistically only the frontal and sagittal plane can be assessed. Krebs et al (1985) report that sagittal plane movements are more reliable than frontal or transverse, and that movements at the larger joints, i.e. hip and knee, are more reliable than at the foot and ankle.

The use of visual cues such as skin markers (removable pen marks or small 1 cm adhesive coloured discs) on bony prominences will assist the observation of joint movement. Specifically, the acromion, anterior superior iliac spine greater trochanter, lateral femoral condyle, lateral malleolus and fifth metatarsal head are the points of choice but additional markers can be placed on the posterior superior iliac spines, anterior thigh and anterior shank to assist observation of rotation (Perry 1992). Obviously, this requires that the patient is suitably undressed and markers should contrast with the skin colour.

Vertical lines, e.g. wall bars or a grid on the wall, may also help with recognizing joint position and the position of the trunk relative to the vertical (Kinsman 1986). The observation of standing posture from the frontal and sagittal planes will help assess the static posture and will indicate any change in spinal postures or deformities caused by dynamic loading such as valgus/varus, hip abduct or weakness (Trendelenburg test) or increased lumbar lordosis.

Patla et al (1987) reported that the majority of the therapists questioned only looked at the stance phase of gait for patients with back, ankle and knee problems, while both stance and swing were evaluated in those with hip problems. This is not recommended and all the limb segments should be observed in both the swing and stance phases of gait. At this point I should repeat that, for you to recognize the specific difficulties at individual joints, knowledge of the phases of gait and the 'normal' values for starting positions and joint ranges during the gait cycle for the specific age groups is essential (Sutherland et al 1980, Whittle 2003, Winter et al 1990).

When observing gait you must think about the limb axes and the position of the limbs relative to each other. Except for the hip joint, the axes will normally be the lines bisecting the length of the bone. Thus as the thigh and lower leg move there

will be a relative change in angle at the knee joint. At initial contact the ankle joint is in the neutral position with the knee in neutral and the hip at 25° of flexion (Rancho Los Amigos Medical Centre 1989), although on observation the ankle may appear dorsiflexed because of the relative knee position. Loading response differs from initial contact because the knee has flexed to 15° and the ankle is now in 10° plantar flexion (Rancho Los Amigos Medical Centre 1989). The ankle looks as if it has not moved from the neutral position but is in plantarflexion because the tibia is still behind the axis of motion (ankle joint) while the foot is in contact with the ground.

The skill of assessing joint motion by observation is to know the normal ranges, to monitor the position of the limbs relative to the joints and to be able to describe the axes of the angles being monitored.

You will need assistance in recognizing the relative motion of the limb segments and video can help with this. By freezing the frame of the video at the point in the gait cycle being assessed, the position of the limb segment can be viewed and compared to a vertical line dropped from the top of the monitor screen. For example, when measuring hip movement in the sagittal plane, if a vertical line is placed near the hip joint centre (approximately the greater trochanter), then the relative positions of the lower limb segments and trunk can be taken from this. This can also be done in the frontal plane view but the vertical line is more difficult to place as there is no definitive point of rotation. This technique is purely to help judge the relative positions of the limb segments, not to measure the actual joint angle.

Limb accelerations Assessing the acceleration or timing of the limb segments is enhanced by video-taping, as the tape can be slowed down to observe more time-specific changes such as foot drop or knee wobble at terminal swing/initial contact. Changes in acceleration or timing of the limb segments are predominantly due to loss (reduction in strength and/or recruitment) or increase (spasm, imbalance or spasticity) of muscle control. Electromyography can be used to help record which muscle is working and the level, timing and extent of muscle activity in the dynamic situation (Perry 1992).

Measure of overall walking disability As a global indicator of the effect an altered walking pattern has on energy expenditure and disability, measures of respiratory function can be used. These are often costly and laboratory-based but indices of overall cardiorespiratory function may be useful. The physiological cost index (PCI) is one such index and can be calculated by the difference of the end of walk to resting heart rate divided by the speed.

PCI = (HR at end of walk – Resting HR)/Speed

(beats/m) = (beats/min) − (beats/min) (m/min)

This gives a global indication of the energy expenditure of walking and does not require expensive equipment. The index is sensitive to change and has been used in both adults (Nene 1993) and children (Butler et al 1984) and validated as a comparative index of energy cost (McGregor 1981).

However this is not a true measure of the disability of walking. One such measure is the 'patient perception' questionnaire used to assess walking disability in patients following stroke (Steadman et al 1997b). This simple questionnaire correlated significantly with walking velocity, Berg balance scores and the results of the Rivermead Mobility Index, indicating that the perceptions of patients with moderate to severe walking disability gave an indication of their overall physical performance (Steadman et al 1997b). Further investigations remain to be done in this field to validate measures of walking disability.

Recording

If objective measures have been recorded (e.g. gait velocity, timing, distance, step length), there is no need for a specific recording format to be used so long as all the parameters are recorded clearly. However, when recording the impressions from observation you can make a choice from a number of recording formats depending on how detailed the observation or measurement has been. Patla et al (1987) questioned 22 therapists on their gait analysis procedures, reporting that 'Unfortunately, after doing such a detailed examination, the final report takes the form of a single comment'. It is easy to make and record a quick simple overall

impression but this does not give a suitable outcome measure, only a subjective qualitative opinion. It may be easy to interpret this information at the time of writing but at a later date the words could be meaningless and the overall interpretation may change. When describing the relevant components therapists tend to look at, and record, the easier global temporal-spatial parameters of 'width of base of support, torso positioning, symmetry and foot placement, stride length and cadence' (Patla et al 1987).

Examples of the charts available for recording these impressions include:

- recording the estimated range of motion overall or at the appropriate phase of gait (Patla et al 1987, Reimers 1972)
- ticking a box if there is a loss or gain of motion, or for specific gait deviations (Rancho Los Amigos Medical Centre 1989)
- using an ordinal scale to record the quality and/or quantity of the gait deviation (e.g. Eastlack et al 1991, Hughes & Bell 1994, Krebs et al 1985, Lord et al 1998, Lower Limb Orthotics 1981)
- Key component charts – using a basic chart format to record when a joint movement is impaired during gait cycle.

Which chart to use will depend on the question asked in the first instance. The simplest format is to record all the phases of the gait cycle and write down the main abnormal components observed. This only gives a global view and is open to misinterpretation if normal gait terminology and facts are not up to date. The observational gait analysis (OGA) form (Rancho Los Amigos Medical Centre 1989) requires that the therapist indicates if there is a gait deformity present at any of the joints, through any phase of the gait cycle. If there is a deformity present then this will indicate either a major or a minor effect on walking ability, and the chart has been colour-coded to help this decision.

The successful use of the Rancho Los Amigos OGA form requires both practice and a complete understanding of the terminology, as it is complex and time-consuming. The team at Rancho Los Amigos has developed a complete observational package and the OGA form is only one part of this. The package helps the therapist to understand the implications of the gait deformities and the causes of these, thus aiding problem solving in gait analysis. This type of recording means that the therapist must have a full understanding of normal kinematic gait data and be up to date with the terminology used in the form.

It may therefore be easier to use a simple box system to note your observations. Figure 10.5 represents a grid format for this, where for each phase of the gait cycle you can record any abnormal event by the main body parts, but there is also a place for the linear and time measures as well.

A patient with a left hip problem may have a chart that looks like Figure 10.6, where there is a lean to the left short and weak side on weight bearing that continues throughout the stance period. This is accompanied by a posterior rotation of the pelvis on the same side, indicating a lack of hip extension, and this again continues through until the pre-swing phase. In the swing phase there is increased pelvic tilt, which indicates greater use of the pelvis because of loss of hip movement and that help is needed to help move the left limb forward. The left step is shorter and the base of support is wider. This chart would represent anyone with a single hip joint problem but things might get more complicated if the problem was more severe or if other joints were involved, as with Mrs White in Chapter 7.

Although this grid is open to criticism, it offers a standardized format for you to record your findings easily.

There are many other methods of recording gait deformity; in particular, the ordinal scale is

	Stance				⇒	Swing		
	Initial contact	Loading response	Mid	Terminal	Pre	Initial	Mid	Terminal
Arms								
Trunk/ pelvis								
Hip								
Knee								
Ankle								
Stride								
BOS								
WA								

BOS = Base of support
WA = Walking aids

Figure 10.5   Key component analysis form.

	Stance					Swing		
	Initial contact	Loading response	Mid stance	Terminal stance	Pre	Initial	Mid	Terminal
Arms								
Trunk/ pelvis		Lean to L ↑ Posterior rotation (L)	⇒ ⇒	⇒ ⇒	⇒	↑ tilt	⇒	⇒
Hip				↓ extension	⇒			
Knee								
Ankle								

Step   R = 0.46 m, L = 0.34 cm   **Time 10 m**
Base of support ↑ to 15 cm
Walking aids   1 stick outdoors or longer distances R hand
Leg length   Left   Right
⇒ indicates that the abnormality continues to the next phase

Figure 10.6   Completed key component analysis form – general hip.

commonly used. The therapist is asked to indicate from a list of possibilities whether a gait deformity is present, and the extent of its presence. Krebs et al (1985) used the symbols 0 for normal gait, + for just noticeably abnormal or ++ for very noticeably abnormal gait. Eastlack et al (1991) used the scale I = inadequate, N = normal, E = excessive. The main problem with these scales is the lack of specific definitions: for example, precisely what does 'just noticeably abnormal' or 'inadequate' mean? Lord et al (1998) developed a form using a four-point ordinal scale and giving very clear definitions of each component of the form. The definitions are based on the normal position of the joint and the therapist records whether the gait deviation is 'normal, mild, moderate, severe' based on the definition. Although not all points on the scale have been defined, there is a standardized definition from which the therapist can make a judgement.

One recording format will not be acceptable in all therapeutic environments but whatever the choice it must represent the answer to the question asked at the start – what are the objectives of this gait assessment?

Case study 10.1: Mrs Stamford

Please read the case study of Mrs Stamford in Case study 7.1 (Chapter 7, page 172).
  Known key points regarding Mrs Stamford's gait:

- Osteoarthrosis left knee
- Walks with one stick (L) hand
- Swollen knee
- Decreased quadriceps bulk
- Quadriceps grade IV
- Knee range of movement:
  – Passive movement (−5°)–90°
  – Active movement (−5°)–80°
  – Varus deformity
  – Full hip and ankle movement R = L.

Table 10.3   Observed gait deformities for Mrs Stamford: sagittal and frontal planes

Physical sign	Gait deviation
Sagittal plane	
Knee flexion deformity, swollen knee	↑ Knee flexion in IC, MS, TS
	↓ Hip extension TS
	↓ Step length
Lack of quadriceps control	↑ Knee wobble on weight bearing in LR, MS, TS
	↑ Hip flexion in TS, PSw
Frontal plane	
Varus deformity	↑ Varus on weight bearing, MS, TS & PSw
	↑ Abduction hip MS & TS
	↑ Pronation foot MS & TS
	↑ Base of support LR, MS, TS
	↑ Adduction in swing, ISw–PSw
Reduced weight bearing on (L) knee	Trunk lateral lean to left side if using a stick or lateral lean to right side if not using a stick
Painful knee (antalgic gait)	Moves off the left foot quickly on weight bearing, hurried left stance phase

IC = Initial contact; ISw = Initial swing; LR = Loading response; MS = Mid-stance; MSw = Mid-swing; PSw = Pre-swing; TS = Terminal stance; TSw = Terminal swing

---

Problem-solving exercise 10.3

After hypothetically observing Mrs Stamford's gait from both the sagittal and frontal planes, what might you expect to see?

(The answer is given in Table 10.3.)

As we cannot see Mrs Stamford it is difficult to be absolutely certain what her gait looks like but the table gives a gross overview of the expectations, given her history as we know it.

The key points from the observation of Mrs Stamford's gait are:

- Reduced left step length
- Decreased stance phase time on left leg

- Increased stance phase time on right leg
- Decreased gait velocity
- Increased knee flexion.

The use of a stick will assist Mrs Stamford in a number of ways:

- Lower cadence – steps/min 90 (with) versus 101 (without)
- Vertical ground reaction force reduced by 25%
- Total vertical force did not exceed 100% – cautious loading on cane
- Anteroposterior shear reduced – 50 N (with) versus 120 N (without)
- Cane backward force very low, indicating may assist in forward propulsion of body
- Reduced joint moments at hip, knee and ankle
- Reduced powers at hip, knee and ankle
- Cane loading begins at initial contact and reduces before pre-swing
- Significant alterations in the loading of upper limb in some gait subphases (Winter et al 1993).

The stick reduces the speed of walking, so the forces required are reduced as the cane is loaded. Likewise, the forces across the lower limb joints are reduced as weight is borne by the stick. Loading of the upper limb joints will increase during the stance phase on the side that the stick is held.

The major issue for Mrs Stamford will be whether she places her stick in the left or right hand.

With her left knee being worse than the right, the stick can go in either hand. Most research papers and texts indicate that the stick should go in the opposite hand to the side affected, but Edwards (1986) found that the stick in the opposite hand to the problem side allowed:

- greater mean step length
- increased cadence
- faster mean walking velocity
- use except when the patient has reduced hip movement

while use of a stick in the same hand to the problem side caused:

- knee joint motion on affected side to be greater
- hip joint motion on affected side to lower
- peak vertical floor reaction forces to be greater.

So for a painful knee there is no set answer to the side for the stick: both have advantages and

	Stance					Swing		
	Initial contact	Loading response	Mid stance	Terminal stance	Pre	Initial	Mid	Terminal
Arms	↓ arm swing	⇒	⇒	⇒	⇒	⇒	⇒	⇒
Trunk/ pelvis		Lean to L	⇒	⇒				
Hip			↑ Abduction	↓ extension ⇒	⇒	↑ Add	⇒	⇒
Knee		↑ Flexion	⇒ ↑ varus ↑ wobble	⇒ ⇒ ⇒	⇒ ⇒			
Ankle			↑ pronation	⇒				

Step   R > L   **Time 10 m**
Base of support: Increased
Walking aids   1 L hand
Leg length   Left   Right
⇒ indicates that the abnormality continues to the next phase

Figure 10.7   Completed key component analysis form – Mrs Stamford (Case study 7.1).

disadvantages and the choice may depend on the patient's preference.

Knee wobble is a recognized term in gait analysis, where the knee control is poor during weight bearing and the knee moves, usually forward and backwards but it can move from side to side depending on knee ligament laxity.

Figure 10.7 gives a graphical overview of the gait problems identified in Table 10.3 and shows how easy it is to put these in chart format.

In Figure 10.6 the gait of someone with a single painful hip was portrayed. If a more complex hip problem is encountered, such as you would expect to find in Mrs White in Case study 7.2 on page 199 (bilateral hip problems), then Figure 10.8 is a better representation. As Mrs White walks with a walking frame it will be difficult to fully assess her gait unless she can manage a few steps without the frame. It would still be valid to assess her walking with the frame but the assistance gained from its use would have to be taken into account.

> **Problem-solving exercise 10.4**
>
> Using Figure 10.8, can you place, in table format (as per Table 10.3), the main issues that would be found for the problems with Mrs White's hips, assuming that she is able to walk a few steps without her frame. If necessary, go back and look at the issues identified for Mrs Stamford.
>
> (Answer at end of chapter.)

The key things and the easiest problems to spot in the observation of Mrs White's gait are:

- Reduced step length
- Reduced base of support with possible cross-over
- Reduced gait velocity
- Increased hip flexion
- Increased trunk flexion
- Increased hip adduction.

	Stance				Swing			
	Initial contact	Loading response	Mid stance	Terminal stance	Pre	Initial	Mid	Terminal
Arms								
Trunk/ pelvis	Trunk flexion	Lean to L ↑ posterior rotation (L) ⇒	⇒ ⇒ ⇒	⇒ ⇒ ⇒	⇒ ⇒	↑ tilt ⇒	⇒ ⇒	⇒ ⇒
Hip			↑ ADD	↓ extension ⇒	⇒ ↑ Ext. Rot.		↑ ADD ⇒	⇒
Knee	↑ flexion		↑ flexion	⇒				
Ankle			? ↑ PFlexion	⇒				

Step   R =, L =   **Time 10 m**
Base of support   Decreased ++
Walking aids   Walking frame, poor upper limb function especially grip
Leg length   Left   Right
⇒ indicates that the abnormality continues to the next phase

Figure 10.8   Completed key component analysis form – Mrs White (Case study 7.2).

patient between a set of parallel bars and observe even one or two steps unaided with the safety of having the bars available to hold on to if necessary.

Problem-solving exercise 10.5

What changes do you think occur in the normal gait cycle when a person walks with an ordinary walking frame?

(Answer at end of chapter.)

Given that increased hip flexion is the biggest problem when walking with a frame, two things should be encouraged to increase hip extension when walking with a walking frame:

- Simultaneous motion of the affected limb and frame
- The higher the frame the more extension gained (Crosbie 1994).

From these questions I hope that you can appreciate how much a walking aid can hide gait deviations and that ideally gait should be observed with and without the use of an aid. If it is not possible for the patient to do so without the walking aid, then an alternative is to place the

SUMMARY

By the end of this chapter I hope you have a much better understanding of normal gait and gait assessment in the 'clinical environment', i.e. wherever physiotherapists assess gait. The case studies give examples of the findings of a gait assessment for two patients and how gait assessment forms can be used. The suggestions given are only one format for documenting gait issues and there are many others available.

ANSWERS TO QUESTIONS AND EXERCISES

Self-assessment question 10.1 (page 293)

- **SAQ 10.1** What are the walking speeds, cadence and stride lengths for males and females ages 18–40 years and over 65 years?

Answer:

	Females		Males	
	18–40 years	>65 years	18–40 years	>65 years
Walking speed (m/s)	0.94–1.66	0.80–1.52	1.10–1.82	0.81–1.61
Cadence (steps/min)	98–138	96–136	91–135	81–125
Stride length (m) (Whittle 2003)	1.06–1.58	0.94–1.46	1.25–1.85	1.11–1.71

Self-assessment question 10.2 (page 294)

- **SAQ 10.2** Using Figure 10.3 and the three points above, discuss why you think these differences occur.

Answer:

Main points	Point in gait cycle	Differences	Causes
Hip joint	Start of the stance	↓ flexion	↓ step length and ↓ push off with less plantar flexion, ↓ gait velocity
	End of the swing	↓ flexion	
Knee joint	Loading response	↑ extension	Need to ensure good foot placement at IC with control of the knee, cannot absorb shock as efficiently
	Through stance	↓ flexion	↓ step length, ↓ plantar flexion control
Ankle joint	Start of the stance	↓ plantar flexion	↓ plantar flexion strength and need to secure balance
	End of the stance	↓ plantar flexion	
	Through-out swing	↑ dorsiflex-ion	Need to ensure toe clearance as reduced hip flex-ion and spinal movement

Problem-solving exercise 10.1 (page 295)

- List the difficulties that need to be overcome when doing gait assessment outside of a labora-tory situation.

Answer:

- Limited space both length and width
- Floor coverings vary: carpet with various thick-ness versus linoleum
- Distractions: other people, pets, etc.
- Limited room for use of walking aids
- Door widths
- Limited turning space.

Problem-solving exercise 10.2 (page 296)

- Take each of the points above (page 296) and work out what might happen to the person's gait if they are observed to have problems with these issues.

Answer:

Question	Gait problem
How do patients interact with their environment?	Do they try to hold on to furniture, walls, etc? The patient may have a wider base of support in an open space versus narrow, indicating a balance problem
Do they walk near the wall?	People with a balance problem or poor vision will walk nearer a wall or look for hand holds wher-ever possible
How do they manoeuvre around obstacles?	Difficulty with changes in speed as required for this type of manoeuvre are associated with poor balance, co-ordination or muscle control
How do they use their walking aid?	In the correct hand Adequate weight bearing Used correctly Correct height
Are they easily distracted?	Poor concentration may mean alteration to foot placement, leading to safety issues, or diffi-culty balancing in single support
Can they handle different environments (outdoors, slopes rough ground, busy streets, etc.)?	Reduction in gait velocity in different environments can indicate poor balance or loss of motor control, strength or co-ordination

Problem-solving exercise 10.3 (page 303)

See Table 10.3 in text.

Problem-solving exercise 10.4 (page 304)

- Using Figure 10.8, can you place, in table format (as per Table 10.3), the main issues that would be found for the problems with Mrs White's hips, assuming that she is able to walk a few steps without her frame. If necessary, go back and look at the issues identified for Mrs Stamford.

Answer: Observed gait deformities for Mrs White: sagittal and frontal planes – left & right legs are affected, so the main issues would apply to both legs (see table next column).

Problem-solving exercise 10.5 (page 305)

- What changes do you think occur in the normal gait cycle when a person walks with an ordinary walking frame?

Answer:

- Narrower base of support in all double support times
- Reduced gait velocity
- Smaller step length
- Reduced hip flexion (IC, LR, TSw)
- Reduced hip extension (MS, TS and PSw)
- Decreased knee extension (MS and TS)
- Decreased knee flexion (PSw, ISw and MSw)
- Reduced plantar flexion movement and strength (TS and PSw)
- Forward lean of the trunk throughout the gait cycle.

Physical sign	Gait deviation
Sagittal plane	
Loss of hip extension	↓ Hip extension TS & PSw
	↑ Posterior pelvic rotation in TS & PSw
	↓ Step length
Increased lumbar lordosis	↑ Hip flexion in IC, LR, MS, TS, PSw
	↑ Pelvic tilt IS, MS
Increased knee flexion	↑ Knee flexion at IC, MS, TS, PSw, Isw
Reduced weight bearing on (L & R) hip	Trunk lateral movement to each side on weight bearing
Stooped gait	↑ Trunk flexion throughout gait cycle
Frontal plane	
Adduction deformity	↑ Adduction hip MS & TS, MSw
	↑ Knee valgus
	↓ Base of support stance phase
Circumduction	↑ In combined hip rotation and abduction in PSw, MSw, TSw
Increased external rotation	
Antalgic gait	Weight moves quickly off the stance leg to other leg, shortened stance phase
Trendelenburg	Shoulders shift to same side in MS, TS, PSw

IC = Initial contact; ISw = Initial swing; LR = Loading response; MS = Mid-stance; MSw = Mid-swing; PSw = Pre-swing; TS = Terminal stance; TSw = Terminal swing.

References

Bowker P, Messenger N 1988 The measurement of gait. Clinical Rehabilitation 2: 89–97

Butland RJ, Pang J, Gross ER et al 1981 Two, six and twelve minute walks compared. Thorax 36: 225

Butler P, Engelbrecht M, Major RE et al 1984 Physiological Cost Index of walking for normal children and its use as an indicator of physical handicap. Developmental Medicine and Child Neurology 26: 607–612

Clarkson BH 1983 Absorbent paper for recording foot placement during gait. Physical Therapy 63: 345–346

Craik R, Oatis C 1985 Gait assessment in the clinic: issues and approaches. In: Rothstein J (ed) Measurement in physical therapy. Churchill Livingstone, New York, ch 6

Crosbie J 1994 Comparative kinematics of two walking frame gaits. Journal of Orthopaedic and Sports Physiotherapy 20: 186–192

Davis RB 1997 Reflections on clinical gait analysis. Journal of Electromyography 7: 251–257

Eastlack ME, Arvidson J, Snyder-Mackler L et al 1991 Inter-rater reliability of videotaped observational gait-analysis assessments. Physical Therapy 71: 465–472

Edwards BG 1986 Contralateral and ipsilateral cane usage by patients with total knee or hip replacements.Archives of Physical Medicine and Rehabilitation 67: 734–740

Elbe RJ, et al 1991 Stride-dependent changes in gait of older people. Journal of Neurology 238: 1–5

Goodkin R, Diller L 1973 Reliability among physical therapists in diagnosis and treatment of gait deviations in hemiplegics. Perception and Motor Skills 37: 727–734

Gulmans VAM, vanVeldhoven NHMJ, deMeer K, Helders PJM 1996 The six-minute walking test in children with cystic fibrosis: reliability and validity. Pediatric Pulmonology 22: 85–89

Hughes KA, Bell F 1994 Visual assessment of hemiplegic gait following stroke – pilot study. Archives of Physical Medicine and Rehabilitation 75: 1100–1107

Kinsman R 1986 Video assessment of the Parkinson patient. Physiotherapy 72: 386–389

Kippen SC 1993 A preliminary assessment of recording the physical dimensions of an inked footprint. Journal of British Pediatric Medicine (May): 74–80

Kopf A, Pawelka S, Kranzl A 1998 Clinical gait analysis – methods, limitations, and indications. Acta Medica Austriaca 25: 27–32

Krebs DE, Edelstein JE, Fishman S 1985 Reliability of observational kinematic gait analysis. Physical Therapy 65: 1027–1033

Law HT, Minns RA 1989 Measurement of the spatial and temporal parameters of gait. Physiotherapy 75: 81–84

Lord SE, Halligan PW, Wade DT 1998 Visual gait analysis: the development of a clinical assessment and scale. Clinical Rehabilitation 12: 107–119

Lower Limb Orthotics 1981 Lower Limb Orthotics, New York. New York University Postgraduate Medical School, Prosthetics and Orthotics

McGregor J 1981 Evaluation of patient performance using long term ambulatory monitoring technique in domestic environment. Physiotherapy 67: 30

McNicol MF, McHardy R, Chalmers J 1980 Exercise testing before and after hip arthroplasty. Journal of Bone and Joint Surgery 62B: 326–331

McNicol MF, Uprichard H, Mitchell GP 1981 Exercise testing after the Chiari pelvic osteotomy. Journal of Bone and Joint Surgery 63B: 48–52

McRae R 1997 Clinical orthopaedic examination, 4th edn. Churchill Livingstone, Edinburgh

Mendeiros J 1984 Automated measurement systems for clinical motion analysis. Physical Therapy 64: 1846–1850

Nene AV 1993 Physiological Cost Index of walking in able-bodied adolescents and adults. Clinical Rehabilitation 7: 319–326

Öberg T, Karaszima A, Öberg K 1993 Basic gait parameters: reference data for normal subjects 10–79 years of age. Journal of Rehabilitation Research and Development 30: 210–223

Patla AE, Proctor J, Morson B 1987 Observations on aspects of visual gait assessment: a questionnaire study. Physiotherapy Canada 39: 311–316

Perry J 1992 Gait analysis: normal and pathological function. Slack, Thorofare, NJ

Prince F, Corriveau H, Hébert R, Winter DA 1997 Gait in elderly. Gait and Posture 5: 128–135

Rancho Los Amigos Medical Centre 1989 Observational gait analysis handbook. Los Amigos Research and Education Institute, Downey, CA

Reimers J 1972 A scoring system for the evaluation of ambulation in cerebral palsy patients. Developmental Medicine and Child Neurology 14: 332–335

Robinson JL, Smidt GL 1981 Quantitative gait evaluation in the clinic. Physical Therapy 61: 351–353

Rose GK 1983 Clinical gait assessment: a personal view. Journal of Medical Engineering and Technology 7: 273–279

Rowe PJ, Nicol AC, Kelly IG 1989 Flexible goniometer computer system for the assessment of hip function. Clinical Biomechanics 4: 68–72

Shores M 1980 Footprint analysis in gait documentation. Physical Therapy 60: 1163–1167

Silvino N, Evanski PM, Waugh TR 1980 The Harris and Beath Footprinting Mat: diagnostic validity and clinical use. Clinical Orthopaedics and Related Research 1551: 265–269

Singh SJ 1992 The use of field walking tests for assessment of functional capacity in patients with chronic airways obstruction. Physiotherapy 78: 102–104

Singh SJ, Morgan MDL, Scott S et al 1992 Development of a shuttle walking test of disability in patients with chronic airways obstruction. Thorax 47: 1019–1024

Smith A 1993 Variability in human locomotion: are repeat trails necessary? Australian Journal of Physiotherapy 39: 115–123

SMS Health Care Ltd 1998 Manufacturer's information, GAITRite Walkway System. SMS Health Care, Harlow, Essex

Steadman J, Archer A, Jackson H et al 1997a Impairment and walking disability following stroke: a multi-centre study. Clinical Rehabilitation 11: 81–89

Steadman J, Archer A, Jackson H et al 1997b Is there a link between patients' perception of their walking and objective walking performance following stroke? Age and Ageing 26(suppl I): 26

Sutherland D, Olshen R, Cooper L, Woo S 1980 The development of mature gait. Journal of Bone and Joint Surgery 62A: 336–353

Volpon JB 1994 Footprint analysis during the growth period. Journal of Pediatric Orthopedics 14: 83–85

Wade D 1992 Measurement in neurological rehabilitation. Oxford University Press, Oxford

Wade D, Wood V, Heller A et al (1987) Walking after stroke. Scandinavian Journal of Rehabilitation Medicine 19: 25–30

Wall JC 1991 Measurement of temporal gait parameters from videotape using a field counting technique. International Rehabilitation Research 14: 344–347

Wall JC, Crosbie J 1996 Accuracy and reliability of temporal gait measurement. Gait and Posture 4: 293–296

Wall JC, Crosbie J 1997 Temporal gait analysis using slow video and a personal computer. Physiotherapy 83: 109–115

Wall JC, Ashburn A, Klenerman L 1981 Gait analysis in the assessment of functional performance before and after total hip replacement. Journal of Biomedical Engineering 3: 121–127

Whittle M 1996 Clinical gait analysis: a review. Human Movement Science 15: 369–387

Whittle M 2003 Gait analysis – an introduction, 3rd edn. Butterworth Heinemann, Oxford

Winter DA 1987 The biomechanics and motor control of human gait. University of Waterloo Press, Waterloo, Ontario

Winter DA, Patla AE, Frank JS, Walt SE 1990 Biomechanical walking pattern changes in the fit and healthy elderly. Physical Therapy 70: 340–347

Winter DA, Deathe AB, Halliday S et al 1993 A technique to analyse the kinetics and energetics of cane assisted gait. Clinical Biomechanics 8: 37–43

Wolfson L, Whipple R, Amerman P, Tobin J 1990 Gait assessment in the elderly: a gait abnormality rating scale and its relationship to falls. Journal of Gerontology 45: M12–M19

Worsfold C, Simpson JM 1996 The repeatability and acceptability of a stopwatch timed 3 metre walk among elderly in-patients. Society for Research in Rehabilitation, London

Yack HJ 1984 Techniques for clinical assessment of human movement. Physical Therapy 64: 1821–1829

Chapter **11**

Hydrotherapy in orthopaedics

Karen Atkinson

OBJECTIVES

By the end of this chapter you should:

- Have an understanding of the relevant hydrostatic and hydrodynamic principles and their application in the development of exercise programmes in water
- Have a basic understanding of the physiological changes that occur in the body as a result of immersion and be able to consider these in relation to safe selection of patients for treatment
- Have a grasp of the therapeutic effects of hydrotherapy
- Be aware of the core aspects of health and safety in relation to working in a pool environment
- Have some understanding of the issues involved in hydrotherapy pool management
- Have an overview of the benefits, disadvantages and appropriate use of hydrotherapy, both generally and within the orthopaedic specialty
- Understand the ways in which hydrotherapy can be used effectively in a range of case scenarios used in other sections of the book.

KEYWORDS

Hydrotherapy, orthopaedics, hydrostatics, hydrodynamics, physiology, immersion, contraindications, health and safety, therapeutic effects, mobilization/strengthening, rehabilitation, exercise programmes, pool management.

Prerequisites

In order to obtain the most benefit from this chapter, it is recommended that you have an overview of the information contained in the introductory chapters (1–4). This is to remind you of the background to the problem-solving approach. You also need to have an overview of the orthopaedic conditions covered in the book, with particular emphasis on the case studies we have presented. We will be relating back to some of these cases when discussing the application of hydrotherapy in a range of client groups and conditions.

INTRODUCTION

Use of water

Some theories of evolution suggest that life began in the oceans and that we existed in a watery environment before emerging on to the land. In general, water still seems to hold an extraordinary fascination for humans (Kuroda 1963). This ranges from the enjoyment of the sight and sound of it in different settings, such as fountains and the seashore, to the great variety of activities it facilitates, including therapy, occupations, sport and leisure. Many people feel at home in the water and swim regularly.

Hydrotherapy in the broadest sense is a treatment that involves the external application of water for therapeutic purposes. This usually means the patients attending a warm pool for exercise and relaxation. The experience of numerous therapists would suggest that the vast majority of patients, even those unable to swim, find hydrotherapy very effective and thoroughly enjoy attending for treatment. For some disabled people, water is the only environment in which they can experience any significant independence in terms of freedom of movement.

One of the major advantages of hydrotherapy for patients with a range of orthopaedic conditions is that it provides a medium in which they are able to exercise. The physical properties of water enable ease of movement. This same level of activity would be impossible on dry land. For someone who is experiencing pain and immobility, water treatment can help to boost morale and increase confidence. Being immersed in a pool also exercises the whole body, there is less focus on one particular area and more of the body can be treated in less time. Large numbers of joints and muscles can be exercised in different planes with minimal change in starting position, which is an advantage for those patients who find changing position on dry land painful or difficult. Movement through water provides much of the resistance and progression is achieved by working from the easy exercises to the most difficult. The advantage here is the self-regulating nature of the exercise, i.e. the harder the patients work the more resistance is experienced, but this will never be more than they can manage. The water allows an almost infinite range of resistance at any stage of a condition. Patients may eventually learn how to swim or become confident enough in the water to continue with exercise at their local swimming baths.

As with many areas of physiotherapy there is a paucity of good-quality research providing hard evidence of the effectiveness of hydrotherapy as a treatment modality. In a recent review by Geytenbeek (2002), however, it was found that there is a balance of high- to moderate-quality evidence supporting the use of hydrotherapy with particular reference to 'pain, function, self efficacy and affect, joint mobility, strength and balance particularly among older adults, subjects with rheumatic conditions and chronic low back pain'. Many of the problems mentioned above are experienced by patients with orthopaedic conditions and so it would seem that hydrotherapy can be a useful modality for us to use in these situations.

You must remember that, even though most of us enjoy the water, it is essentially an alien environment for humans. As a physiotherapist working in the hydrotherapy setting you need to be conscious of this fact at all times. If you are to work safely and effectively in this area, you need an additional set of knowledge and experience to that which you might gain in any other area of physiotherapy practice. The knowledge underpinning hydrotherapy can be broken down into a number of themes:

- Physical principles of water (hydrostatics/ hydrodynamics) and how they are used in treatment
- Physiological effects of immersion
- Therapeutic effects
- Contraindications to pool treatment
- Health and Safety issues in the pool environment
- Pool management
- Advantages and disadvantages of pool therapy.

The rest of the chapter will now take you through these themes, applying them to the orthopaedic setting as appropriate.

PHYSICAL PRINCIPLES

When treating patients in a pool, you need a clear understanding of hydrostatic and hydrodynamic principles as these underpin every activity and exercise. It is not appropriate to transfer land-based exercises into the pool, as this neglects the unique properties of water and consequently will not produce optimum results. It is vital that you appreciate the difference between exercise carried out on land and that performed in water.

This section does not cover all aspects of physics that come into play when you enter the water: for these we recommend that you refer to a basic physics text. The aim here is to introduce you to those physical principles that will enable you to plan and explain the rationale behind a reasoned pool treatment. This includes the progression of exercise, which differs to that on dry land because of the additional factors involved with your patients being immersed in another medium.

Buoyancy

An immediately obvious effect when entering the water is that of buoyancy – the apparent reduction in the weight going through our lower limbs. Gravity acts downwards on body mass and the resultant effect is our perception of weight. The buoyancy or upthrust we experience when in the water supports the body and acts to counterbalance gravity, so we feel lighter.

Archimedes' principle states: When a body is partially or wholly immersed in a fluid, it will experience an upthrust that is equal to the weight of the fluid displaced.

Density and specific gravity

Density (the relationship between the mass of an object and its volume) and specific gravity (SG) (which allows comparison of the densities of different substances, with water as the standard at a SG of 1) are important in relation to Archimedes' principle. If an object is placed in water and it comes to rest in a position where its weight is neutralized by the upthrust and part of it remains above the water line, then it has a SG of less than 1. The greater the proportion of the object below the water, the nearer its SG approaches to 1. If the whole object sinks, then its SG is greater than 1.

These factors apply to the human body but, as we are varied in our make-up – i.e. different percentages of fat (less dense) and muscle (more dense) – some people float better than others. Various parts of the body have different SGs: the thorax includes the lungs, which reduces overall SG; the legs tend to be more muscular, which increases the SG. This means that the legs usually float lower in the water than the trunk. On average, the SG of the human body is between 0.95 and 0.97, but there are natural 'sinkers' and 'floaters'. Do you know which you are? Many people do float but with the majority of the body below the surface. This may be inappropriate for treatment and so you can add floats to bring the appropriate parts higher in the water.

The SG of the body varies with age. In general children have a lower SG and so float well. Young people, who have a greater ratio of muscle to fat and a higher bone density, have a higher SG and so may tend to be natural 'sinkers'. Later in the life cycle we often have a larger ratio of fat to muscle. This, along with reduced bone density, decreases the overall SG, so older people tend to be better 'floaters'.

Self-assessment question

- **SAQ 11.1** Why is it inappropriate to use land exercises in the pool?

Percentage weight bearing during immersion

As mentioned earlier, we feel lighter when standing in the water. Harrison & Bulstrode (1987) found that percentage weight bearing when immersed in water is as shown in Table 11.1.

The percentage weight bearing at the different levels of immersion will vary slightly from person to person and does differ a little in men and women, but it is a good rule of thumb. It is extremely useful when you treat patients who are partial or non-weight-bearing, e.g. following lower limb fracture or knee/hip replacement. They can move more easily in the pool and will be able to use a reciprocal gait pattern earlier than would be possible on dry land. If your pool has different depths, the weight passing through the patient's lower limbs can be progressed in a controlled manner (Reid Campion 1990). The risk (and fear) of falling is also reduced because of the support of the water and this can greatly improve confidence.

General uses of buoyancy in hydrotherapy

Support. Because of the effect of the upthrust as described above, buoyancy can be used as a support. This can be global support of body weight in standing or float lying or it can be local support of a particular part of the body during specific exercises.

Resistance. If you push down in the water against the upward force of buoyancy you can feel the resistance to your movement. This can be used as a resistance during strengthening exercises. The effect of the upthrust, i.e. the amount of resistance, can be modified by changing the length of the lever (shorter lever = less resistance; longer lever = more resistance) and/or by adding floats.

Assistance. Conversely, the upthrust can be used as an assistive force to enable greater amounts of movement. This can be used in mobilizing exercises for patients with stiff joints and/or where they have decreased muscle strength. Care needs to be exercised here to ensure that the upward force of buoyancy does not take the patient beyond available range, i.e. a forced passive movement. You need to bear this in mind, especially if you add a float to the part.

Self-assessment question

- SAQ 11.2
  a. Approximately how much weight goes through the lower limbs when a person is immersed to C7, the xiphisternum and the anterior superior iliac spines respectively?
  b. How can this reduction in body weight be used to advantage in patients with orthopaedic problems?

Table 11.1 Percentage weight bearing when immersed to different levels in standing

Level of immersion	% weight bearing
C7	Approximately 10
Xiphisternum	Approximately 30
Anterior superior iliac spines	Approximately 50

Moment of buoyancy

A moment is a measure of a force that tends to rotate the body on which it is acting. If a force is applied to a body that has a pivoting point through which the line of force does not pass, then the body will tend to rotate about that point. Buoyancy is a force that acts on bodies immersed in water and the moment of buoyancy will result in rotatory movements of the limbs or segments of limbs around the joints, which act as the pivot points. This is an important principle to be aware of when you work in the pool, in both treatment and safety contexts.

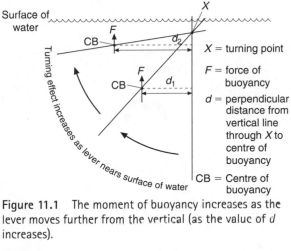

Figure 11.1   The moment of buoyancy increases as the lever moves further from the vertical (as the value of d increases).

Figure 11.2   Moment of buoyancy in shoulder abduction.

The moment of buoyancy can be represented by an equation:

$$\text{Moment of buoyancy} = F \times d,$$

where F = force of buoyancy (upthrust) and d = perpendicular distance from a vertical line through X (X = point about which turning effect is exerted) to a vertical line through the point at which the force is exerted (e.g. the line of force; Fig. 11.1).

Given that the upthrust remains constant (unless a float is added) it is the perpendicular distance (d) between the vertical line through X and the line of force that has the most influence on the magnitude of the turning effect. For instance, during shoulder abduction, as the arm moves away from the side of the body, d increases (Fig. 11.2). In this case, as the arm gets nearer to the surface of the water the turning effect increases. This would provide either more assistance to the shoulder abductors as the arm nears 90° or, conversely, more resistance to the adductors.

The effect of the turning force can be modified in two ways. First, you can change the length of the lever, e.g. bending the elbow, so decreasing d, which consequently decreases the magnitude of the turning effect (Fig. 11.3). Second, you can add a float, which increases the amount of upthrust both by increasing the value of F in the equation

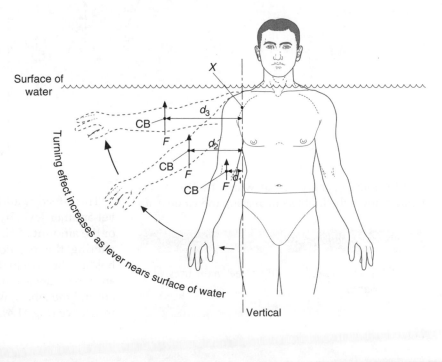

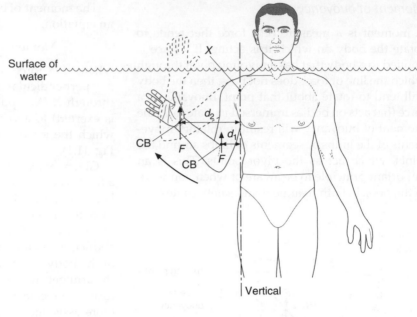

Figure 11.3 Shortening the lever (bending the elbow) decreases the value of d so reducing the magnitude of the turning effect.

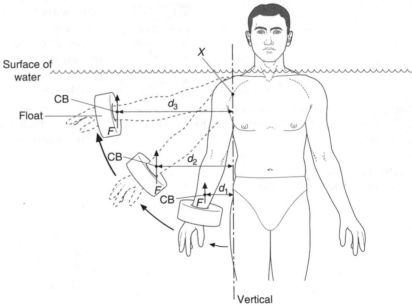

Figure 11.4 Adding a float moves the point at which the force acts further down the limb so increasing the value of d and consequently the magnitude of the turning effect.

and by moving the point at which the force acts further down the limb, so increasing the value of d.

Self-assessment question

- SAQ 11.3 What are the three main uses of buoyancy?

The effect of adding floats can be modified at yet another level by changing the size of the float or the amount of air that you put into it and/or by altering the position of the float. For example, holding the float in the hand provides greater assistance/resistance to movement than putting the float around the elbow, which provides less assistance/resistance (Fig.11.4).

Figure 11.5 Because of the increase in magnitude of the turning effect with an increase in the value of *d*, the hip adductors work six times harder when the hip is in 45° of abduction than when it is abducted only 5°.

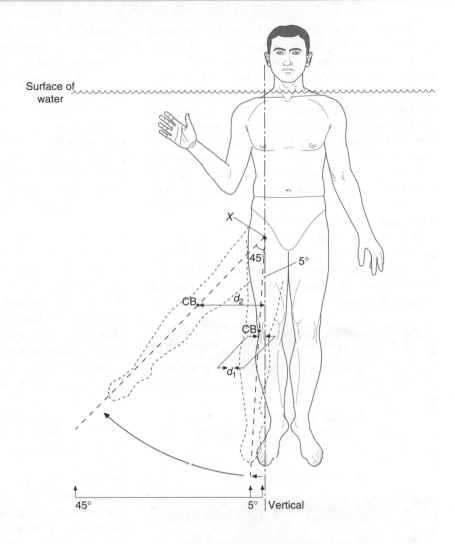

Practical implications

This has a number of implications in the treatment setting. First, when moving the body or body segment up and down in the water, the amount of assistance/resistance varies depending on where in range the part or segment is positioned. Using hip abduction as an example, because of the increase in *d* as the leg moves away from neutral, the adductors will need to work approximately six times as hard to hold the leg in position at 45° of abduction as they would at 5° of abduction (Fig. 11.5). Second, using changes in lever length and floats of different sizes or containing different amounts of air, and placing those floats in different positions on the limb, you can provide an almost limitless variation in the amount of assistance or resistance you provide to particular movements.

It is important to note that progression of assisted movements with regard to lever length is opposite to that on dry land. A long lever provides more assistance so the exercise is easier and a short lever provides less assistance so is slightly harder. With respect to buoyancy-resisted exercises the principle is the same as on dry land, i.e. a longer lever provides more resistance.

Purely buoyancy-assisted/resisted movements are quite slow. As soon as you ask the patient to move more quickly through the water, you are introducing increased levels of resistance into the equation because of the effects of turbulence – see later.

The effect of buoyancy can be used to carry out hold–relax techniques to increase range of movement in joints where there are shortened structures. As an example, if knee extension is limited, a patient can be positioned in sitting with a float on the foot. The patient is instructed to allow the float to extend the knee to its maximum extent. The foot is then pushed down slightly into the water to carry out a static contraction against the upthrust. This position is held for 2 seconds and then the muscles are relaxed for 6 seconds. The float will then take the knee further into extension as the tight structures reciprocally relax.

It is essential that you ensure that you do not provide excessive buoyancy assistance/resistance, particularly when using floats. This could take the patient's joint and soft tissues beyond the safe and comfortable range.

Self-assessment questions

- SAQ 11.4 How can you modify the effect of the turning force produced by the moment of buoyancy?
- SAQ 11.5 What happens when you introduce more speed into buoyancy-assisted/resisted movements?

Problem-solving exercise 11.1

Imagine a patient who has reduced range of hip abduction. How could you use buoyancy in a progressive manner to increase abduction?

Metacentre

The metacentric principle concerns balance in the water. As we mentioned earlier, a body immersed in water is acted upon by two opposing forces – gravity acting downwards through the body's centre of gravity and buoyancy acting upwards through the centre of buoyancy (this is located at the centre of the body of water that has been displaced by the immersed object). If these two forces are equal and opposite then the body is balanced and there is no movement. If the two forces are unequal and out of alignment, however, then movement occurs. The movement is always rotatory and continues until a state of balance is once again achieved, i.e. when the two forces are back in alignment.

This applies to ourselves and our patients. Imagine a patient floating in a symmetrical position with arms by the side and legs together. This is a position of balance, with no movement occurring. If the patient changes the position of part of the body, whether above or below the surface of the water, rotation will occur because the centres of gravity and buoyancy are no longer in alignment. For example: if the left hand is lifted out of the water, the patient will roll to the left; if the head is turned to the right the patient will roll that way (both horizontal rotations); if the head is lifted out of the water the feet will sink (vertical rotation). Alterations in shape due to disability can also cause rotation, e.g. an amputation or the limbs being held in a particular position because of spasticity.

During activity in water, therefore, it is important that you are aware of these rotational effects and are able to act to control them if necessary. As you assess your patient prior to treatment, pay some attention to body symmetry and shape so that you are aware of any rotation that may occur and can be ready to instruct the patient in ways to counteract rotational effects (Reid Campion 1990).

Conversely, you can use the small movements that cause misalignment of the centres of gravity and buoyancy in order to teach people how to initiate movement in the water. The Association of Swimming Therapy (AST) uses rotation in the water as a basis for much of their input with disabled swimmers. Teaching balance in the water, how to regain safe breathing positions and to use rotation to initiate movement form the foundation for good water confidence, independence in the water and eventually swimming. The AST promote all aspects of swimming for disabled people and use the Halliwick method to achieve these results (Association of Swimming Therapy 1992).

Problem-solving exercise 11.2

Next time you go swimming or have a moment to spare in the hydrotherapy pool, experiment with changes in body shape. See what happens when you move part of the body out of the water or away from the trunk; try bending one arm or knee; lift your head.

Can you control the rotation?

If so how do you do it?

How safe do you feel?

How do you think this might affect the patient's level of confidence?

How do you think you might be able to use these effects in treatment?

Hydrostatic pressure

'Fluid pressure is exerted equally on all surface areas of an immersed body at rest at a given depth' (Pascal's law).

Hydrostatic pressure represents the weight of the column of water from the point in question to the surface. The pressure exerted on the body at a given depth is equal and opposite in all directions but it increases both with depth and with the density of the medium.

Probably the most important implication of hydrostatic pressure is that it causes a redistribution of the fluid volume within the body. In standing, a person of average height immersed to neck level will be subjected to a pressure of around $120 \, g/cm^2$ at mid-calf. Because of this greater pressure on the lower limbs, approximately 700 ml of fluid is redistributed from this region into the thorax. This effect is responsible for most of the profound physiological effects that occur during head-out water immersion (HOWI; see later).

Self-assessment question

• SAQ 11.6 What is the metacentric effect?

The pressure exerted on the calf by the water is between two and nine times greater than the pressure that is exerted by a crepe bandage newly applied to the same area (Davis & Harrison 1988). This means, therefore, that oedema may be reduced by the pressure but only during the immersion period. This temporary reduction may, however, enable the patient to exercise more effectively while in the pool, causing a longer-term reduction in swelling and subsequently aiding mobility.

The thorax and abdomen are also subjected to an increase in pressure (around $30 \, g/cm^2$ and $40 \, g/cm^2$ respectively) during immersion, resulting in some increase in resistance to anteroposterior, transverse and vertical chest expansion. This, coupled with a slight internal increase in pressure due to the redistribution of approximately 700 ml of fluid from the legs to the thorax, will result in a small decrease in vital capacity. While this decrease undoubtedly takes place, its clinical significance should not be exaggerated. You should remember to carefully monitor patients with low vital capacity in case of problems but this is by no means a contraindication to treatment in the pool (Davis & Harrison 1988, HACP 2000).

Movement through water

This is the basis of most pool therapy and it is therefore essential that you are familiar with the physical principles that govern it. When you move in water you meet resistance to that movement. The total resistance comprises a number of factors but the two that are of most importance to you when treating patients are the bow wave and the wake.

The bow wave is positive pressure that builds up in front of a moving object as a result of the displacement of the water. This makes up approximately 10% of the overall resistance. The wake is an area of negative pressure that forms behind the object and causes a drag effect. The negative pressure is produced by turbulent water flowing into the area immediately behind the object, causing eddy currents (see below). The wake makes up approximately 90% of the resistance to movement (Fig. 11.6).

The other factors involved in offering resistance to movement through the water are friction, the viscosity of the fluid and the cohesive and adhesive forces that occur at the skin–water interface. The effects of these components of resistance are, however, minimal when compared to the total.

Turbulence

Bernoulli's theorem defines the relationship between fluid velocity and fluid pressure along a

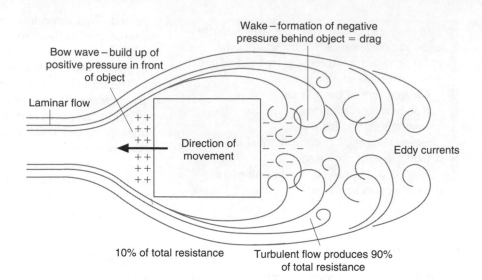

Figure 11.6   Resistance to movement through water.

streamline in the steady flow of a frictionless fluid that has a constant density. Part of this theorem addresses the relationship between the various types of energy contained within a water particle. The total energy of the particle is a sum of three types of energy:

- Pressure energy
- Potential energy
- Kinetic energy (Reid Campion 1990).

The amount of energy in the universe has always been the same – energy cannot be created or destroyed. When we say that energy is used, it does not disappear, it is just converted into other forms of energy and these conversions or changes are occurring all the time (Oxlade & Parker 1999). In relation to water particles, therefore, if the level of one of the energies increases, then the level of the others must decrease. The two of most relevance to us in relation to water movement are kinetic and pressure energy.

Turbulence is the term used to describe the eddy currents that follow an object that is moving through the water. The degree of turbulence depends partly on the speed of movement; in other words, faster movement creates more turbulence, slower movement creates less turbulence and the flow of water is more streamlined. Faster movement, with many eddy currents being formed behind the object as it moves through the water, indicates the presence of high levels of kinetic

energy in the water particles. As a result of this the level of pressure energy goes down, so causing an area of low pressure behind the object, resulting in the drag.

There are three variables that can affect the amount of turbulence produced by an object moving through the water; these are:

- Speed
- Shape
- Size.

You can change the shape and size by altering the length of lever, changing the aspect of the limb that is leading the movement (e.g. the edge of the hand produces a more streamlined flow than the flat of the hand) and/or by adding apparatus (e.g. bats, flippers, webbed gloves). In general terms these changes increase or decrease the surface area that is presented to the water. But, as you can see from the equation below, the most significant factor here is the speed of movement:

$$\text{Drag} \propto \text{area} \times \text{speed}^2.$$

The drag is proportional to the area of the object leading the movement multiplied by the speed of movement squared.

You can use streamlining and increase in turbulence to vary resistance to exercises and so produce a progressive exercise programme.

Drag can be used to both resist and assist movement in the water. You can use changes in shape, size and speed, either in isolation or combination, to increase the difficulty of a movement. You can, however, also assist a patient's movement. In the same way that a mother duck uses the drag she creates while swimming to draw her ducklings along behind her, you can create turbulence in the water in front of the patient or part of the body to enable easier movement. You can create this turbulence either by using your hands or by moving through the water in front of the patient. For example, you walk together; you going backwards so you can observe and steady the patient if necessary and the patient walking forwards. This same technique of creating turbulence can be used to resist movement or to encourage stability. To increase resistance, add your turbulence behind the moving part. For stabilization, ask the patient to maintain a particular position while you produce turbulence in different areas of the water around the body.

Remember that, as described above, when you move through the water you produce turbulence and drag. If you move past a patient who is unstable it could cause a loss of balance. Coping with the effects of turbulence demands co-ordination and balance. You can utilize these principles when designing treatment programmes to develop co-ordination and balance skills in appropriate patients.

Self-assessment question

• SAQ 11.7 Why are the effects of hydrostatic pressure important?

Problem–solving exercise 11.3

Describe a progressive strengthening programme for weak knee flexors using buoyancy and movement through the water.

Refraction

Refraction occurs whenever light passes from one transparent medium to another. The rays are bent or refracted at a certain angle from the normal depending on the two types of media. As light passes from water (more dense) to air (less dense), the rays bend away from the normal. The effect of this is to make anything in the water appear nearer than it actually is.

This physical property of water has two implications for us. First, it is important to warn patients that the floor of the pool and any steps will look nearer than they actually are, so care needs to be taken. Second, it is not recommended that you attempt to assess the patient's movement while in the pool. There is distortion as you look into the water and you will see the 'apparent' image as opposed to the 'real' image. Your assessment is likely to be incorrect – do it on dry land.

Problem–solving exercise 11.4

You were introduced to Mr Kingston in Case study 5.2 in Chapter 5. He sustained a fractured shaft of femur that was treated with internal fixation. He was discharged non-weight-bearing. How could you use hydrotherapy in his rehabilitation?

PHYSIOLOGICAL EFFECTS OF IMMERSION

Immersion in water has marked physiological effects, many of which are due to the hydrostatic pressure. As mentioned earlier, these pressure gradients cause a redistribution of fluid that shifts 500–700 ml of the blood pooling in the legs to the cardiothoracic space. This in effect causes an increase in blood returning to the heart. The relative hypervolaemia stimulates cardiopulmonary receptors, which go on to provoke a series of physiological reactions. Much of the initial work in this area was carried out by NASA, as immersion is the nearest that we can get on Earth to the weightlessness of outer space. This environment was used for both experimental procedures and astronaut training. Most of the work on HOWI has been carried out in thermoneutral water (35°C) with subjects seated with the water to the level of the sternal notch. This temperature of water has no effect on the core temperature of the body. Any increase in water temperature can cause substantial alterations in circulation (Hall et al 1990).

Cardiovascular system

In the cardiovascular system, the increased venous return to the heart seems to be the basis for all of the physiological changes associated with immersion (Hall et al 1990). Cardiac output, described as a function of stroke volume (the amount of blood ejected from the left ventricle each time the heart contracts) and heart rate, increases by 34% in thermoneutral water but the heart rate remains fairly stable, or occasionally a slight bradycardia occurs. With water at higher temperatures the effect on cardiac output is more pronounced and the heart rate tends to rise, with tachycardia occurring when the water reaches 37°C. In water at 39°C cardiac output rises as much as 120% and heart rate can increase to 113 beats per minute (Weston et al 1987). The general effect on the blood pressure is that it either remains the same or falls during immersion, which suggests a decrease in peripheral resistance (Davis & Harrison 1988, Hall et al 1990). These cardiovascular changes also occur when a subject is in the supine position, but to a slightly lesser extent.

It is important for you to be aware that these changes are occurring in the cardiovascular system, not just in your patients' bodies but in yours as well. This is prior to any exercise being undertaken. The temperature of hydrotherapy pools used to regularly exceed the thermoneutral temperature

stated above (some still do) but the Chartered Society of Physiotherapy Service Standards (CSP 2001) now recommend that 'the pool water temperature is maintained within a range 32–36°C, with the optimum being thermoneutral, i.e. 34–35.5°C'. If the pool you work in is maintained to the recommended standard, therefore, neither you nor your patients will experience the magnified physiological effects of immersion at higher temperatures.

Haemodilution

It has been noted that, during the first 30 minutes of immersion, haemodilution occurs, but this generally returns to normal over the following 2 hours. It has been speculated that this haemodilution effect could be of use in diseases, such as rheumatoid arthritis, where blood viscosity is higher than usual (O'Hare et al 1984). You will usually take patients into the pool for periods of 20–30 minutes and so this effect may be of help to some of your rheumatology patients.

Renal function

Immersion has a marked effect on renal function, particularly a profound diuresis due to the suppression of antidiuretic hormone. This causes the distal tubules and collecting ducts of the kidney to become less permeable to water, so less is reabsorbed, resulting in more urine being produced. The kidney usually filters 120 ml/minute and produces 1 ml of urine. When immersed the rate of urine production increases up to 7 ml/minute after 3 hours. Along with the increased urine production there is an increase in the excretion of sodium and to a lesser degree potassium, calcium and phosphate.

The natriuresis is thought to be brought about by the increased amount of atrial natriuretic peptide released by the atrial muscle fibres of the heart in response to the hypervolaemia (Hall et al 1990).

It is therefore not just 'all in the mind' when you feel you need to go to the loo after being in the pool for a while. This is due to actual physiological changes occurring in the body. It is a good idea therefore to ensure that you and the patients use the toilet before entering the pool and also that you drink regularly to avoid becoming dehydrated.

Self-assessment question

• **SAQ 11.10** What happens to your cardiac output during head-out water immersion in thermoneutral water? How is this modified in water that is warmer than thermoneutral?

Stress and anxiety

There is some evidence to suggest that blood levels of stress hormones (such as noradrenaline (norepinephrine)) are reduced during immersion. It is also hypothesized that there is a reduction of sympathetic nervous system activity (Coruzzi et al 1988). This may provide some explanation for the reports of improved mood after swimming. Berger et al (1983) reported significantly less tension-anxiety, depression, anger and confusion in subjects after swimming. Levine (1984) noted reduction in anxiety in subjects after they had participated in hydrotherapy sessions. More work is being carried out on the blood levels of stress hormones during immersion. If evidence shows reduction in these levels, this could be an exciting development for hydrotherapy, especially in the treatment of patients with chronic disorders who experience stress and anxiety as a result of the nature of their disease. It could also be important for patients with conditions such as mental health problems, fibromyalgia or chronic fatigue syndrome.

Exercise in water

Relatively little work has been carried out on the physiological effects of exercise in water. Of those

studies that have been done, most have concentrated on the cardiovascular effects. It was thought that exercise would dissipate the central hypervolaemia that occurs during immersion but in fact the end-diastolic volume of the left ventricle remains larger during mild to moderate activity in water, when compared with similar exercise on land. This does not, however, seem to alter the normal cardiovascular adaptation to aerobic exercise training (Sheldahl 1986). Kirby et al (1984) also found that oxygen consumption during graduated exercise in a heated pool increased similarly to that during activity on land. They suggest that the more vigorous exercises stress aerobic capacity heavily but not excessively. Hall et al (1990), however, cite studies showing that increased depth of water causes subjects to experience more resistance, resulting in greater energy expenditure. When comparing walking on a treadmill on land to doing the same in water, heart rate and oxygen consumption responses were significantly greater during the immersion exercise.

These studies were all carried out on healthy subjects. When in the pool, therefore, you should keep this extra energy expenditure in mind, as patients are often debilitated because of their condition. It is advisable to begin treatment with short sessions including only a few exercises in order to gauge each person's reaction to being in the water.

Self-assessment questions

• **SAQ 11.11** Why do you feel that you need to go to the loo after being in the pool for a period of time?
• **SAQ 11.12** Why might hydrotherapy be helpful for patients who experience stress and anxiety?

THERAPEUTIC EFFECTS OF HYDROTHERAPY

Hydrotherapy is an extremely versatile treatment modality and is used for a wide variety of conditions. The most important point in today's climate, which is firmly focused on finance and outcomes, is to use the pool to treat those patients who will benefit the most. It is still the case that some patients are only referred for hydrotherapy as a 'last resort' treatment when all other ideas have been exhausted. This is unfortunate, as often these are the patients who would benefit from the particular qualities offered by pool therapy.

As we have emphasized in other parts of the book in relation to the management of patients with orthopaedic conditions, the principles and effects being employed in each of the treatments in hydrotherapy are very similar but it is vital to apply them appropriately for individual patients.

Pain relief

Pain relief is probably the most obvious effect to patients as they enter the water. This is due to two factors. First the warmth of the water desensitizes the nerve endings and second the buoyancy reduces the amount of weight going through the joints. This is particularly useful for patients, such as those with arthritis, who find that weight bearing increases their pain. It is important to remember, however, that the pain relief is only a temporary effect. You must use this time to encourage patients to gently increase their mobility and strength while in the water.

We would, however, like to add a note of caution here. Ensure that patients do not do too much. Movement is so much easier because of the warmth and weight relief that they could inadvertently cause an increase in pain after treatment.

Pain relief is particularly helpful in orthopaedics as pain is an issue for most patients, e.g. following injury, either soft tissue or fracture; arthritis and other disease processes affecting the musculoskeletal system; or post-surgery. Many patients are reluctant to move because of pain and because movement is difficult. As you know, this leads to stiffness, muscle weakness and reduced function. The patients will be able to work on these problems early on if we can provide an environment such as the pool where pain is reduced and movement is easier.

Decreased muscle spasm

Because of the warmth of the water and the decrease in pain experienced by the patients, muscle spasm also tends to decrease. This is another factor that enables movement while in the pool.

Relaxation

Patients describe feeling more relaxed when in the pool (Jackson 1996). This has two elements: local and general physical relaxation and mental relaxation. This will depend on the patient's attitude to water; if they are afraid of coming into the pool they will be less able to relax. In most cases, however, this does not become an issue as staff members are able to support and reassure patients so that they feel safe and confident in the water. As mentioned earlier, some research has shown that immersion can decrease activity in the sympathetic nervous system and reduce the levels of stress hormones in the blood, which will have an effect on the patient's ability to relax.

Maintain/increase range of movement

Because of the decrease in pain, ease of movement and reduction in spasm experienced in the water, patients are able to exercise further into range. You can also make use of the physical principles of buoyancy and movement through the water to help to increase range by using floats or other equipment and by encouraging changes in speed and direction of movement.

It is possible to carry out a wide variety of stretching techniques in the water and these can be very effective in increasing range of movement. This can be done in two ways, either hands-on hold–relax or using buoyancy.

Strengthen and re-educate muscle

It is possible to strengthen and re-educate muscle using similar principles as for increasing range of movement. It is important to realize, however, that in many instances the principles are applied differently. A very simple example is as follows.

To increase range of shoulder abduction you could use buoyancy-assisted work in standing starting with a long lever and then moving to a short lever (think back to moment of buoyancy) and turbulence (drag) could be used to increase range in float lying. You would only use this technique in muscle strengthening, however, if the abductors were extremely weak. To strengthen the abductors in standing or float lying you could ask the patient to move faster through the water so using turbulence as a resistance with first a short lever, then a long lever and then holding a bat in the hand or you could position the patient in side float lying to use buoyancy as a resistance. The effect of the buoyancy could then be increased by lengthening the lever and/or using floats.

One advantage of using these hydrodynamic effects is that the resistance is self limiting. In other words, the harder the patients work the more resistance is encountered but it will never be more than they can manage. Exercises can range from very easy assisted work through to extremely difficult resisted work depending on the patient's ability.

Exercise in water can be used to develop both muscular and cardiovascular power and endurance. Some sports teams now incorporate pool sessions into their training regimens and players or athletes returning to activity following injury often do their initial training in the water to avoid too much stress being placed on the injured structures.

Increase circulation

We talked about the profound physiological effects that occur in the cardiovascular system just from being immersed in water. Peripheral resistance decreases because of dilatation of the arterioles so bringing more blood to the periphery. This effect will be magnified by the warmth of the water (especially if it is above thermoneutral) and by increased activity. This could help to improve skin condition, especially if a patient has been immobilized in a cast, and may also help to reduce oedema. The latter effect will of course only occur during immersion but again the increased activity that is possible in the water could extend any reduction in oedema achieved during treatment.

Improve balance and co-ordination

When patients are in the water they have to get used to balancing and co-ordinating the body while moving in a denser medium. If other patients and therapists are moving around them, they will also be automatically correcting for the changes in the flow of the water around them. You can use turbulence and the metacentric effect to work on balance and co-ordination in different starting positions in the pool such as standing and float lying. For example, if you position the patient in

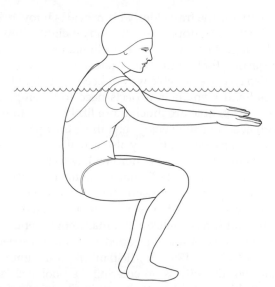

Figure 11.7   The box position.

float lying and then you produce turbulence under the shoulder or pelvic region, the trunk muscles have to work hard to maintain the floating posture. You can also use the metacentric effect. For example, ask the patient to take up the 'box' position (Fig. 11.7) and then to lift one arm out of the water. Again, the muscles have to work hard to prevent rotation occurring.

Psychological effects

As mentioned earlier, there is evidence to suggest a link between exercise in water and mood elevation, reduction in anxiety and depression. Some studies have looked more generally at the effect of exercise in water in an elderly population. This is a group that tends to be more sedentary for a variety of reasons. Weinstein (1986) found that the subjects she interviewed, who all participated in swimming or exercise in water, reported many positive benefits. Many of them were unable to exercise on land and could do much more in the water, finding it 'invigorating' and 'relaxing and good for the circulation'. They also reported that they felt better and that it reduced their aches and pains. There was a strong social aspect as they met and talked to others with similar interests. They found this encouraging and motivating.

Rissel (1987) goes so far as to suggest that 'gentle water exercise is the most appropriate form of activity for the frail elderly'. It provides buoyancy that acts as a support for the body weight, allows full range of movement and eliminates much of the jarring that occurs with exercise on dry land. It is also a very enjoyable way of keeping active. The social and enjoyment aspects need to be emphasized, as people are much more likely to continue with activities they enjoy than those they perceive to be unrewarding. If they also actually feel better afterwards they will be more willing to repeat the experience. Rissel (1987) notes that the majority of subjects reported increased fitness, improved body tone, decreased stiffness, were more relaxed and calm, had fun, socialized and made new friends.

These results are supported in a study carried out by Jackson (1996). Participants reported immediate positive effects on entering the pool such as being able to do things that were impossible on dry land, finding it easier to relax and being more confident. Communication and the social aspects were again important to the patients. Overall, patients felt that hydrotherapy enabled them to cope better and to feel more in control of their bodies and lives. There were physical, psychological and functional improvements.

Treatment of whole patient

The pool is an excellent medium for treatment of the generally debilitated or immobile patient as the whole body is immersed. Independence is immediately enhanced. Although you will often teach patients exercises that relate to particular areas, depending on their specific problems, the whole body still moves through the water and there is not such a focus on one area as there often is with dry-land treatments. As mentioned in the previous paragraph, there are also psychological benefits that can be gained from treatment in the pool, so it could be described as an excellent 'all round' modality resulting in improved function, increased levels of well being and better quality of life.

Problem-solving exercise 11.6

John Brown, a 24-year-old man with a sprain of the medial collateral ligament of the knee and James Low, a 46-year-old man with a total rupture of the lateral ligaments of his ankle are both discussed in the Chapter 6 (Case studies 6.1 and 6.3). Review these cases and think about why you might use hydrotherapy with these patients as part of their rehabilitation.

CONTRAINDICATIONS TO POOL THERAPY

As discussed earlier, treating patients in the pool demands a specific set of knowledge with which you need to be familiar in order to be safe and effective. This also applies to the contraindications to pool therapy. Most contraindications to hydrotherapy are relative and should be determined on the basis of informed assessment findings. If you have any doubts about whether a particular patient is suitable to come into the pool, then you should exercise caution. The Hydrotherapy Association of Chartered Physiotherapists standards of practice state that 'the physiotherapist has knowledge and understanding of contraindications to hydrotherapy and has the ability to identify them' (HACP 2001). This indicates that, if you are working in the pool environment, you need to be aware of the factors that might preclude a patient from entering the pool and you must be able to identify these during your assessment. But this does not mean that you are not able to check out your thoughts with the physiotherapist who manages the pool, or contact the HACP if you have any doubts. This is especially the case if you are a student or newly qualified.

Absolute contraindications

The following situations are considered to be absolute contraindications to pool therapy:

- Uncontrolled cardiac failure – the patient is unable to lie flat without becoming dyspnoeic
- Resting angina
- Shortness of breath at rest
- Medical instability following an acute episode, e.g. cerebrovascular accident, deep vein thrombosis, pulmonary embolus, status asthmaticus
- Acute vomiting and/or diarrhoea
- Proven chlorine sensitivity.

Relative contraindications

Patients with the following problems may be considered for hydrotherapy if it is felt that the benefits of treatment outweigh the small amount of risk involved. These decisions should be made by senior therapists with input from the medical team if this was felt necessary. Patients should be closely monitored while in the pool with follow up to ensure no ill effects.

Open infected wounds

This type of wound may benefit from immersion in the disinfected water. Often, physiotherapists place waterproof dressings over such wounds but these rarely keep all the moisture out. If you are concerned about the risk of infection to others, however, you could treat the patient at the end of a morning or afternoon session. Pool turnover time is usually 1–1.5 hours, so this would allow the pool water to go through the disinfection and filtration systems prior to other patients being immersed. This is usually only necessary if there are particularly vulnerable patients being treated at the same time.

Poorly controlled epilepsy

It is important that you make sure the patient is monitored while in the water. If a patient experiences a seizure when in the pool it is less of a risk to them to leave them in the water as long as they are in a safe breathing position. It is easier to evacuate them from the pool once the seizure has passed.

Acute systemic illness/pyrexia

It would be unlikely that you would want to take patients into the pool who are feeling so ill. The heat and humidity would probably add to their discomfort and so it might be advisable to wait until symptoms have diminished.

Radiotherapy

Some patients are not taken into the pool during a course of radiotherapy if the irradiated area of skin is to be immersed. The practices regarding hydrotherapy treatment of patients undergoing radiotherapy vary from place to place. If the hydrotherapy is felt to be particularly beneficial, it may be possible to treat the patient. This is often negotiated with the local oncologist and radiotherapist.

Unstable diabetes

Patients with diabetes are often taken into the pool. If, from your assessment, you are aware that a particular patient is prone to collapse (e.g. hypoglycaemic attack) but you also feel that hydrotherapy is the treatment of choice, it is advisable to monitor this person closely and perhaps even to carry out one-to-one treatment to guard against unexpected submersion.

Known aneurysm

This situation may need to be carefully considered given the cardiovascular changes that occur during immersion. Individual cases need to be considered with regard to how useful you feel hydrotherapy would be in the circumstances. If, during your assessment, you discover that the patient has regularly been swimming with no ill effects there should be no reason for excluding them from hydrotherapy. The reason that patients are referred to the pool may have no connection with their vascular condition.

Situations where precautions should be taken

If you discover any of the following problems when you assess patients presenting for hydrotherapy, they should not be excluded from pool treatment.

- *Hypertension/hypotension*: monitor
- *Epilepsy*: as previous section
- *Haemophilia*: gentle exercise, protect from unexpected knocks and bumps
- *Poor skin integrity*: careful handling and not too long in the water to avoid waterlogging of skin

- *Impaired sensation*: careful introduction to pool, monitor either until you decide the patient is safe or at all times depending on the situation
- *Widespread methicillin-resistant Staphylococcus aureus (MRSA) infection*: pool disinfection can cope with this microorganism. If necessary see the patient at the end of a pool session as described under 'Open infected wounds'
- *Invasive tubes in situ*: ensure tubes are clamped off securely
- *Behavioural problems*: you will need to assess each situation individually. You may need to see the patient at a quiet time and you might need a one-to-one session. Conversely, some patients respond better in a group setting
- *Fear of water*: this does not usually stop patients coming for hydrotherapy; most will gain confidence with your support and reassurance. You will discover any acute fear of water during your assessment and it may be necessary to refer the patient elsewhere
- *Gross obesity*: monitor the patient for ill effects from immersion. If the patient is uncomfortable about appearing publicly in a swimsuit it may be possible to offer a time when there are fewer patients in the pool at the beginning or end of a session
- *Incontinence of urine/faeces*: pool disinfection can cope with urine and formed stools being released into the pool. Stools can be removed easily with a net and disposed of appropriately
- *Hearing aids/grommets*: the patient should not put the head into the water. If the hearing aid is removed it may make communication more difficult
- *Contact lenses*: patients should be notified if you intend to carry out exercises where you might expect them to immerse their faces. This will enable them to remove the lenses if they wish.

Self-assessment question

- SAQ 11.13 Review the absolute contraindications to hydrotherapy treatment.

Problem–solving exercise 11.7

Steve Morris (Chapter 6, Case study 6.6) has a long history of back pain and eventually has an operation to decompress his S1 nerve root. Read about his problems on assessment and how he is after surgery. How might hydrotherapy be of use in this case?

HEALTH AND SAFETY

As mentioned earlier in the chapter, water is an alien environment for humans and as such has various inherent dangers. Because of this, guidelines for safety in and around water are essential in each situation. As a physiotherapist you have a duty of care towards all patients under your supervision and one aspect of this is the responsibility to make sure that they are safe at all times. This is why you must be familiar with safety and legal issues, as there are particular environmental points to be addressed. Although in general the patient is the focus for this, it is also important to remember that other staff working in the area, such as inexperienced physiotherapists, students, assistants or porters, need to be aware of safety matters and risk situations, in order to protect both themselves and any patients with whom they interact.

The plant room, where the heating, filtration and disinfection of the pool water are carried out, is another area that needs to be considered. The day-to-day running and maintenance of the plant machinery and the handling of potentially dangerous chemicals must be closely monitored. The amount of time that individual physiotherapists spend in the plant room varies greatly depending on the local arrangements. It is, however, extremely important that you have at least outline knowledge of the procedures and possible risks to health and safety that can occur in this area.

There is no doubt that there are hazards inherent in working in a hydrotherapy/pool department but, if care is taken and the recommended guidelines followed, both staff and patients can operate safely in this setting. Detailed guidelines can be found in specific publications from the Health and Safety Commission (responsible for developing the law and formulating general policy on health and safety matters) and the Health and Safety Executive (a separate body appointed by the Commission to implement policy and enforce legal requirements).

Self–assessment question

- **SAQ 11.14** With regard to contraindications to hydrotherapy treatment, in what situations might you need to monitor patients while they are in the pool and why?

When you start work in a hydrotherapy department, your senior therapist or the local health and safety representative should provide information on general and local safety issues. Your employer has an obligation to ensure your health, safety and welfare but you will find it useful to have prior knowledge of the general risks associated with working in this environment. These can be considered in three sections: patient related, staff related and general issues.

Patient related

Accidental submersion

Accidental submersion occurs rarely. Even so, everything possible must be done to avoid this, as it can be very frightening for all concerned. At the least, being unexpectedly submerged could severely affect the patient's confidence and at worst it could result in drowning. It is therefore a very important issue for you to address. The following precautions should help to avoid accidental submersion:

- During the land-based assessment, you should routinely ask patients pertinent questions about any medical condition that could cause distress during treatment. If you are concerned then you might consider it more appropriate to refer them for land-based therapy.

- Patients found suitable for pool therapy should be supervised at all times while in the water. Depending on your professional judgement (including the type of patients and their particular conditions) this supervision may range from one-to-one contact with patients throughout

treatment sessions to you being present at the pool side during group work.

- Flotation equipment must be used appropriately and checked regularly for faults.

- Your knowledge will avoid the occurrence of unwanted hydrodynamic effects, e.g. drag from turbulence that could accidentally disturb the equilibrium of the patient.

Acute fear of water

This can be a contraindication to treatment in the pool if patients are so nervous that they find it impossible to co-operate with you. Patients should be asked how they feel about going into the pool during the assessment, and this should avoid potential problems. If a patient does enter the pool in a state of high anxiety it could constitute a hazard. In this case a dry-land approach would probably be more appropriate. Often, patients' fears can be overcome with reassurance and careful handling.

If patients tell you they are afraid of water but, in your opinion, hydrotherapy would be an invaluable treatment, it may be possible to have short, supervised trial sessions to see how they cope.

In general, many patients are apprehensive when first attending for hydrotherapy. On first treatments you should remain with patients throughout if necessary. If they are very apprehensive, it may be wise to use standing holding on to the bar as the initial starting position and only move on to less stable positions such as sitting and float lying in subsequent sessions when confidence has increased. This is not always possible, especially if patients enter the water lying on a hoist stretcher. To reduce anxiety and for ease of handling, some floats can be put on before getting into the water and you must be there to receive the patient. You should provide extra reassurance and manual support until patients feel more confident.

At first you should assist patients to take up different starting positions. Help may be necessary in putting on and removing floats, flippers and other equipment. You should carry out these manoeuvres slowly, using firm, supportive grips. Later on, once confidence is gained, patients will probably be able to perform these tasks independently. Before leaving patients in new starting positions, you should ensure that they feel comfortable and safe and know how to attract attention in case of difficulty. If these simple precautions are followed, patients will be safeguarded against mishap or injury in this treatment environment.

Slips and falls poolside

This is a hazard in all areas of physiotherapy but particularly in hydrotherapy because of the added risk of water pooling on the floor surfaces. The following precautions should mitigate the problem:

- Supervise patients at all times, with staff present to support if necessary
- Provide advice to patients on the safe use of walking aids
- Check walking aids, especially the ferrules
- Use handrails wherever available
- Inspect the pool and surrounding areas regularly for accident hazards such as slippery or rough surfaces
- Ensure that the pool concourse is kept dry and clear of obstacles
- If you have any doubts about patients' ability to walk safely to and from the pool, you should ensure that they are supervised or that a wheeled chair or trolley is used.

Fainting and fitting in the pool

The likelihood of fainting or fitting can be minimized by careful screening during assessment. This rules out a percentage of people who may be at risk. It is important to avoid patients fainting or fitting while in the pool as it could lead to accidental submersion. Aside from screening, the most important safety precaution is to ensure that all staff members are familiar with emergency evacuation procedures and that these are practised regularly. Resuscitation equipment should be available and easily accessible in case of need and there must always be at least two members of staff present in the pool area.

Cardiac arrest in the pool

Because of the profound physiological changes that occur during immersion, there is a small risk of cardiac arrest in some patients who have cardiovascular disease. You should carefully screen all patients to check for any contraindications that could predispose them to cardiac arrest during treatment in the pool. As before, all staff members must be prepared for emergency evacuation and resuscitation procedures. They should also be aware of the position of the alarms and know what they sound like. If the alarms do not automatically alert the crash team (in the hospital situation) the number must be displayed in prominent positions near the telephones. Pool rescue drills must be conducted at least four times a year for staff likely to be involved in the emergency procedures (HACP 1992).

As mentioned in the section on contraindications, many patients with problems such as high blood pressure, diabetes, epilepsy or cardiac disease who could in some circumstances be distressed by exercise in water are not totally excluded from pool therapy. If these conditions are well controlled there should be no reason for barring the patient from hydrotherapy, particularly if you feel that it would be particularly beneficial. This decision does depend on your professional opinion, which in turn will depend on your level of experience. If you have any doubts you should check with more senior colleagues, medical staff or the clinical interest group (Hydrotherapy Association of Physiotherapists) before taking a patient into the water.

Spread of infection

The hydrotherapy pool is an ideal environment for the proliferation of bacteria and fungi – wet, warm and humid. The filters in the plant room through which the pool water passes can harbour pockets of bacteria. Patients and staff can also bring infection into the hydrotherapy area. The disinfection process normally deals with these bacteria and levels are insignificant. The following precautions should be taken to ensure low risk of the spread of infection:

- Regular microbiological testing
- Correct pool disinfection
- Assessment of all patients prior to treatment.

All wounds should be checked for signs of infection. It will be your decision as to whether patients with infected wounds should be allowed in the pool. As mentioned earlier, if you feel that hydrotherapy is particularly important then they can be taken in at the end of a session when the other patients have vacated the water. This means that the water will have passed through the disinfection system many times overnight before anyone enters the pool the next day. An alternative is to temporarily boost the amount of disinfection to combat the presence of any microorganisms.

Plantar warts (verrucas) and athlete's foot do not preclude patients from treatment. In the case of verrucas they should be asked to wear verruca socks. For athlete's foot they should wear flip-flops and not walk barefoot on the poolside and surrounding areas. This avoids skin flakes from the affected area coming into contact with other patients' skin, so reducing the risk of spread. The verruca sock/ flip-flops are kept specifically for each patient and disinfected as necessary. Patients can also be advised on appropriate foot hygiene.

Patients who are HIV-positive or are known to have hepatitis can attend for hydrotherapy as long as they have no open wounds.

Fatigue

The heat and humidity levels in the hydrotherapy department are very tiring. Patients may be debilitated before coming to the pool and performing activities in the water may add to their fatigue. To avoid any risks, patients should be supervised at all times during treatment to ensure that they adhere to set time limits and only exercise as you instruct them.

Unfamiliarity with the pool surroundings

There are marked differences between land and pool settings. In order to reduce the risks, patients should be informed of and shown the pool geography, including the location of toilets, showers and handrails. They must be shown how to safely enter and exit the pool under supervision and warned about the effects of refraction. The edges of any steps should be clearly marked.

Staff related

Storage and handling of chemicals

In the UK the Control of Substances Hazardous to Health Regulations 1988 (COSHH) are in place and must be strictly followed. All chemicals and hazardous substances must be stored and handled in accordance with these regulations (CSP 1994). COSHH does not set out specific requirements for each separate circumstance but gives a basic system for managing risk to health. You may not come into direct contact with the chemicals used for pool disinfection, as generally the maintenance/ engineering department will deal with all functioning of the plant room. In some situations, however, you may be responsible for part or all of the pool dosing. In either circumstance it is strongly advisable that you have a working knowledge of the regulations governing the safe handling of chemicals, and you need enough information to be able to discuss issues regarding the overall management of the pool.

In summary, the regulations cover the following points:

- A COSHH assessment must be carried out and reviewed on a regular basis. Changes in procedures should then be made as necessary as a result of the assessment or review.
- All chemicals must be stored and handled separately in strict accordance with COSHH.
- Chemicals must never be mixed as some combinations are explosive or can produce toxic gases.
- Inhalation of chemicals and contact with the skin should be avoided. If any chemicals do come into contact with the skin, anyone administering first aid must avoid contamination. Any clothing not stuck to the skin should be removed and the area flushed with clean, cool water for 10–15 minutes. A sterilized dressing should be applied to exposed, damaged skin and the person should be sent to hospital for treatment (Health and Safety Executive 1991).
- Any chemical spillage should be flushed with water immediately.

Fatigue

Staff in the hydrotherapy department can easily be fatigued as they are working in a warm, humid environment. There is no specific legislation regarding working in high temperatures or humidity. The following precautions should be taken, however, to avoid risks to both staff and patients as a result of fatigue:

- Staff working in the pool on a daily basis should not be immersed for longer than 2 hours in one session or 3 hours in one day
- Breaks should be taken and drinks must be available to avoid dehydration
- If the water temperature is higher than 35–36°C or the humidity above 60%, then both breaks and drinks should be taken more frequently.

Staff members working poolside should be advised to wear light clothing, in natural fibres if possible (i.e. low thermal resistance, which allows sweating) and to take rests whenever practicable. This will reduce activity levels, which in turn will reduce the internal heat production in the body.

Skin problems – dry skin, irritation and rashes

For staff working in the hydrotherapy pool, the main problem when it comes to skin irritation is that we are immersed for long periods. We need water that is as kind as possible to the skin but safe for immunocompromised people. There are a number of predisposing factors to be taken into consideration but 'wetting' is one of the most important.

Problems with this are related to the frequency and duration of wetting of the skin. Frequency is in fact the more important issue, in that four immersions of 1 hour each is a worse situation than one immersion of 4 hours. Frequent wetting/drying cycles are stressful for the skin. The pool water also degreases the skin and chlorine contributes to this. The skin is not designed to be immersed for long periods, there is a limit to the amount of wetting it can take and it has a cumulative effect. People with fair hair and skin are affected more. Younger skin can deal with effects of wetting better than older skin but generally you should only be immersed for a maximum of 3 hours per day. After immersion, you must let the water dry out of your skin before regreasing, otherwise the creams (E45/Nivea/emollient cream) will just seal the water into the skin.

Self–assessment question

- SAQ 11.15 What are the main patient-related health and safety risks when in the pool environment?

The Chartered Society of Physiotherapy (2001) recommend the following as best practice for staff working in hydrotherapy:

- Limited immersion (as above)
- Early reporting of any rash symptoms. A visit to the GP or occupational health may result in therapists being advised to stop immersion for a period of time although they could still work poolside
- Shower effectively and remoisturize regularly
- Shower before entering the pool. Unless there is a pre-existing skin condition there should be no need to pre-grease the skin
- Wash thoroughly with a moisturizing agent at the end of hydrotherapy sessions, dry thoroughly and apply a non-perfumed moisturizer (this should be provided by the employer)
- Treat any rash that develops with a mild steroid cream.

General

Poorly maintained/incorrect pool chemistry

The pool should be a safe and comfortable environment for everyone entering the water. This will only be the case if the chemical balance is correct and maintained properly. A poorly maintained pool can lead to a variety of problems ranging from spread of infection and skin irritation to turbid water and corrosion of metal fittings. The correct parameters for hydrotherapy pools are covered briefly in the next section. The following precautions should be followed to avoid any risks to health and safety:

- All staff must have a working knowledge of the recommended parameters for correct chemical balance specific to their own pool
- Chemical parameters (disinfection and pH levels) must be tested daily to ensure the maintenance of

safe chemical levels. All results of tests must then be noted in a log book to act as a record, which can be referred to as necessary. If a physiotherapy assistant, engineer, maintenance worker or student physiotherapist performs these tests then the physiotherapist in charge of the pool should check the levels or be informed if they are outside acceptable limits. If they are, this may have a bearing on whether staff and patients will be allowed into the water.

Generally all chemical parameters should be within acceptable limits, with occasional exceptions. If there are recurrent problems then the dosing of the pool should be investigated thoroughly to pinpoint the fault.

Poorly maintained pool environment

If the overall pool environment is poorly maintained then again there could be risks to health and safety such as spread of infection. If you are in charge of the pool it will be your responsibility to ensure that the whole pool environment is macroscopically clean. This includes all areas: toilets, kitchen, storage area, showering facilities, changing and waiting areas, the pool concourse and the pool itself. This may involve liaison with cleaning and maintenance staff to ensure that the correct cleaning methods are used. You will also need to ensure that other users of the pool (such as physiotherapists bringing in their own patients from other areas or outside user groups) follow correct pool procedures, e.g. use of overshoes, hosing down of the pool concourse, patients showering before entering the water.

Poorly maintained equipment

This could be a risk to both staff and patients. Faulty flotation equipment may cause distress for patients while in the water and could result in accidental submersion. For staff, if the hoist is not functioning this will add unnecessary strain to any manual handling operations when helping patients in and out of the pool.

In order to prevent such problems occurring, equipment must be regularly checked for faults.

Defective flotation equipment must be discarded and replaced. It is advisable to have maintenance contracts in place for the hoists and alarm systems – if this is not possible, then they should at least be tested regularly and any faults rectified immediately.

POOL MANAGEMENT

The most important point to make is that an effective team approach is necessary to keep a pool functioning well. A senior physiotherapist should have overall responsibility for the pool, but it is essential that all physiotherapists working in the environment have background knowledge of the factors involved in keeping the water quality high and the pool safe for both staff and patients. It is also a good idea to visit the plant room and to liaise regularly with the engineer and/or any other staff involved in controlling and monitoring the pool.

Pollutants

Various forms of pollution are introduced into the pool almost continually. If left untreated, these pollutants build up in the water, increasing the risk of infection from bacteria and other microorganisms. There is also a reduction in safety through loss of clarity of the water due to suspended particulate matter.

Pollution from bathers

Many substances are introduced into water by bathers, both staff and patients. These pollutants include:

- Material from bathers such as mucus, saliva, sweat, hair, skin flakes, urine and faecal matter
- Material collecting on the body before bathing, such as general dirt
- Materials such as powders, creams, lotions and oils applied to the body before bathing.

It is difficult to entirely avoid these pollutants but pre-cleansing facilities and good hygiene on the part of bathers can help to reduce the amount going into the pool.

Pollution not derived from bathers

A number of products may contaminate the pool, particularly cleaning materials from the surrounds. Care should be taken in the use of such products and ideally the pool surrounds should drain away to waste or to the circulation system of the pool prior to filtration to minimize the possibility of contamination.

Self-assessment question

- **SAQ 11.16** What are the main staff-related health and safety risks when working in the pool environment?

Pool plant and maintenance

The aim of pool maintenance is to provide high-quality water for maximum safety and protection of bathers in accordance with valid regulations. The pool should be safe and pleasant to use. It should be clean, should look inviting and be free from irritant/toxic substances, algae and micro-organisms. In order to achieve this, attention must be given to physical (macroscopic) and biological (microscopic) cleanliness.

This is dependent upon filtration and disinfection, which need to be adequate to deal with the likely levels of pollution/contamination. The systems put in place will avoid accumulation of pollutants that can be a risk to health and/or make the pool look unsightly.

Filtration

This is the absorption and retention of mechanically removable particles from the water by some sort of filtration system. Pool water cannot be regarded as satisfactory for use, however well disinfected, if it lacks clarity because of excess turbidity. This can be caused by:

- excessive pollution from bathers
- inadequate filtration and circulation
- contamination from external sources
- inadequate disinfection

- incorrect use of water treatment chemicals
- bubbles of air.

Filtration reduces turbidity by removing particles. A good test is to drop a coin into the centre of the pool. If your water is of an acceptable level of clarity you should be able to see the face of the coin from all angles and positions around the pool. If not, you probably need to look at your filtration system.

In the filter, water passes through a permeable membrane and solid particles are removed by progressive dilution. The effectiveness of the filter depends on:

- the size of the particles of the filter bed
- pool turnover rate, i.e. how long it takes for the whole volume of water in the pool to pass through the filters once. In a public pool this is approximately 2–4 hours, in a therapy pool approximately 1–2 hours and in a whirlpool approximately 0.5–1 hour.

Backwashing

This is an important process that cleans the filter medium by reversing the flow of water through the filter. The water used goes to waste along with the particles it removes from the filter. The backwashing is determined by the pressure in the filter bed and it can be manual or automatic. In many pools now, it is automatic.

There is a 'sight glass' in the waste water line and through this you can see the water going to waste after it comes from the filter. This can indicate the cleanliness of the water, i.e. when the majority of trapped particles have gone.

Pool pipework

This is high-density PVC; the only metal is in the heating coils. The changes in acidity/alkalinity (pH) of the water can have a corrosive effect on metal so it is not suitable. The pipe sizes should be determined by a hydraulic engineer to ensure that the flow rate matches the pump size and filter.

Water should drain out from the top of the pool via skimmer boxes, scum channels or ideally a wet deck. The placement of water return lines should be through the floor of the pool or in the walls at different levels to ensure there are no 'dead spots' in the water.

Disinfection systems

The pool water is treated with a disinfectant agent maintained at a level that protects bathers from microorganisms (CSP 2000).

Chlorine

The most common type of disinfectant agent is chlorine, through the use of liquid sodium hypochlorite. This method is economic and effective and it can be used in manual or automated systems. Calcium hypochlorite granules and tablets are also available, but these are not suitable for all pool systems. Stabilized chlorine – chlorinated isocyanurates – are not as effective and there is a problem with the build up of cyanuric acid. Salt chlorination provides chlorine by means of an electrolytic chlorine generator.

Hypochlorous acid is the most effective sanitizing agent. Bathers introduce pollutants into the water. Oxidation occurs, which transforms these pollutants into harmless, inactive substances and the disinfection kills pathogens. The result of the reaction of the hypochlorous acid with the nitrogenous compounds in the water (i.e. the pollutants) causes the formation of chloramines. These are poor sanitizers and are irritants. The most common are the monochloramines and then the dichloramines. These two compounds react to release nitrogen. If further chlorine is added then trichloramines are formed. Trichloramines have a characteristic chlorine-like odour, are aerated out of the water by agitation and are responsible for eye irritation. The formation of the trichloramines is most pronounced if there is a low pH (i.e. if the water is more acidic). It is important to note that the odour and eye irritation are often thought to be due to the chlorine levels – this is not the case: they are due to high levels of trichloramines, i.e. in a pool with a poorly controlled disinfection system. It is more difficult to keep the levels of trichloramines low if there is an increased bathing load.

The bathing load relates to a number of factors:

- Number of bathers using the pool at any one time
- The volume and surface area of the pool
- The pool turnover time
- The pollutants released by individual bathers.

Disinfection should be calculated to accommodate bather load and fluctuations in the numbers of bathers.

Ozone

Ozone is the best oxidizer and it is a disinfectant. It has a short active life in water and it is toxic in excess of $0.1 \, mg/l$ (above this the level is illegal). An ozone generator with chlorine residual gives the best water quality levels. Less chlorine is necessary and the water 'feels good'. The drawback with this system is that it doubles the cost!

Bromine

Over the last few years the Chartered Society of Physiotherapy has received an increasing number of calls relating to physiotherapists having skin problems when working in brominated pools. There is concern over the possible link between the use of bromine as a cleaning agent and skin rash amongst pool users, especially hydrotherapists, who spend more time in the water (CSP 2001). The Pool Water Treatment Advisory Group (1995) describes skin rash as a 'complicated subject' with it being difficult to tell whether a rash is due to the water and its disinfectant or whether other factors in the individual's physical make-up and environment are contributing factors. It does, however, make reference to 'bromine itch', where some people develop an 'intensely itching contact dermatitis' after immersion in a brominated pool. This is unusual in children and more common in bathers over 50 years of age. It is also described as being 'more frequent and severe with prolonged exposure' and so hydrotherapists may be concerned about this (Pool Water Treatment Advisory Group 1995). For more information on this issue you can refer to the Chartered Society of Physiotherapy's Health and Safety Briefing Pack no 12: *Hazards in Hydrotherapy Pools*.

Self-assessment question
• **SAQ 11.17** What is the reason for backwashing?

Pool chemistry

We shall only consider chlorine here as this is the disinfection system you are most likely to come across in clinical practice. You should test the pool for disinfection levels and pH two or three times a day (Table 11.2). If disinfected using chlorine only, the levels are as follows:

- Free chlorine (i.e. that available to combine with pollutants) should be within the range 1–4 parts per million (ppm)
- Total chlorine should be within the range 1.5–5.0 ppm
- Combined chlorine should never be more than 1.0 ppm.

There should always be two to three times more free chlorine than combined.

If the pool is being disinfected with ozone and chlorine residual or ultraviolet and chlorine, the levels do differ and you will need to learn about these locally.

pH control

It is extremely important that you have good control of the pH of the water, as it involves a number of factors:

- Protection of the pool plant
- Bather comfort
- Effectiveness of the disinfection system.

Table 11.2 Tests carried out on pool water, the reagent used and frequency

Tests	Reagent	Frequency
Free chlorine	DPD 1	2 × daily
Combined chlorine	DPD 3	
Total chlorine	DPD 1 + 3	3 × daily (hand dosed)
pH	Phenol red	2 × daily
TA	Acid solution	Weekly
CH	Standardized reagent	Weekly
TDS	Electronically tested	Monthly
Bacteriological	Laboratory	Weekly

CH = calcium hardness; TA = total alkalinity; TDS = total dissolved solids.

The optimum range is 7.2–7.8 (pH is a logarithmic scale from 0–14. 7 is neutral, so pH 6 is 10 times more acidic, pH 5 is 100 times more acidic, pH 8 is 10 times more alkaline, pH 9 is 100 times more alkaline, etc.).

pH below 7.0 (acidic). There is the possibility of rapid loss of chlorine, eye irritation due to the rapid formation of chloramines, destruction of cement grouting and corrosion of metal components. The water will feel uncomfortable, sometimes described as 'prickly', as it takes minerals from the skin.

pH above 7.8 (alkaline). There is the possibility of reduced chlorine efficiency and so a need for increased chlorine, eye irritation and dry skin, cloudy water and scale formation in plant and pool.

Total alkalinity

Total alkalinity (TA) is a measure of the total amount of dissolved alkaline compounds in the pool water. This acts as a pH buffer without which it is difficult to balance the pH (pH bounce). If TA is low you can add sodium bicarbonate.

Calcium hardness

Calcium hardness (CH) is a measure of the amount of dissolved calcium compounds in the water. If it is low, add calcium carbonate.

Self-assessment question

- SAQ 11.18 Why might there be a strong chlorine odour in the pool area and why is this a negative sign?

Total dissolved solids

Total dissolved solids (TDS) is a measure of the amount of dissolved solids in the water. If the TDS is increased there is a loss of sparkle, with flat, dull-looking water. To adjust this, empty or partly empty the pool and refill with fresh water.

Recommended values

- TA: 100–150 mg/l
- CH: 100–300 mg/l
- TDS: <1250 mg/l (indoor).

Water balance tests

Langelier index: $pH + TF + CF + AF = 12.1 \pm 0.5$. If the index is increased then the water is scale-forming and if the index is decreased then the water is corrosive.

Taylor's watergram

This illustrates the relationship between total alkalinity, pH and calcium hardness. It assumes conditions of temperature $27°C + 5°C$ and TDS <1000 mg/l.

Emptying schedule

There are situations in which hydrotherapy pools may need to be partially or totally emptied. If there are excessively high levels of chloramines or TDS then the pool can be partly or totally emptied as required. The pool would need to be totally emptied if the water was contaminated or for major maintenance.

On emptying a number of routine and maintenance checks can be carried out:

- Check functioning of the hydrostatic valve
- Disinfect the main drain
- Check rails, tiles, steps
- Descale, scrub floor/walls.

Note: If there is no hydrostatic valve there is a risk of structural damage from the pressure of the surrounding earth fill. When empty, the natural water table pressure may dislodge the whole pool.

> **Self-assessment question**
>
> - **SAQ 11.19** What is the importance of having pool water at the correct pH level?

ADVANTAGES AND DISADVANTAGES OF HYDROTHERAPY

Advantages

- The warmth of the water has the effect of decreasing pain and so helps to decrease muscle spasm and promote relaxation. The warmth is also present throughout treatment and not just before or after exercise, as with many other pain-relieving modalities.

- The whole body is actively involved in the treatment and there is less focus on one particular area. It is also very useful for patients with wide-ranging problems and many weak muscles. More of the body can be treated in less time. Large numbers of joints and muscles can be exercised in different planes with minimal change in starting position, which is a definite advantage for patients who find changing position on dry land difficult or painful.

- Buoyancy supports the body and decreases weight bearing. Walking re-education can begin sooner than on dry land and the patient will be able to do more especially if weight bearing causes pain under normal circumstances. Buoyancy can be used to support starting positions and to assist or resist movement. It also means that movement is much easier in the pool, not only giving the patient more freedom but also making it much easier for you to handle and manoeuvre the non-mobile patient.

- There is no pressure on bony points and no friction to cause damage to the skin.

- Water allows an infinite range of resistance and is therefore suitable for patients at any stage.

- Generally the patient can do more in the water than on dry land, which may boost morale and increase confidence.

- Hydrotherapy has a social aspect, as there are usually several patients in the pool at one time or there may be classes of patients with similar problems. This allows for interaction and mutual support and the treatment is more enjoyable.

- Patients may learn how to swim or become confident enough in the water to then continue with the exercise at their local swimming baths.

Disadvantages

- The main disadvantage of hydrotherapy in today's financial climate is the great expense of the installation and upkeep of the facilities. As well as the pool room itself, other areas are necessary for waiting, changing, examination, resting, storage of linen/towels, washing and drying of costumes and so on. Office space is also required for administrative activities. This all adds to the cost, as does the day-to-day running of the pool and plant room. Staffing is also a factor. For safety reasons there must always be at least two members of staff present in case of emergencies. There should be a senior physiotherapist and an assistant or porter available at all times.

- As explained in earlier sections of the chapter, the hydrotherapy department is a potentially dangerous environment and so safety standards must be extremely rigorous.

- Occasionally the more debilitated patients find that, with travel to and from the pool, they are too tired to benefit fully from the treatment.

- Because of the effects of buoyancy it is occasionally difficult to gain adequate fixation to isolate particular movements.

- Because movement in water is very different from that on dry land, final rehabilitation may need to be carried out either on the ward or in the physiotherapy department. This is not always necessary, however, if the patient is given a comprehensive set of home exercises to carry out as an adjunct to pool treatment. This will of course depend on individual patients and their particular problems.

- Patients sometimes become very dependent on the pool as they are able to do so much more in the water.

- As with any type of physiotherapy treatment, there are contraindications, but those for hydrotherapy rarely apply anywhere else. These issues have been discussed previously but, as you will remember, there are few absolute contraindications to pool treatment.

Self-assessment question

- SAQ 11.20 Which tests of pool chemistry need to be carried out and how often are they done?

Problem-solving exercise 11.8

After briefly reviewing the case studies in Chapter 7, formulate a list of reasons why you might use hydrotherapy in the management of patients with rheumatic conditions. Are there any disadvantages?

How would hydrotherapy for a patient with rheumatoid arthritis vary from that for a patient with ankylosing spondylitis?

Problem-solving exercise 11.9

In Chapter 9 (Case study 9.1) you were introduced to Mrs Bell, a 58-year-old lady with osteoporosis. Review her case and think about how hydrotherapy might be used as part of her management.

SUMMARY

This chapter has given you an overview of hydrotherapy and its application with patients who have orthopaedic conditions. It includes relevant hydrostatic and hydrodynamic principles and their application in the development of exercise programmes in water, physiological changes that occur in the body as a result of immersion, contraindications to pool therapy, therapeutic effects, health and safety issues, pool management, the benefits, disadvantages and appropriate use of hydrotherapy.

It is impossible to cover all aspects of hydrotherapy in one chapter, but by now you should feel that you have a basic understanding of the important elements. This is, of course, all theoretical. The best advice we can give you is to get into a pool to try out the principles we have discussed for yourself.

Above all, remember to use the water, do not transfer your land-based exercises into the pool.

As emphasized in many chapters of the book, this chapter has covered the principles of hydrotherapy intervention and has given some specific examples. These illustrate that a sound understanding of the treatment modality you are using and competence in your patient assessment will enable you to apply the principles successfully. Again it is your decision-making process that is the key to effective patient management.

On reading this summary, do you feel you have grasped the above points? If not, perhaps you should go back and re-read any appropriate parts of the chapter before moving on.

ANSWERS TO QUESTIONS AND EXERCISES

Self-assessment question 11.1 (page 314)

- **SAQ 11.1** Why is it inappropriate to use land exercises in the pool?

Answer: It is not appropriate to transfer land-based exercises into the pool, as this neglects the unique properties of the water and consequently will not produce optimum results.

Self-assessment questions 11.2 (page 314)

- **SAQ 11.2**
  a. Approximately how much weight goes through the lower limbs when a person is immersed to C7, the xiphisternum and the anterior superior iliac spines respectively?
  b. How can this reduction in body weight be used to advantage in patients with orthopaedic problems?

Answer:
a. C7 – 10%
   Xiphisternum – 30%
   Anterior superior iliac spines – 50%.
b. In two main ways. First, if a patient experiences pain on weight bearing then this reduction in body weight will relieve the pain and make movement much easier while in the water. Second, if a patient is partially or non-weight-bearing then exercise can be carried out in the water to improve the reciprocal gait pattern before this could be done on dry

land. If the pool has a range of depths then weight bearing can be gradually progressed.

Self-assessment question 11.3 (page 316)

- **SAQ 11.3** What are the three main uses of buoyancy?

Answer: Assistance to movement, support of the body or body segments and resistance to movement.

Self-assessment question 11.4 (page 318)

- **SAQ 11.4** How can you modify the effect of the turning force produced by the moment of buoyancy?

Answer: This can be modified in a number of ways (remember the equation: moment of buoyancy = force (F) × distance (d) and d is the most significant because F remains constant):

1. Change the length of the lever
2. Add a float
3. Change the amount of air in the float
4. Change the position of the float, i.e. move it nearer to or further from the body
5. Change the position of the part in relation to the surface, i.e. nearer the surface = greater turning effect.

Self-assessment question 11.5 (page 318)

- **SAQ 11.5** What happens when you introduce more speed into buoyancy-assisted/resisted movements?

Answer: Purely buoyancy-assisted/resisted movements are quite slow. As soon as you ask the patient to move more quickly through the water, you are introducing increased levels of resistance into the equation because of the effects of turbulence. This means that you need to think carefully about your progressions of exercise and about exactly what you are asking the patient to do. The best way to check it out is to carry out the movements yourself.

Problem-solving exercise 11.1 (page 318)

- Imagine a patient who has reduced range of hip abduction. How could you use buoyancy in a progressive manner to increase abduction?

Answer: After your assessment you will have a good idea of how much hip abduction the patient has and what the reduction in range is caused by. We will assume that it is due to stiffness and shortened structures on the inner aspect of the thigh and that there is minimal pain (obviously, if the patient was experiencing pain, you would modify your treatment accordingly). Repetition should be used in each step described below.

1. In standing (facing side of pool, holding bar) with legs straight, allow buoyancy to lift the affected leg to the side (ensure toes point forward and the hip does not go into flexion or extension).

2. Place a float around the limb, start with a small amount of air and the float positioned more proximally. Perform the movement as in step 1 but because of the float there will be more assistance. If this is comfortable you can progress by adding more air to the float and then moving it more distally to gradually increase the turning effect of buoyancy. This might need to be done with caution as the float could take the leg further into range than is comfortable.

3. In the same position, instruct the patient in hold–relax using the upthrust as resistance to the isometric contraction. On relaxation the patient allows the float to take the leg further into abduction.

You may be able to move through these stages in one treatment session or you may need to spread them over a number of sessions as part of an exercise programme.

Problem-solving exercise 11.2 (page 318)

- Next time you go swimming or have a moment to spare in the hydrotherapy pool, experiment with changes in body shape. See what happens when you move part of the body out of the water or away from the trunk; try bending one arm or knee; lift your head.
  Can you control the rotation?
  If so how do you do it?
  How safe do you feel?
  How do you think this might affect the patient's level of confidence?

How do you think you might be able to use these effects in treatment?

Answer: As suggested above, the best way to carry out this exercise is in a practical setting – in the water. As described in the text, it is very useful to teach patients to control their movement and rotation in the pool – if you feel this yourself you will be able to teach it much more effectively.

You will notice that even a very small asymmetry can cause you to work hard to maintain your position. If you don't work hard to stop the movement, you will roll. As you may imagine, this can make patients feel rather unstable and apprehensive. This is why you need to be able to reassure them and show them how to work with the water. They can actively use the rotation to get into another position in the water, correct the rotation and so maintain equilibrium, or use isometric muscle work to prevent the rotation from occurring. If patients can grasp these basics then they will feel much more confident when in the pool. Of course, many patients will already be water-confident and will be doing some of these things automatically, but you can still use the principles to improve balance and co-ordination or as stabilization techniques.

Self-assessment question 11.6 (page 319)

- **SAQ 11.6** What is the metacentric effect?

  Answer: The metacentric principle concerns balance in the water. A body immersed in water is acted upon by two opposing forces – gravity acting downwards through the body's centre of gravity and buoyancy acting upwards through the centre of buoyancy (this is located at the centre of the body of water that has been displaced by the immersed object). If these two forces are equal and opposite, then the body is balanced and there is no movement. If the two forces are unequal and out of alignment, however, then movement occurs. The movement is always rotatory and continues until a state of balance is once again achieved, i.e. when the two forces are back in alignment.

Self-assessment question 11.7 (page 321)

- **SAQ 11.7** Why are the effects of hydrostatic pressure important?

  Answer: Probably the most important implication of hydrostatic pressure is that it causes a redistribution of the fluid volume within the body. In standing, a person of average height immersed to neck level will be subjected to a pressure of around $120\,g/cm^2$ at mid-calf. Because of this greater pressure on the lower limbs, approximately 700 ml of fluid is redistributed from this region into the thorax. This effect is responsible for most of the profound physiological effects that occur during head-out water immersion.

Problem-solving exercise 11.3 (page 321)

- Describe a progressive strengthening programme for weak knee flexors using buoyancy and movement through the water.

  Answer: For this problem we will assume there is full range of movement in the knee.

1. If the muscles are extremely weak you can use buoyancy as assistance. With the patient in standing, facing the side of the pool and holding the bar, ask him/her to take the heel to the buttock (keeping the hip in extension). Buoyancy will assist the movement. If more assistance is necessary, a float could be added. In this case you must ensure that the knee extensors are strong enough to extend the knee back to the starting position against the resistance of the float.

   To progress, take air out of the float and then remove the float altogether.

2. To make the exercise a little harder you can then use buoyancy as a resistance. Place the patient in sitting with the leg outstretched. The heel is pushed down into the water so bending the knee against the upthrust. A float can then be applied proximally and subsequently moved distally to increase resistance, and more air added as necessary. In this position you can only get the patient working against resistance up to 90° of flexion. After this point buoyancy starts to assist the movement as the heel moves up towards the buttock (this can however, be useful if you are working on both strengthening and mobilizing which is often the case).

   Remember that these movements should be performed slowly in order to be resisted only by buoyancy. As soon as you increase the speed, turbulence is produced and this increases the resistance to movement.

3. To provide the greatest resistance in the sitting position you could add a float and a flipper to the foot and ask the patient to perform the movement quickly, thus working against both buoyancy and turbulence. Flexion with a float and flipper in this position can be a very strong exercise but again only up to 90° of flexion. Because the patient is working hard you will need to give some attention to fixation to ensure you are getting the action you require.

4. You can now position the patient in side lying, either in floats or on a half plinth. The heel is taken towards the buttock, slowly at first so producing little turbulence and then the movement is speeded up to increase the amount of resistance. To progress further a flipper can be applied to the foot – this will produce even more resistance – and then add speed.

An advantage of this position is that the patient can move further into the range of knee flexion and still be working against the full resistance. This is unlike the sitting position, where the resistance offered varies depending on where in range the joint is. A disadvantage of side lying is that it is more difficult to stabilize the movement so you may need to use your hands to fix the thigh/hip region.

When you try these exercises out for yourself you will notice that there is some overlap: the last exercise we described in the sitting position (with float and flipper) is actually harder than the first exercises against turbulence that we described in side lying. So for a pure progression you may need to alternate the patient's starting position.

Although, for clarity we have talked about buoyancy and turbulence separately and strengthening and mobilizing as separate techniques, in reality you will often be using the principles in tandem and, as mentioned earlier, many patients need help to both strengthen and mobilize an area.

Problem-solving exercise 11.4 (page 321)

- You were introduced to Mr Kingston in Case study 5.2 in Chapter 5. He sustained a fractured shaft of femur that was treated with internal fixation. He was discharged non-weight-bearing. How could you use hydrotherapy in his rehabilitation?

Answer: This patient was required to have active knee range from 0–70° and grade III strength in the quadriceps prior to discharge. If hydrotherapy was available while he was an inpatient, this would be an ideal environment in which to work on these areas, especially as he was non-weight-bearing. Depending on his ability, Mr Kingston might be able to get into the pool independently using the handrails or you might need to lower him in using the hoist. As mentioned a number of times, the whole body is treated while the patient is in the pool and this helps with general fitness and can stave off the negative effects of bed rest and the relative immobility of the inpatient environment.

On looking back at the treatment objectives for Mr Kingston, hydrotherapy can be used to address many of these:

- Increase range of movement using buoyancy and turbulence in an active exercise programme using a wide range of starting positions.

- Strengthen knee flexors/extensors and muscles around the hip (as well as general strengthening and fitness) through strong but non-weight-bearing exercises and pool circuit training using the principles mentioned above.

- Regain full soft tissue length through the exercises above, specific stretching exercises and hold–relax techniques. The pain relief and general/local relaxation that occurs while in the pool may also help with this problem.

- Gait and locomotor activities can be worked on in the weight-free environment of the water, concentrating on reciprocal activities that can be performed more easily in the pool than on dry land. Once partial weight bearing is allowed at 6 weeks, progression can occur in the pool with the patient working in shallower water to increase the percentage of weight going through the lower limbs.

- Return to playing football – the patient can carry out medium- to high-intensity exercise in the pool while still non-weight-bearing and so will return to full fitness more quickly once weight bearing on dry land commences.

- In conjunction with hydrotherapy, Mr Kingston should be carrying out a comprehensive set of home exercises and may also be attending the physiotherapy gym, depending on available resources. Final rehabilitation will need to be carried out on dry land.

Self-assessment question 11.8 (page 322)

- **SAQ 11.8**
  a. What factors offer resistance when moving through the water?

  Answer:
- Bow wave (positive pressure in front of the object)
- Wake (turbulence producing negative pressure/drag behind the object)
- Viscosity of the water
- Friction
- Adhesive/cohesive forces.

  b. Why does turbulence produce resistance?

  Answer: Turbulence is the term used to describe the eddy currents that follow an object that is moving through the water. The degree of turbulence depends partly on the speed of movement, i.e. faster movement creates more turbulence, slower movement creates less turbulence and the flow of water is more streamlined. Faster movement with many eddy currents being formed behind the object as it moves through the water indicates the presence of high levels of kinetic energy in the water particles. As a result of this, the level of pressure energy goes down, so causing an area of low pressure behind the object resulting in the drag.

  c. What are the variables that can affect the amount of turbulence produced by an object moving through the water? Which of these is the most significant?

  Answer: Three variables affect the amount of turbulence produced by an object moving through the water, speed, shape and size. The most significant is the speed of movement – Drag $\propto$ area $\times$ speed^2.

Self-assessment question 11.9 (page 322)

- **SAQ 11.9** Why do you need to know about refraction?

  Answer:
- Safety – it is important to warn the patients that the floor of the pool and any steps will look

nearer than they actually are, so care needs to be taken

- Incorrect assessment – it is not recommended that you attempt to assess the patient's movement while in the pool. There is distortion as you look into the water and you will see the 'apparent' image as opposed to the 'real' image. Your assessment is likely to be incorrect – do it on dry land.

Problem-solving exercise 11.5 (page 322)

- Mrs Jones is the 77-year-old lady with a fractured neck of femur treated with a dynamic hip screw (Case study 5.3 in Chapter 5). How do you think that management of this patient in the hydrotherapy pool would vary from that you decided upon for Mr Kingston?

Answer: As noted in Chapter 5, the main focus for Mrs Jones is her return to functional independence. The more specific range of motion and strength around the hip is the secondary consideration. Given the differences in function between the two patients prior to injury, Mrs Jones will not need to increase strength and range of motion to the same extent as Mr Kingston.

You may need to provide more support and reassurance for this lady when she first comes to the pool. It is possible that she may not ever have been swimming, or at least not for a very long time. It is also important to remember that her injury occurred as the result of a fall and so she may be nervous, particularly in the very different environment of the pool. If this is an issue you could bring her into the pool area using a wheeled chair and lower her into the pool using the hoist. She may also feel rather self-conscious about appearing in front of others in a swimsuit. You can check these points out in your assessment and modify your approach accordingly.

Your treatment programme needs to be less vigorous than that of Mr Kingston. Start with gentle exercises for the hip in standing, checking for compensatory movements. If she has enough confidence in you, you may be able to put Mrs Jones in float lying or on to the half plinth in order to carry out hip and knee movements (e.g. alternate knee/hip flexion/extension, gentle cycling action, bilateral abduction, hip extension against buoyancy). For the more functional activities you can ask the patient to walk in the pool – forwards, backwards, sideways, gradually increasing stride length. She can practise sitting to standing and, if you have steps in the pool, she can do step-ups – buoyancy will assist these activities.

Depending on the patient's progress you might go on to use floats and flippers to increase resistance.

Being in the water and moving around will improve general mobility, flexibility, fitness and endurance. Mrs Jones will be able to move more easily than on dry land and this will help to improve her confidence and her ability to cope. Coming to the pool will also provide the opportunity to meet others, so providing social interaction.

Self-assessment question 11.10 (page 323)

- **SAQ 11.10** What happens to your cardiac output during head-out water immersion in thermoneutral water? How is this modified in water that is warmer than thermoneutral?

Answer: Cardiac output increases by 34% in thermoneutral water but the heart rate remains fairly stable, or occasionally a slight bradycardia occurs. With water at higher temperatures the effect on cardiac output is more pronounced and the heart rate tends to rise, with tachycardia occurring when the water reaches 37°C. In water at 39°C cardiac output rises as much as 120% and heart rate can increase to 113 beats per minute.

Self-assessment question 11.11 (page 323)

- **SAQ 11.11** Why do you feel that you need to go to the loo after being in the pool for a period of time?

Answer: Immersion has a marked effect on renal function, particularly a profound diuresis due to the suppression of antidiuretic hormone. This causes the distal tubules and collecting ducts of the kidney to become less permeable to water, so less is reabsorbed, resulting in more urine being produced. The kidney usually filters 120 ml/minute and produces 1 ml of urine. After 3 hours of immersion the rate of urine production increases up to 7 ml/minute.

Self-assessment question 11.12 (page 323)

- **SAQ 11.12** Why might hydrotherapy be helpful for patients who experience stress and anxiety?

Answer: There is some evidence to suggest that blood levels of stress hormones (such as noradrenaline (norepinephrine)) are reduced during immersion. It is also hypothesized that there is a reduction of sympathetic nervous system activity. This may provide some explanation for the reports of improved mood after swimming.

Problem–solving exercise 11.6 (page 326)

- John Brown, a 24-year-old man with a sprain of the medial collateral ligament of the knee and James Low, a 46-year-old man with a total rupture of the lateral ligaments of his ankle are both discussed in the Chapter 6 (Case studies 6.1 and 6.3). Review these cases and think about why you might use hydrotherapy with these patients as part of their rehabilitation.

Answer: John Brown injured the medial collateral ligament of his knee while playing football. He is a keen sportsman and so will want to get back to activity as soon as possible. It is noted in the case study that he is perhaps not as fit as he could be. As with the other case studies mentioned, hydrotherapy can be used in order to allow earlier exercise in a warm, weight-relieving environment. Both the reduction in weight and the warmth of the water will reduce discomfort and enable greater activity levels.

Fitness levels can be worked on both in the pool and on dry land, but it may be easier to carry out vigorous exercise initially in the water. Some examples of exercises are given below:

Sports therapy rehabilitation

- Sitting on float – pelvic control. Add breaststroke with arms forward and backward while sitting on board. Progress by creating more turbulence and then change the patient's position to kneeling on the board and finally to standing on it while performing the same arm movements
- Supported by floats or swim jacket – cycling movements and deep water running
- Jumping to walk standing, jump together, jump feet apart, jump together. Add floats to feet and repeat
- Stand on one leg (with or without float on foot). Move other leg in all directions, then switch to other leg. Good exercise for stabilizing stance knee. Can add floats for extra resistance
- Barbell in each hand, hold down in water (using latissimus dorsi). Kick legs from the hips. Progress by adding flippers to feet
- Jumping with arms raised above the head (so the patient cannot use the arms to do the work) in deep water and progress to shallower water. Change from right leg to both legs to left leg in different order. Jump for 2 minutes then have 30-second rest. Add moving forward, backward and sideways. Emphasize quick response time
- Jogging forward, backward, to right and left, and then add diagonal directions
- Jumping with skiing action on either side of line on bottom of pool. Add posture control
- Large kickboard – doing 'kickboard clocks'. Can keep foot on board by adding two rubber bands and sliding the foot underneath them
- 6 o'clock and 12 o'clock – dorsiflexion and plantar flexion
- 3 o'clock and 9 o'clock – inversion and eversion
- Progress by adding in the diagonals and progress further by asking patient to move to all 12 points of the clock
- Can use repetitions and/or changes in speed to progress further
- Cool down – walking or jogging.

These are some examples that will help with general fitness and lower limb strength and mobility. You can think up more for yourself.

James Low has ruptured the lateral ligament of his ankle joint and has been in plaster for 4 weeks. His main problems are swelling, decreased range of movement and decreased mobility. Hydrotherapy will enable him to carry out early reciprocal lower limb activities, especially as he is initially partial weight bearing.

The hydrostatic pressure may help to reduce the swelling around the ankle. He could do lots of walking activities in different directions, practise going up and down the steps in the pool, active ankle and foot movements while wearing a flipper, balance work – e.g. patient stands on the affected leg while you produce turbulence in different places around him and he has to maintain his position, or he has to maintain his balance while carrying out strong movements with the arms. In this way it is possible to work on range of movement and strength in the ankle region to a certain extent, although this would need to be augmented by a land-based programme. The 'kickboard clocks' exercise described above would be helpful in increasing range of movement, concentrating particularly on inversion and plantar flexion.

Generally, Mr Low is unfit and unused to using his body because of his sedentary lifestyle. The hydrotherapy pool is the ideal environment to introduce him to gentle all-round exercise. Depending on his progress he could move on to some or all of the above sports therapy rehabilitation exercises to improve his fitness and then possibly to swimming, which he could continue on his own at his local pool.

You will need to modify your approach to patients depending on their priorities. In the end, if Mr Low is unwilling to exercise beyond the rehabilitation of his ankle problem then that is his choice – you can only offer advice and support.

Self-assessment question 11.13 (page 328)

- **SAQ 11.13** Review the absolute contraindications to hydrotherapy treatment

  Answer: Absolute contraindications:

- Uncontrolled cardiac failure – the patient is unable to lie flat without becoming dyspnoeic
- Resting angina
- Shortness of breath at rest
- Medically unstable following an acute episode e.g. cerebrovascular accident, deep vein thrombosis, pulmonary embolus, status asthmaticus
- Acute vomiting and/or diarrhoea
- Proven chlorine sensitivity.

Problem-solving exercise 11.7 (page 328)

- Steve Morris (Chapter 6, Case study 6.5) has a long history of back pain and eventually has an operation to decompress his S1 nerve root. Read about his problems on assessment and how he is after surgery. How might hydrotherapy be of use in this case?

  Answer: It is well recognized that the effects of warm water and the gravity-free environment assist in promoting generalized relaxation. In addition, the suppression of the sympathetic nervous system leads to a reduction in muscle tone, a reduction in level of pain and an elongation of the spinal column. These benefits of immersion, combined with the variety of principles we can use to mobilize joints, stretch tight structures and strengthen muscles, all contribute to creating an ideal medium in which to treat back pain.

As with any exercise programme, the regimen you design for Mr Morris should be developed on an individual basis following a full assessment on land. There are numerous ways in which we can treat low back pain, but even those experiencing more acute pain can benefit from relaxation and isometric exercises in the pool. This patient should be finding that the acute pain has diminished but he will be feeling stiff and sore after the operation and bed rest. Because of the long-standing nature of his back problem, Mr Morris will probably be generally deconditioned.

The following exercises are a sample of those that can be used in this context:

1. Relaxation

Starting position – supine, supported in floats

Exercise/activity: 'Seaweeding' through the water. The therapist walks backwards supporting the patient at the chest or between the patient's knees at the same time slowly moving the patient's body from side to side so it moves like a piece of seaweed in the water. This provides excellent therapist control and an ability to determine the degree of specific and generalized relaxation.

Starting position – in deeper water in vertical supported by a buoyancy vest or by a ring under each arm

Activity: Passive 'hanging'. This activity can be performed independently.

2. Isometric exercises

Starting position – supine, supported by floats

a. *Exercise for abdominals*: Apply pressure on both shoulders in a downward direction, graded to gain contraction without movement.
b. *Exercise for obliques*: Apply pressure on one shoulder at a time. This can also be done by

applying pressure on one hip at a time. This exercise can be used to detect unilateral weakness and determine muscle balance.

c. *Exercise for erector spinae*: Apply pressure under both scapulae to lift the body upwards.

With all of these the patient is asked to resist the pressure applied by the therapist.

Starting position – supine, supported by floats

d. *Exercise for obliques*: Patient is asked to lift one hand out of the water while maintaining the trunk in a straight position (resist the resultant body roll). Alternate with the other hand.

e. *Exercise for side flexors*: With the therapist standing between the patient's knees, hands on the outer aspect of the thighs or hips, patient is moved from side to side and has to maintain the trunk in a straight line. Progress to therapist holding between the patient's feet. Further progression can be provided by standing at the patient's head with hands under scapulae and around thorax so holding at chest level. Increasing the speed of the turn will also increase the difficulty.

f. *Exercise for trunk rotators and extensors*: As above with the patient's legs rotated to the right or the left.

All the above exercises utilize drag to obtain an isometric contraction.

g. *Exercise for extensors*: With a float on both feet, depress the float into the water and hold the position.

h. *Exercise for abdominals*: Turn into prone. With a float on both feet, depress the float into the water and hold the position. Repeat this with the legs rotated to left or right to exercise the obliques.

These exercises use buoyancy to gain an isometric contraction.

3. Mobilizing exercises

Starting position – supine, supported in floats holding the rail with both hands

a. *Rotation*: With bent knees and thighs under the water, turn the feet from side to side, bringing the ankle towards the surface on each side alternately.

b. *Side flexion*: With straight knees, take both legs together to one side and then the other, by bending at the waist. Rotation can be added by turning the legs to the left or right before taking them from side to side.

Starting position – facing the rail, no floats, hold rail with forearms (front of body against pool side), bend knees, keeping hips in extension

c. *Rotation*: Keeping the body vertical (do not side flex), turn the ankles from side to side to bring alternate lateral malleoli towards the wall.

d. *Rotation with flexion*: Bend the hips and knees while bringing them up to the left-hand side of the body, push the hips down into extension and repeat to the opposite side by bending at the hips and bringing the knees up on the right-hand side of the body.

e. *Side flexion*: Keeping the knees bent and the hips in extension, bend at the waist, allowing the water to lift the legs to the side. Repeat to the other side.

Starting position – standing at the rail holding with both hands

f. *Extension*: Facing the rail, take one leg back as far as possible without leaning forwards. Repeat with the other leg.

g. With back to the rail, push hips forwards and rise on to toes, allowing the buoyancy to lift into lumbar extension. A small float can be used in the hollow of the back.

h. Flexion – with back to the rail as above, lift both knees towards the chest. A small float can be used under both feet. This would increase the mobilizing effect of buoyancy but also add strengthening activity for the extensors when returning to the starting position.

4. Strengthening exercises

The isometric exercises described above become strengthening exercises through range when movement is added, rather than maintaining a static hold.

5. Mobilization of the nervous system

Starting position – standing at the rail and holding the rail with both hands

a. *Sciatic nerve*: With back to the rail, with straight knee, lift leg forwards as far as possible (a small float can be used on the foot). Flex the head forward and then lift head up.
   Caution: before attempting this, the degree of irritability must be assessed on land.
b. *Femoral nerve*: Facing the rail, take the leg into hip extension and bend the knee. Take head into flexion.
   Caution: as above.

Other components with either of these nerve stretches can be added as in land-based treatments.

6. Posture and balance

a. Use turbulence in different places to facilitate the use of abdominals or back extensors, or maintain pelvic tilt. Varying the depth of water will increase the difficulty. The deeper the water the greater muscle effort is required to maintain a position. Patients can create their own turbulence by moving their arms forwards and backwards.
b. Balance on one foot with and without turbulence.
c. Balance on one foot while holding a float under the other foot just above the floor of the pool. Move the foot with the float in different directions, keeping it just off the floor at all times. Repeat with the other foot.

7. Functional activities

Activities such as walking in different directions, exaggerated reciprocal walking, and using steps. Increase the walking difficulty by increasing the speed and/or by adding bats in the hands to unstreamline the body and increase the resistance to movement.

The above exercises/activities are not exhaustive. There are many others that can be included in a back treatment programme.

Consideration should also be given to general fitness activities that could be done in the pool, as improving fitness is known to improve self-esteem.

Many patients report benefits in terms of improved well-being and self-efficacy. The psychosocial aspects of exercising in a pool cannot be ignored, particularly when exercising in a group.

It is therefore important to design a programme that will ultimately allow Mr Morris to take control of his own treatment and carry out the exercises without supervision.

Self-assessment question 11.14 (page 329)

- **SAQ 11.14** With regard to contraindications to hydrotherapy treatment, in what situations might you need to monitor patients while they are in the pool and why?

  Answer: Open infected wounds, poorly controlled epilepsy, unstable diabetes, known aneurysm, gross obesity. Patients should be closely monitored while in the pool, with follow-up to ensure no ill effects. This is particularly important with those patients where there is a slight risk of collapse in the pool, which could lead to accidental submersion.

Self-assessment question 11.15 (page 332)

- **SAQ 11.15** What are the main patient-related health and safety risks when in the pool environment?

  Answer:
- Accidental submersion
- Acute fear of water
- Slips and falls poolside
- Fainting and fitting in the pool
- Cardiac arrest in the pool
- Spread of infection
- Fatigue
- Unfamiliarity with the pool surroundings.

Self-assessment question 11.16 (page 334)

- **SAQ 11.16** What are the main staff-related health and safety risks when working in the pool environment?

  Answer:
- Storage and handling of chemicals
- Fatigue
- Skin problems – dry skin, irritation and rashes.

Self-assessment question 11.17 (page 335)

- **SAQ 11.17** What is the reason for backwashing?

Answer: This is an important process that cleans the filter medium by reversing the flow of water through the filter.

Self-assessment question 11.18 (page 336)

- **SAQ 11.18** Why might there be a strong chlorine odour in the pool area and why is this a negative sign?

Answer: The result of the reaction of the hypochlorous acid with the nitrogenous compounds in the water (i.e. the pollutants) causes the formation of chloramines. These are poor sanitizers and are irritants. The most common are the monochloramines and then the dichloramines. These two compounds react to release nitrogen. If further chlorine is added then trichloramines are formed. Trichloramines have a characteristic chlorine-like odour, are aerated out of the water by agitation and are responsible for eye irritation. The formation of the trichloramines is most pronounced if there is low pH (i.e. if the water is more acidic). It is important to note that the odour and eye irritation are often thought to be due to the chlorine levels – this is not the case, they are due to high levels of trichloramines, i.e. in a pool with a poorly controlled disinfection system.

Self-assessment question 11.19 (page 337)

- **SAQ 11.19** What is the importance of having pool water at the correct pH level?

Answer: It is extremely important that you have good control of the pH of the water as it ensures: protection of the pool plant, bather comfort and effectiveness of the disinfection system. With pH below 7.0 (acidic), there is the possibility of rapid loss of chlorine, eye irritation due to the rapid formation of chloramines, destruction of cement grouting and corrosion of metal components. The water will feel uncomfortable, sometimes described as 'prickly' as it takes minerals from the skin. With pH above 7.8 (alkaline), there is the possibility of reduced chlorine efficiency and so a need for increased chlorine, eye irritation and dry skin, cloudy water and scale formation in plant and pool.

Self-assessment question 11.20 (page 338)

- **SAQ 11.20** Which tests of pool chemistry need to be carried out and how often are they done?

Answer: See Table 11.2.

Problem-solving exercise 11.8 (page 338)

- After briefly reviewing the case studies in Chapter 7, formulate a list of reasons why you might use hydrotherapy in the management of patients with rheumatic conditions. Are there any disadvantages?
- How would hydrotherapy for a patient with rheumatoid arthritis vary from that for a patient with ankylosing spondylitis?

Answer: Reasons might include:

- *Pain relief*: All patients with rheumatic conditions will have some degree of pain because of the disease process in general, often more specifically on weight bearing. The warmth and weight relief are helpful therapeutic effects enabling greater freedom of movement because of decreased pain and spasm. The pain relief, although temporary, is present throughout the treatment, unlike many other modalities.

- *Whole-body treatment*: Many patients with rheumatic conditions have widespread problems. When moving in the water, the whole body is treated and there is less focus on a specific area – again unlike other modalities used in physiotherapy. This is particularly important for both Mrs White (RA) and Mr Smith (AS), who both have widespread problems. Large numbers of joints can be treated in less time. Different planes of movement can be used with minimal change in starting position, which is an advantage for those patients who find changing position on dry land painful or difficult.

- Gait can be re-educated earlier in the pool. This will be helpful to Mrs Stamford (OA knee) and more particularly to Mr Nicholls after his total knee replacement.

- Patients with RA often have delicate skin. In the water there is no friction to cause damage. There is also no pressure on bony points, so this could be important for a patient who is very immobile such as Mr Nicholls. Movement and exercise in the water will help to reduce problems over pressure points that may have arisen during periods of bed rest.

- As water provides an almost limitless range of resistance to movement, patients at any stage and with a wide variety of problems can still be treated effectively in the pool. The resistance will never be more than they can manage if you choose your exercise programme carefully and tailor it to the individual patient.

- Rheumatic conditions are chronic and so have associated psychosocial problems. The greater freedom of movement in the water can boost morale and increase confidence. The social aspect of the treatment can also help to lift mood and provide mutual support. Patients report physical, functional and psychological improvement, better quality of life and feelings of increased well-being.

- *Lack of major adverse effects*: This is quite different from other forms of therapy that many of these patients have to undergo, especially drug treatments.

Possible disadvantages:

- Fatigue
- Dependence on treatment
- Doing too much in the water and experiencing post treatment pain. This should be avoided with careful monitoring of the patient's activity levels.

The main difference in hydrotherapy for the patient with RA and that for the patient with AS would be the intensity of the exercise. For Mrs White the treatment would be gentler, taking note of pain and not pushing too far into range. This is to avoid aggravating symptoms and to prevent further joint damage. You would ask her to perform low- to medium-intensity exercises and functional activities.

For Mr Smith the pool treatment would be much more vigorous as exercise is necessary to improve the pain and stiffness experienced as a result of the condition. The following exercises are examples of those that can be used in the management of AS.

Supine lying

Neck collar; hip float; ankle float (some patients prefer not to wear a collar and this may in fact allow more cervical extension). Ensure correct posture in float lying and ensure that you keep giving posture reminders throughout the session.

- With feet together and legs straight, rotate legs so that lateral (outer) surface of thigh is uppermost and then rotate to the other side. Avoid hip flexion by pulling heels back.
- Hip hitching, keeping legs straight.
- Pendulum swing both legs from the right to the left with knees straight and at the surface of the water. Stabilize the pelvis as needed.
- Press right leg down into the water, keeping the left leg just under the surface of the water to help stabilize the pelvis. Repeat with the other leg.
- Abduction of hips with legs straight and heels just under the water. Add hold–relax technique as necessary.
- Alternate knee bends with ankles at 90°.
- Extend back and hips by pushing heels down into the water with both legs together, knees straight.
- Bend knees towards the chest and roll both knees from side to side. Stabilize the pelvis as needed.
- Floating free of the bar, arms out sideways, palms up. Press arms down into water then relax as they return to the surface (could float with toes tucked under bar, head to centre of pool to give some stability).

While neck and shoulders are warmed, the patient should stand with back to the wall with shoulders under the water, start with shoulder muscle relaxation exercises and then do neck exercises.

Standing

Ankle floats as necessary. Repeat exercises on both sides.

- Facing side of pool, both hands on bar starting with body in an inclined position – press-ups.
- Standing sideways to wall, keeping ankle float slightly behind the knee, bend the knee up and then press the foot downwards to the floor trying to get the knee as straight as possible.

- With the leg straight, take forward and up towards the surface then draw leg backwards with the heel leading (ensuring that there is minimal movement in the trunk), then pull leg strongly forward and up, keeping both knees straight. Add hold–relax technique as necessary.
- With knee straight, take leg into abduction going as high as possible (keep toes pointing forwards). Add hold–relax as necessary.
- Stand with back to the wall, bend right knee and rest right foot on to left knee. Take right knee round towards the wall and then across to the left as far as possible.
- Squat with feet wide apart, holding a float in both hands, push the float round to the right and then the left. Maintain neck retraction throughout.
- Feet wide apart, keeping arms straight and out to the side just under the surface of the water, thumbs pointing to the ceiling. Bring palms together in front of body and then push arms back to try and touch wall behind.
- Position as before, arms at shoulder level and at side, push palms down into water to touch body and return to starting position.
- Stand facing the wall, with the right arm straight holding on to the bar. With a float in the left hand, push it down from the surface of the water to sweep under the right arm and across to try and surface on the other side. Control the movement at all times.
- Strides across pool, backwards, forwards and sideways, aiming to decrease the number of strides taken each time.
- Blowing a float across the pool.

As you can see, these exercises focus on rotation and extension using active movements, isometric contraction and stretching but being aware of correct posture at all times. You can also work on improving vital capacity by doing aerobic work and encouraging swimming underwater if the patient is able.

Problem-solving exercise 11.9 (page 338)

- In Chapter 9 (Case study 9.1) you were introduced to Mrs Bell, a 58-year-old lady with osteoporosis. Review her case and think about how hydrotherapy might be used as part of her management.

Answer: There are a number of factors that make hydrotherapy a suitable treatment modality for patients with osteoporosis.

- Patients feel safe, as there is no fear of falling. This is important for confidence, as some of these patients may have sustained fractures or other injuries as a result of falls
- Relaxation caused by the support and warmth of the water helps to reduce pain
- The reduction in pain plus the support of the water enables both active and static muscle contraction
- As the level of exercise tolerance increases, the pull of muscle on bone promotes bone strengthening
- There are many ways of statically strengthening the anterior and posterior spinal muscles in the pool
- Activities in the pool can facilitate normal movement
- Re-education of functional movement in the pool can lead to increased dry land activity
- It is possible to use the water to increase cardiovascular and respiratory fitness levels
- Improvement in postural control
- Improvement in thoracic expansion and respiratory function
- Many patients report psychological effects such as an improvement in well-being when undergoing pool therapy and exercise
- Group social interaction
- The pool can be used to prevent associated problems once fractures have occurred.

A regimen of hydrotherapy is performed with repetitions gradually increasing from 15 to 30 over a 6-week period. The regimen used is very precise and specific, needing correction and input from the physiotherapist. Treatment does however, take place in a group situation – thus it is cost-effective.

Stability trunk exercises for the pool

Begin all exercises with a gentle warm up of walking either on the spot or through the water. All exercises should be done with water at shoulder height if possible. Begin with 10–15 repetitions of each exercise and gradually build up to a maximum of 30.

- Standing – hold float in front of you resting it on the water. Press float into water with both arms so the water just passes over top of float. Keep posture upright. Hold for 5 seconds.
- Standing – hold float to side with one arm and press into water at side as above. Keep posture upright. Hold for 5 seconds and repeat with the other side.
- Standing – hold float behind you in the water with both arms straight. Press on float with arms and hold, then relax but do not let arms bend up.
- Sit into water – hold float vertically in front of you, push it away and pull back. Keep body posture as upright as possible in the sitting position. Keep movement flowing forwards and backwards as long as you don't fall over.
- Sit into water – hold float vertically in front of you and move it side to side – small movements. Keep body stable.
- Standing – face the side of the pool and hold on with finger tips keeping both legs straight. Move one leg forwards and backwards in a small arc of movement. Repeat with the other leg. The aim is to be able to do this exercise without holding on to the side of the pool.
- Standing – stand sideways on to the side of the pool, hold on with fingertips of one hand. Keep legs straight and move one leg out to side and back – small movements. Again aim to do exercise without holding on to the side.
- Standing – position as for exercise above. Bend one hip and knee up in front and stretch leg out straight behind. Repeat with other leg.
- Sit into water – push both arms up and out to side and then pull back down and in towards the body. Repeat with speed. Do not let body move out of the water.
- Sit into water – start with both arms up to the surface at the side. Take arms across surface of water until hands meet in the middle and then back out to the side. Repeat with speed. Do not allow body to move in the water.
- Stride standing – swing both arms in opposite directions backwards and forwards at side with speed. Keep body as still as possible, do not twist.
- Standing – face wall as described earlier and hold on to bar. Feet approximately 15 cm away from wall. Keeping elbows in position, push hips forward to touch the wall then let the rest of the body follow. Relax and return to starting position, then repeat.
- Standing – position as above. Keeping legs straight, push one leg behind you as far as you can and return to starting position. Do not allow your trunk to move forward as your leg moves back.

References

Association of Swimming Therapy (1992) Swimming for people with disabilities, 2nd edn. A & C Black, London

Berger BG, Owen E, Owen DR (1983) Mood alteration with swimming – swimmers really do 'feel better'. Psychosomatic Medicine 45: 425–433

Coruzzi P, Ravanetti C, Musiari L et al (1988) Circulating opioid peptides during water immersion in normal man. Clinical Science 74: 133–136

CSP 1994 Health and safety: safety representatives' information manual. Chartered Society of Physiotherapy Industrial Relations Department, London

CSP 2000 Standards of Physiotherapy Practice. Chartered Society of Physiotherapy, London

CSP 2001 Hazards in hydrotherapy pools. Health and Safety Briefing Pack 12. Chartered Society of Physiotherapy Industrial Relations Department, London

Davis BC, Harrison RA 1988 Hydrotherapy in practice. Churchill Livingstone, Edinburgh

Geytenbeek J 2002 Evidence for effective hydrotherapy. Physiotherapy 88: 514–529

HACP 1992 Hydrotherapy. Standards of good practice. (Hydrotherapy Association of Chartered Physiotherapists.) Chartered Society of Physiotherapy, London

HACP 2001 Contraindications to hydrotherapy. Hydrotherapy Association of Chartered Physiotherapists, London

Hall J, Bisson D, O'Hare P 1990 The physiology of immersion. Physiotherapy 76: 517–521

Harrison RA, Bulstrode S (1987) Percentage weight bearing during partial immersion in the hydrotherapy pool. Physiotherapy Practice 3: 60–63

Health and Safety Executive 1991 First aid at work – Health and Safety (First Aid) Regulations 1981. HMSO, London

Jackson A 1996 Hydrotherapy as experienced by outpatients in a general hospital. British Journal of Therapy and Rehabilitation 3: 601–608

Kuroda PK 1963 What is water? In: Licht S (ed) Medical hydrology. Elizabeth Licht, Connecticut, p 1–23

Levine BA 1984 The use of hydrotherapy in reduction of anxiety. Psychological Reports 55: 526

O'Hare P, Heywood A, Dodds P et al 1984 Water immersion in rheumatoid arthritis. British Journal of Rheumatology 23: 117–118

Oxlade C, Parker S 1999 Pocket science. Parragon, Bath

Pool Water Treatment Advisory Group (1995) Pool Water Guide. Greenhouse Publishing, Diss, Norfolk

Reid Campion M (1990) Adult hydrotherapy: a practical approach. Heinemann Medical, Oxford

Rissel C 1987 Water exercises for the frail elderly: a pilot study. Australian Journal of Physiotherapy 33: 226–232

Sheldahl LM, Tristani FE, Clifford PS et al (1986) Effect of head-out water immersion on response to exercise training. Journal of Applied Physiology 60: 1878–1881

Weinstein LB 1986 The benefits of aquatic activity. Journal of Gerontological Nursing 12: 6–11

Weston DFM, O'Hare JP, Evans JM, Corrall RJM 1987 Haemodynamic changes in man during immersion in water at different temperatures. Clinical Science 73: 613–616

Index

Page numbers ending in b refer to boxed text; page numbers in **bold** refer to major discussions; page numbers in *italics* refer to figures or tables.